Clinical Care Classification (CCC) System, Version 2.5

Virginia K. Saba, EdD, Honorary PhD, DSN, DScN, RN, FAAN, FACMI, LL, president and chief executive officer of SabaCare, Inc., pioneered for over 40 years the integration of computer technology in the nursing profession. Dr. Saba continues to serve as an active member on several national committees for electronic healthcare information technology (HIT) systems standards sponsored by the Office of the National Coordinator (ONC) for implementing meaningful use requirements. Dr. Saba spearheaded the Nursing Informatics movement, integrated computer technology in nursing, promoted distant learning technologies, and developed computer-based information systems for community health as well as the Clinical Care Classification (CCC) System. She is an Informatics Consultant and has served as a faculty member in academia and as a Nurse Officer in the U.S. Public Health Service (PHS).

In 1997, Dr. Saba received the title of Distinguished Scholar from Georgetown University School of Nursing (GUSON). During her 15-year tenure in the GUSON, she taught and integrated computer technology in the graduate and undergraduate programs, supervised the faculty and student computer laboratories, and served as liaison to campuswide computer committees. She conducted a federally funded national research study known as (Home Care Project), which focused on community health patient care and produced the CCC System.

Dr. Saba also served as a full professor at the Uniformed Services University of the Health Sciences (USUHS), where she taught and integrated computer technology in the Graduate School of Nursing Research Program. At USUHS, she designed and coordinated a distance learning project between the Department of Defense (DoD) and the Veterans Administration (VA). The project was the prototype for an adult nurse practitioner (ANP) program using interactive video technology with participating VA Medical Centers. In Autumn of 1997, students from eight VA Medical Centers across the nation participated in a Post-Masters Certificate ANP Program culminating with its first USUHS/VA Virtual Graduation in June 1999.

She has received numerous professional awards, including the American Academy of Nursing Living Legend Award, the American Medical Informatics Association (AMIA) Nursing Informatics Working Group Appreciation Award for her seminal work in nursing informatics and professional leadership in promoting the development of the field, the USUHS Award for spearheading the DoD/VA Distance Learning Project, the GUSON Faculty Distinguished Service Award for her dedication to the school, the first Sigma Theta Tau International Information Resources Information Award for her dedication and commitment to the advancement of nursing through information systems and computer technology, the Excellence in Nursing Informatics Awards from the American Nurses Association and Rutgers Colleges of Nursing, and the PHS Commendation Medal for her contribution in manpower and management information system studies.

Dr. Saba is a past Chair of the Nursing Informatics Special Interest Group of the International Medical Informatics Association and was Chair of the Steering Committee of the International Organization for Standardization Technical Committee: Health Informatics (ISO/TC215) Workgroup (WG3) Reference Terminology Model for Nursing. She served as a consultant for the creation of the Excelsior College Distance Learning Informatics Program. Dr. Saba has authored several books, chapters, and articles, and served on the original editorial board of *Computers in Nursing Journal* and other healthcare technology journals. She is a fellow of American Academy of Nursing (FAAN) and the American College of Medical Informatics (FACMI) and a member of the Sigma Theta Tau International Honor Society and the Academy of Medicine of Washington, DC.

Dr. Virginia K. Saba is a graduate of the Skidmore College Baccalaureate Nursing Program and earned a Master of Nursing Arts at Teachers College, Columbia University. She received a Master of Science in Computer Technology of Management and a Doctorate of Education in Educational Administration and Scientific and Technical Information Science at American University, Washington, DC. She holds honorary doctorates from the University of Maryland (DSN, 5/2008), Excelsior College in New York (DScN, 7/2005), and University of Athens, Greece (PhD, 6/2000).

Clinical Care Classification (CCC) System, Version 2.5

User's Guide, 2nd Edition

Virginia K. Saba, EdD, DSN, DScN, RN, FAAN, FACMI, LL

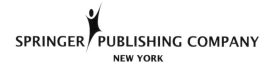

SPRINGER / PUBLISHING COMPANY
NEW YORK

Springer Publishing Company, LLC
11 West 42nd Street
New York, NY 10036
www.springerpub.com

Acquisitions Editor: Allan Graubard
Production Editor: Michael O'Connor
Composition: The Manila Typesetting Company

ISBN: 978-0-8261-0985-9
E-book ISBN: 978-0-8261-0986-6

12 13 14 15/ 5 4 3 2 1

Clinical Care Classification (CCC) System, Version 2.5 [previously known as: (a) Clinical Care Classification (CCC) System, Version 2.0, Copyright© 2004; and (b) Home Health Care Classification (HHCC) System, Version 1.0, Copyright© 1994] pending Copyright© 2012 by Virginia K. Saba, EdD, RN, FAAN, FACMI, LL, may be used ONLY with written Permission by Dr. Virginia K. Saba. (Permission Form available from Web Site http://www.sabacare.com)

The author and the publisher of this Work have made every effort to use sources believed to be reliable to provide information that is accurate and compatible with the standards generally accepted at the time of publication. Because medical science is continually advancing, our knowledge base continues to expand. Therefore, as new information becomes available, changes in procedures become necessary. We recommend that the reader always consult current research and specific institutional policies before performing any clinical procedure. The author and publisher shall not be liable for any special, consequential, or exemplary damages resulting, in whole or in part, from the readers' use of, or reliance on, the information contained in this book. The publisher has no responsibility for the persistence or accuracy of URLs for external or third-party Internet Web sites referred to in this publication and does not guarantee that any content on such Web sites is, or will remain, accurate or appropriate.

Library of Congress Cataloging-in-Publication Data

Saba, Virginia K.
  Clinical care classification (CCC) system, version 2.5 : user's guide / Virginia K. Saba. — 2nd ed.
    p. ; cm.
  Rev. ed. of: Clinical care classification (CCC) system manual / Virginia K. Saba. c2007.
  Includes bibliographical references and index.
  ISBN 978-0-8261-0985-9—ISBN 978-0-8261-0986-6 (e-book)
  I. Saba, Virginia K. Clinical care classification (CCC) system manual. II. Title.
  [DNLM: 1. Nursing Records—classification. 2. Clinical Coding—classification. 3. Electronic Health Records—classification. 4. Nursing Process—classification. WY 100.5]
  651.5'04261—dc23
                                                                                    2012009724

Special discounts on bulk quantities of our books are available to corporations, professional associations, pharmaceutical companies, health care organizations, and other qualifying groups.

If you are interested in a custom book, including chapters from more than one of our titles, we can provide that service as well.

For details, please contact:
Special Sales Department, Springer Publishing Company, LLC
11 West 42nd Street, 15th Floor, New York, NY 10036-8002s
Phone: 877-687-7476 or 212-431-4370; Fax: 212-941-7842
Email: sales@springerpub.com

Printed in the United States of America by Bradford & Bigelow

Contents

PART IV: APPENDICES

Contributors

Amy Coenen, PhD, RN, FAAN
Director, International Classification of Nursing
Practice (ICNP) Programme
International Council of Nurses
Geneva, Switzerland

Patricia C. Dykes, DNSc, RN, FAAN
Corporate Manager
Nursing Informatics and Research
Partners Healthcare
Wellesley, MD

Veronica D. Feeg, PhD, RN, FAAN
Professor, Division of Nursing
Associate Dean, PhD Program
Molloy College
Rockville Centre, NY

Deborah Konicek, MSN, RN, BC
Managing Director
SNOMED Terminology Solutions™
Chicago, IL

Cynthia B. Lundberg, BSN, RN
Clinical Informatics Consultant
CAP-STS
Chicago, IL

Virginia K. Saba, EdD, RN, FAAN, FACMI
President and CEO
SabaCare, Inc.
Arlington, VA

Sheryl Taylor, BSN, RN
Former Senior Consultant
Farrell Associates
San Francisco, CA

Luann Whittenburg, PhD, RN
Chief Nursing Informatics Officer
Medicomp Systems
Chantilly, VA

EXHIBITORS

Kelly Aldrich, DNP, RN

Deborah Ariosto, PhD, RN

Livio Ciacciarelli, EN, BN, DGMA

Jane Englebright, PhD, RN

Anneli Ensio, PhD, RN

George Grayson, EMT-P

Amber Greer, RNC

Ulla-Mari Kinnunen, MHSc, RN, PhD Student

Minna Mykkanen, MHSc, RN, PhD Student

Debbie Raposo, BSN, RN

Edith Vick, BSN, RN, NCSN

Luann Whittenburg, PhD, RN

Foreword

The Clinical Care Classification (CCC) System was published in 1991 by Dr. Virginia K. Saba and her colleagues at Georgetown University for use in computerized patient records. During the more than two decades since its introduction, research has proven the CCC System to be a robust set of standardized, coded patient-care terminologies for electronic health records (EHRs) in both acute care and ambulatory care settings. Realizing that the healthcare information technology (HIT) industry required assistance in standard deployment of standardized terminologies, Dr. Saba created a manual to provide guidance for use of the CCC System.

The CCC System Manual, published in 2007, provided an overview of the CCC System, Version 2.0, and explained how to implement the terminologies in a computerized plan of care and clinical documentation applications. Subsequent to that publication, numerous comments and critiques about the CCC System, Version, 2.0 were received from hospital-based EHR implementation teams as well as from EHR vendors using the CCC System. Additionally, the CCC System's National Scientific Advisory Board convened for over a year, reviewed every CCC concept—including new concepts that were submitted by users—and reached consensus regarding which concepts would be added, retired, or modified. The need was identified for an abridged, easy-to-use guide that would help clinicians learn about the CCC System, Version 2.5, quickly to expedite their development of CCC-based plans of care.

As the CCC System addresses a requirement recognized by nursing leaders, this guide will facilitate meeting that requirement. In her *Notes on Nursing* (1860), Florence Nightingale wrote: "It has been said and written scores of times that every woman makes a good nurse. I believe, on the contrary, that the very elements of nursing are all but unknown." Nearly 140 years, later Dr. Norma Lang stated, "If you can't name it, you can't control it, finance it, research it, teach it or put it into public policy" (Clark & Lang, 1992). With the CCC System, Ms. Nightingale's "elements of nursing" have been identified, classified, and coded, and Dr. Lang's call for being able to "name it" can be realized, empowering the profession to control, finance, research, and teach those elements of nursing as well as to influence public policy that affects nursing practice.

The value proposition of using standardized terminologies like the CCC System in EHRs is now being acknowledged by people with power and resources. Congress passed the Health Information Technology for Economic and Clinical Health Act (HITECH) as part of the economic stimulus package called the American Recovery and Reinvestment Act of 2009 (ARRA). The HITECH includes a major HIT initiative that currently is underway—a federally funded, multiyear, mandated program referred to generally as "EHR meaningful use" and intended to promote widespread adoption and use of EHR technologies that meet specific certification criteria. Managed under the Department of Health and Human Services (HHS), the initial phase of this program included requirements and payment incentives that have an impact on acute care and ambulatory care settings and on physicians as well as nurses and other clinicians. The incentive payments to providers and hospitals are projected by the Congressional Budget Office to total $34 billion.

The certification criteria, which delineated features and functions required for meaningful use of EHR technology, also named required standards that EHRs must support—coded terminology standards, which include Systematized Nomenclature of Medicine Clinical Terms (SNOMED CT) and Logical Observation Identifiers Names and Codes (LOINC) along with interoperability standards (e.g., Health Level Seven and the Continuity of Care Document [CCD]) specification. Inclusion of these standards in the EHR certification criteria is an indication of the value the federal government places on the capture of uniquely identified healthcare data in the EHR.

The authors of these criteria recognized that standardized, coded terminology enables patient data to be used for real-time clinical decision support at the point of care; to be exchanged among disparate EHRs without loss of meaning or accuracy; and to be used in healthcare research for identifying the elements of care provided by clinicians and for measuring patient outcomes. Composed of carefully researched, coded, discrete elements of nursing practice, CCC is positioned to contribute to this effort. The CCC System is integrated into SNOMED and LOINC and is already being leveraged on its own as a key component of 21st-century EHR technology.

In addition to mandating vocabulary and interoperability standards for use in certified EHR technologies as part of HITECH, HHS announced in July 2011 that $71.3 million in federal grants has been allocated to strengthen the nursing workforce through expanding "nursing education, training and diversity." Secretary Sebelius stated, "These awards reflect the critical role of nurses in our healthcare system, and our ongoing commitment to attract and retain highly-skilled nurses in the profession" ("HHS Awards," 2011). Under the current economic and budgetary constraints, assigning this amount of federal funding to the nursing profession is concrete affirmation of the contribution nurses make to the health and well being of the nation. Nursing researchers must continue to study nursing actions and patient-care outcomes to outcomes to generate the evidence that forms the basis for rational nursing practice and to encourage ongoing governmental financial support for nursing education.

The CCC System is a standardized set of terminologies that enables the patient-care activities performed by nurses to be identified and studied by naming, classifying, and coding nursing diagnoses and interventions at the atomic level. This guide provides guidance for implementing the CCC System, enabling discrete, coded patient-care data to be captured in EHRs.

Sheryl L. Taylor

● **References**

Clark, J., & Lang, N. (1992). Nursing's next advance: An international classification for nursing practice. *International Nursing Review, 39,* 109–112.

HHS awards $71.3 million to strengthen nursing workforce. (2011, July 29). HHS.gov News Release. Retrieved from http://www.hhs.gov/news/press/2011pres/07/20110729a.html

Nightingale, F. (1860). *Notes on nursing: What it is, and what it is not.* New York: D. Appleton and Company [First American Edition].

Swan, B. A., Lang, N. M., & McGinley, A. M. (2004). Access to quality health care: Links between evidence, nursing language, and informatics. *Nursing Economics, 22*(6), 325–332.

Preface

Welcome to the *Clinical Care Classification (CCC) System User's Guide, 2nd Edition*—which provides an overview of the CCC System updates, Version 2.5. The CCC System is designed to document nursing practice in electronic health record (EHR) and healthcare information technology (HIT) Systems. The CCC System consists of two interrelated terminologies, CCC of Nursing Diagnoses and Outcomes and CCC of Nursing Interventions/ Actions, which form a single system classified by 21 Care Components. The CCC System Guide presents Version 2.5 of the CCC System and the current updates to the two terminologies.

The CCC National Scientific Advisory Board spent 2 years to create, edit, review, and revise the CCC System for Version 2.5. The Board reviewed a substantial number of concepts submitted by CCC System clients as well as each concept, code, and definition from the Version 2.0 terminologies. The CCC System Version 2.5 changes are listed in Tables in Appendix A and are summarized below:

Care Components: 1 Revised Name and 2 Revised Definitions

CCC Diagnoses: 4 New Concepts, 10 Retired Concepts, and 16 Revised Definitions

CCC Interventions: 14 New Concepts, 11 Retired Concepts, and 25 Revised Definitions

The guide is a print version of the CCC System, Version 2.5, which is also presented on the CCC System Web site (http://www.sabacare.com or http://www.clinicalcareclassification.com).

This guide is divided into three parts: Part I: Overview; Part II: Overview and Uses; and Part III: Terminology Tables. Part I has three chapters, with Chapter 1 providing background that sets the stage for why the CCC System, a nursing terminology is needed for the emerging electronic health record (EHR) and healthcare information technology (HIT) systems. Chapter 2 provides an overview and a developmental history as well as current uses of the CCC System in nursing practice, education, research, and administration. The chronological history (2012–1988) has been updated from the previous edition and placed in Appendix B. Chapter 2 provides a description of the features, standards, and policies of the CCC System. Since the previous edition, many EHR/HIT standards organizations have emerged that influence and support the use of the CCC System. Also in Chapter 2, you will find the CCC System maintenance policy, copyright, and trademark. A sample CCC System Permission Form is included for requesting permission to use the CCC System. A complete bibliography of major articles and key publications about the CCC System by nursing informatics experts and researchers found in Appendix C.

Part II has three chapters and highlights selected uses of the CCC System. Chapter 4 highlights the CCC System collaboration with the Systemized Nomenclature of Medicine Clinical Terms (SNOMED CT) as well as the International Classification for Nursing Practice (ICNP). Lundberg and Konicek describe federal requirements to use SNOMED CT as the interoperable terminology for healthcare documentation. In the chapter, Dykes provides a theory on a direct concept mapping process from the CCC System to SNOMED CT; Whittenburg provides a case study of mapping demonstrating the interoperability of the CCC System with SNOMED CT; and Coenen identifies how the CCC System concepts are represented in ICNP. Chapter 5 lists EHR/HIT applications that have implemented the CCC System: four in-hospital applications, one commercial EHR knowledge base vendor, one student school health nursing application, and two international applications. Part II concludes with Chapter 6 by Mannino and Feeg, presenting a nursing education application using the CCC System for student education documentation of their clinical experiences.

Part III contains two chapters. Chapter 7 presents "getting ready" strategies for implementing nursing documentation or plans of care (POCs) using the CCC System. The chapter includes sample POCs as well as coding strategies. Chapter 8 presents 15 CCC System terminology tables outlining the framework and structure of the CCC, the CCC of Nursing Diagnoses and Outcomes, and the CCC of Nursing Interventions/Actions. The terminology tables provide ready access to the CCC System for anyone who is coding and documenting nursing care electronically. The Appendix section includes three tables: Appendix A lists the new concepts, retired concepts, and revised definitions from CCC System terminologies, Version 2.0; Appendix B provides the CCC System Milestones: and Appendix C the CCC System Bibliography of Major Articles.

This guide is an indispensable resource for anyone who is documenting nursing care or implementing nursing documentation and plans of care using the CCC System in an EHR. The CCC System supports the electronic capture of discrete patient-care data for documenting the "**essence of care**" and measuring the relationship of nursing care to patient outcomes.

Virginia K. Saba

Acknowledgments

The authoring of the *Clinical Care Classification (CCC) System, Version 2.5, User's Guide* has taken the time and effort of many colleagues who assisted in production of this publication. First, I wish to thank Dr. Luann Whittenburg, who played a major role in editing and crafting this Guide with her creative ideas, knowledgeable assistance, and technical support. She gave of her time freely to ensure that the Guide accurately depicted the value and usefulness of the CCC System. Second, I want to thank the contributors of the chapters, exhibits, and information pieces, who added their personal experiences with the CCC System for this updated guide.

I should acknowledge the ongoing work of the CCC System National Scientific Advisory Board members: Pattie Dykes, Rosemary Kennedy, Jackie Moss, Bonnie Westra, Barbara Van der Castle, and Luann Whittenberg; the ad hoc members: Susanne Bakken and Connie Delaney; and the consultant, Amy Jacobs, who reviewed and edited the CCC System revisions and codes. All of these experts donated their time and provided their expertise to review the concepts in the CCC System, Version 2.0, as well as evaluate the proposed concepts and revisions for inclusion into this updated CCC System, Version 2.5, Guide. The suggested contributions from CCC System users, educators, and researchers demonstrated the continued growth of the CCC System. I also need to thank my sister, Bernice Scully, as well as other members of my extended family for their support.

I also wish to acknowledge the original research team of the federally funded Home Care Project (1989–1991) conducted at Georgetown University School of Nursing from which the Home Health Care Classification (HHCC) System Version 1.0 emerged. It consisted of myself as principal Investigator, Jennifer Boondas, Eugene Levine, David Oatway, Patricia O'Hare, Willian Scanlon, and Alan Zuckerman, two graduate students (Irene Reyes and Sheila Nveva), and an office manager (Andrew McLaughlin).

I also wish to recognize all of my nursing informatics colleagues and clinicians from around the world who have endorsed, promoted, and continued to support the implementation of the CCC System for documenting nursing practice. They believe, as do I, that the CCC System is a standardized national nursing terminology that documents the "**essence of care**" and demonstrates that nursing practice makes a difference.

Clinical Care Classification (CCC) System, Version 2.5

Background 1

The documents of nurses are the window to a diary of care given to patients. It is obvious that a CCC embedded into an EHR improves the legacy of the contribution of the nurse in care. —Kathleen McCormick, PhD, RN, Vice President, SAIC–Frederick, MD

For over 50 years, computers have been an important component of the electronic health technology revolution in the healthcare industry. Computers have transformed healthcare delivery and the nursing profession. Healthcare is now one of the largest computer technology industries in this country. Also, technology in healthcare is no longer a luxury. Computer and software applications are a business necessity in healthcare facilities, academic institutions, research centers, and other healthcare settings that support and involve nursing.

Today, nurses are concerned with nursing informatics (NI), which is defined as the integration of computer science (hardware), information science (software), and nursing science. Nursing informatics involves the processing of data into information, knowledge, and ultimately, wisdom (ANA, 2008). Today, nurses are also involved in the electronic health record (EHR) and/or healthcare information technology (HIT) systems. Nurses are converting from paper patient healthcare records with handwritten nurses' notes to electronic structured plans of care using a coded computer-based national nursing standard nursing terminology—Clinical Care Classification (CCC) System— (e.g., specifically designed for computer processing) which is the focus of this Users Guide.

● Nursing Advances

The documentation of nursing practice started with the systematic evaluation of care by Florence Nightingale. The "Lady with the Lamp," in her study of ways in which nursing care can be provided to improve patient care, identified though data analysis the impact of hygiene and sanitation on outcomes. Nightingale identified the first nursing standard, which she called her six cannons of nursing care (Nightingale, 1992). Another 100 years would elapse before nursing theorist Virginia Henderson identified and described another significant nursing practice standard. Henderson maintained that nursing was a true profession and indicated that nurses were independent professionals who were responsible for the nursing care they provided as well as carrying out physician orders. She, similar to several nursing theorists of her time, identified and described nursing practice using new nursing code sets, such as Henderson's 14 Activities of Daily Living, Abdellah's 21 nursing problems, or Orem's 6 universal self-care deficits (Flynn & Heffron, 1984).

During this time frame, the Nursing Process standard was described as the philosophical foundation for nursing that serves as a theoretical framework for professional nursing practice. In 1970, the Nursing Process was recognized by the American Nurses Association (ANA) as the standard framework for professional nursing practice and continues to be the framework for nursing practice today (ANA, 2010).

American Nurses Association Involvement

The ANA was the first major professional nursing organization to recognize and promote the use of computer technology for nursing. In 1986, the ANA approved of the formation of the Council on Computer Applications in Nursing (CCAIN), with the focus of promoting the integration of computer technology in nursing. During this period, the CCAIN conducted several promotional activities at the ANA conventions, such as workshops, computer exchanges, and computer software demonstrations for nurses. The CCAIN also submitted several resolutions to the ANA Congress on Nursing Practice dealing with the promotion of computer technology in nursing.

Nursing Minimum Data Set

In 1988 to 1990, Harriet Werley established the Nursing Minimum Data Set, which consisted of 12 variables: 8 variables focused on patient demographics and the remaining 4 focused on nursing practice—(a) nursing diagnoses, (b) nursing interventions, (c) nursing outcomes, and (d) nursing intensity. The Nursing Minimum Data Set became the basis for the nursing classification standards recognized by the ANA (Werley & Lang, 1988). In 1990, the CCAIN was renamed the Database Steering Committee and continued to promote nursing technologies focusing on nursing standards, databases, and terminologies.

Nursing Informatics—A New Nursing Specialty

In 1991, the Database Steering Committee submitted to the Congress on Nursing Practice the resolution that NI be adopted as a new nursing specialty, which was accepted. This led to the development of the *Nursing Informatics: Scope and Standards of Practice* (ANA, 2008) and the certification of NI specialists. In 1992, the Database Steering Committee developed the criteria and recognized the first 4 of 12 nursing classifications/terminologies, one of which was the CCC System, previously known as the Home Health Care Classification System, as nursing standards for the documentation of nursing practice using computer technology systems (Saba, 2011). The ANA subsequently submitted the four of six classifications/terminologies to the National Library of Medicine for input into its developing Unified Medical Language System's (UMLS) Metathesaurus (McCormick et al., 1994).

Database Steering Committee

In the following two decades, 1990 and 2000, the ANA Database Steering Committee conducted national conferences and workshops; published handbooks on the uses of technology in practice, education, research, and management; and promoted numerous professional resolutions for the advancement of NI as a new nursing specialty. The ANA employed an NI consultant who was responsible for servicing the specialty committee, including activities such as presenting testimony on behalf of the ANA, and who continues to be a supporter and promoter of NI today.

● **Nursing Informatics Activities**

Technology Informatics Guiding Education Reform Initiative

In the past decade, the increasing numbers of experts in NI have raised the visibility of nursing practice in EHR/HIT systems. The NI experts have expanded the scope of nursing practice to include health information systems (HITs), created professional NI organizations such as the American Nursing Informatics Association, expanded nursing education to include NI courses as part of the core nursing curriculum, conducted workshops and tutorials, and expanded the expectation and demand for the electronic documentation of nursing practice using a standardized nursing terminology—the CCC System. Also during this time, the Technology Informatics Guiding Education Reform (TIGER) Initiative established workgroups to interweave technologies into nursing practice and education (Troseth, 2011). These initiatives by informatics nurses have helped to define and determine the HIT policies and standards necessary and crucial for the current and sustained implementation of the Health Information Technology for Economic and Clinical Health (HITECH) Act of 2009.

● Medical Advances

Technology would not have advanced HIT as known today if it were not for several events that promoted EHR systems. The impetus for the implementation of the EHR started in 1991 with the Institute of Medicine's report entitled *The Computer-Based Patient Record* (Dick & Steen, 1991), which recommended the need for computer-based patient records. This report gave the federal government the impetus to address the requirements needed to promote EHR and HIT systems.

Office of the National Coordinator

It was another 10 years before the Secretary of Health and Human Services initiated a call to action and, in 2004, established the Office of the National Coordinator for Health Information Technology and appointed Dr. David Brailer as the first national coordinator (Executive Order No. 13335), Dr. Brailer created a strategic plan for the national adoption of HIT, which included the formation of the Healthcare Information Technology Standards Panel (HITSP), with the mandate to identify national terminology standards for the electronic documentation and transfer of patient care data across healthcare systems and facilities (Sensmeier, 2011).

In 2006, President George W. Bush issued an Executive Order (No. 13410) that every person in the country should have an EHR by 2014. In 2007/2008, the Healthcare Information Technology Standards Panel selected and recommended the Clinical Care Classification (CCC) System© as the first national nursing terminology interoperable for the exchange of information between and among HIT systems. The CCC System was one of the standards in the first set of 55 national standards approved for use in the EHR by the Department of Health and Human Services (AHIC, 2006) and the only national nursing terminology standard.

HITECH Act of 2009

In 2009, President Obama, who was also supportive of an EHR system, initiated and passed the American Recovery and Reinvestment Act of 2009, which included the HITECH Act of 2009, which focused on and funded the adoption of EHR systems. The Act promoted the widespread adoption of the EHR and authorized federal funds as incentives for hospitals and healthcare providers to adopt HIT. President Obama established that governmental healthcare programs, such as Medicare/Medicaid, required EHR systems for the electronic reimbursement of healthcare services (Murphy & Johnson, 2011).

Meaningful Use

The HITECH Act initiated two national advisory committees, one for HIT policy and one for HIT standards, which initiated a three-part strategic plan. The Committees were designed to guide the nationwide implementation of interoperable EHR and/or HIT Systems in public and private healthcare sectors to reduce medical error, improve quality, and produce greater value for healthcare funding. The HITECH Act requires the achievement of specific 2011, 2013, and 2015 milestones in the implementation of "meaningful use." The first 2011 milestone requires the implementation of computerized provider order entry as well as the implementation of an exchanged list of patient problems on admission into a hospital. Other milestones are being proposed for 2013, such as quality indicators and patient care plans. (Whittenburg, 2009).

Current Status of EHR and HIT Systems

With the federal mandate for every person in the country to have an EHR, the need for nursing to be included in the legislative initiatives and milestones is apparent. These mandates are an important opportunity for expanding the focus of nursing practice in the healthcare industry. There is an immediate need to integrate a nursing terminology standard, such as the CCC System, a recognized national nursing terminology for EHR information exchange, into the meaningful use milestones. Nursing integrated patient plans of care are needed for the documentation of patient care in the implementation of computerized provider order entry and future HITECH/meaningful use milestone requirements for quality indicators and patient outcomes. In using the CCC System, a coded standardized nursing terminology standard and framework for documenting patient care, nursing will be able to determine workload, resources, and outcome measures as well as other indicators that impact patient care.

Thus, this CCC System Guide provides the processes nurses need for documenting nursing practice in the EHR and HIT systems and becoming active members of the electronic revolution in healthcare.

● References

American Health Information Community (AHIC). (2006, October 31). Meeting minutes. Retrieved from http://www.hhs.gov/healthit/community/meetings/m20061031.html

American Nurses Association. (2010). *Nursing: Scope and Standards of Practice.* Sliver Spring, MD: ANA.

American Nurses Association. (2008). *Nursing Informatics: Scope and Standards of Practice.* Sliver Spring, MD: ANA.

Dick, R. S., & Steen, E. B. (1991). *The Computer-Based Patient Record: An Essential Technology for Change.* Washington, DC: Institute of Medicine.

Flynn, J. M., & Heffron, P. B. (1984). *Nursing: From Concept to Practice.* Bowie, MD: R. J. Brady Communications Co.

McCormick K. A., Lang, N., Zielstorff, R., Milholland, D. K., Saba, V. K. & Jacox, A. (1994). Towards standards classification schemes for nursing language: Recommendations of the American Nurses Association Database Steering Committee to Support Nursing Practice. *Journal of American Medical Informatics Association, 1,* 422–427.

Murphy, J., & Johnson, E. (2011). Nursing informatics and healthcare policy. In V. K. Saba & K. A. McCormick (Eds.), *Essentials of nursing informatics* (5th ed., pp. 247–263). New York, NY: McGraw–Hill.

Nightingale, F. (1992). *Notes on nursing: What it is and what it is not* (commemorative ed.). Philadelphia, PA: J. B. Lippincott Co.

Saba, V. K. (2011). Overview of the Clinical Care Classification: A national nursing standard coded terminology. In V. K. Saba, & K. A. McCormick (Eds.), *Essentials of nursing informatics* (5th ed., pp. 217–229). New York, NY: McGraw–Hill.

Sensmeier, J. (2011). Health data standards: Development, harmonization, and interoperability. In V. K. Saba, & K. A. McCormick (Eds.), *Essentials of nursing informatics* (5th ed., pp. 233–245). New York, NY: McGraw–Hill.

Troseth, M. (2011). The TIGER Initiative. In V. K. Saba & K. A. McCormick (Eds.), *Essentials of nursing informatics* (5th ed., pp. 633–640). New York, NY: McGraw–Hill.

Werley, H., & Lang, N. (1988). *Identification of the Nursing Minimum Data Set (NMDS).* New York, NY: Springer Publishing.

Whittenburg, L. (2009). Nursing terminology documentation of quality outcomes. *Journal of Health Information Management, 23*(3), 51–5.

Overview, History, and Uses   2

● Overview

This chapter provides an overview of the Clinical Care Classification (CCC) System in three sections and sets the stage for this publication. The first section illustrates the framework of the CCC System and how the CCC framework levels are linked together. The second section provides an overview of the history of the original CCC System research and how the CCC System was developed, including the development of the concepts and coding structure. The final section summarizes the major applied uses of the CCC System in all areas of nursing practice: clinical practice, nursing education, nursing research, and nursing administration. The historical highlights of the CCC System with the dates and events from inception in 1991 to the present are listed in Appendix B.

The CCC System, Version 2.5, is an update of CCC System, Version 2.0. The CCC System is a coded, standardized nursing terminology standard and framework designed to document nursing practice in the electronic health record (EHR) and healthcare information technology (HIT) systems. The CCC System captures discrete patient care concepts (data/elements) for electronically documenting the "**essence of care**" following the nursing process (see Figure 2.1) and for measuring the relationship of nursing care to patient outcomes (http://en.wikipedia.org/wiki/Clinical_Care_Classification_System; www.sabacare.com; Taylor, 2007).

The CCC was approved as the first national nursing terminology standard by the Secretary of the Department of Health and Human Services as an interoperable standard for the exchange of information in EHR systems in 2007 (HHS, 2007). The CCC System was empirically developed from live patient care data from a federally funded national nursing research study and is a standardized approach for documenting nursing and allied healthcare and organizing and exchanging nursing plan of care (POC) data. The CCC System consists of two interrelated nursing terminologies, the CCC of Nursing Diagnoses and Outcomes and the CCC of Nursing Interventions/Actions, which together form a single system (the CCC System) for linking nursing diagnoses to nursing interventions and to nursing outcomes.

Hierarchy

The CCC System provides a standardized hierarchy for the two CCC nursing terminologies (classifications/vocabularies/knowledgebase), which consists of four levels. The first and highest level of the CCC System consists of four healthcare patterns: physiological, functional, psychological, and health behavioral. (See Figure 2.2.) Each of the four healthcare patterns consists of a different set of care components, which represent the second level of the terminology hierarchy. There are 21 care components used to classify the CCC System's two nursing terminologies. Each care component represents a cluster of data/elements that characterize the four healthcare patterns. The care components are a holistic approach to providing patient care and provide the coding framework for the electronic processing of the care data. (See Figure 2.3.)

The third level consists of the two nursing terminologies: the CCC of Nursing Diagnoses and Outcomes and the CCC of Nursing Intervention/Actions. The CCC of Nursing Diagnoses consists of 176 nursing diagnoses (60 major diagnoses representing concrete conditions or problems and 116 subcategories providing more precise, granular concepts describing the specific variations of the major diagnoses). The CCC of Nursing Diagnoses represents patient conditions and problems requiring clinical care by nurses and allied health providers.

FIGURE 2.1 ▦ Six steps/ standards of nursing process.
Source: American Nurses Association. (2010). *Nursing: Scope and standards of practice* (p. 8). Silver Spring, MD: ANA.

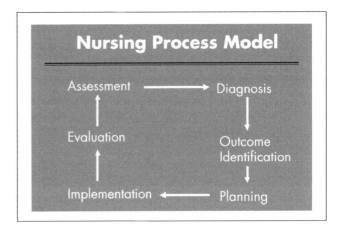

The CCC of Nursing Diagnoses is also used to provide 528 nursing outcomes, which are derived from 176 nursing diagnoses; each of which is combined with one of three outcome qualifiers. The outcome qualifiers are the fourth level of the CCC framework: (a) improve, (b) stabilize, or (c) deteriorate. They are used for documenting the expected outcomes (goals) and/or actual outcomes (resolved nursing diagnoses). The Nursing outcomes represent the diagnosis results of the nursing and patient care processes during the hospitalization, on discharge, or any episode of illness.

The third level also consists of 804 nursing interventions actions: 201 core nursing interventions (77 major and 124 subcategories), each of which is always combined with one of four Action Type qualifiers. The Action Type qualifiers are also the fourth level of the CCC framework, and they include the following: (a) assess, (b) perform, (c) teach, and (d) manage. The nursing interventions are used to document the "**essence of care**" provided by nurses or allied health professionals treating and caring for the assessed nursing diagnoses, medical conditions, or problems.

The 201 core nursing interventions represent 77 major intervention concepts, and the 124 subcategories represent more precise, granular concepts. A nursing intervention represents a single nursing action to achieve an outcome for a nursing and/or medical diagnosis for which the nurse is accountable (Saba, Moss, & Whittenburg, 2011). However, by combining a core nursing intervention with an Action Type qualifier, a new concept is formed, with a new meaning. The Action Types define a specific dimension for each core nursing intervention with codes that can then be used to measure outcomes, workload, resources, and/or cost.

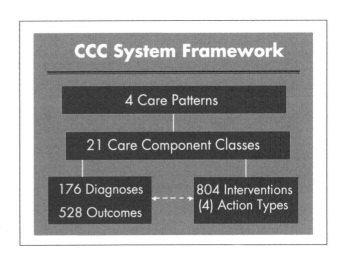

FIGURE 2.2 ▦ Four-level framework of CCC System.

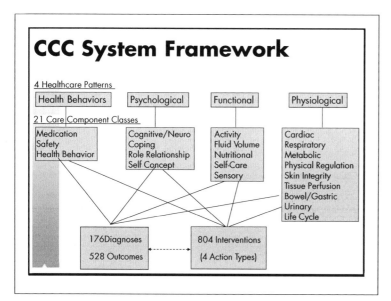

FIGURE 2.3 ▨ Four Healthcare Patterns and 21 Care Components of CCC System.

● Developmental History

Research Study

The CCC System, Version 2.5 augments the 1988–1991 research study conducted by Dr. Virginia K. Saba and a research team at the Georgetown University School of Nursing, Washington, DC, through a contract (#17C-98983/3) with the Health Care Financing Administration (HCFA), currently known as the Centers for Medicare and Medicaid Services. The CCC System, originally known as the Home Health Care Classification (HHCC) System, is a product developed from government-sponsored research designed "to develop and demonstrate a method for classifying patients to predict resources and measure outcomes." The design of this national research study was based on a conceptual framework, literature review, and a pilot study. The research findings were based on actual live resource data that were objectively collected and measured (Saba, 1991).

Research Sample

The research sample consisted of data collected from 8,967 records of recently discharged patients from a national sample of 646 Medicare-certified healthcare facilities, randomly stratified by staff size, type of ownership, and geographic location. The research findings consisted of demographic data and patient care findings, which were collected from recorded narrative notes. The patient care findings depicted the "**essence of care**" recorded by nurses and other healthcare providers. Two sets of statements from the narrative notes were collected from the study records: (a) one set consisting of approximately 40,381 patient problems and/or nursing diagnoses and (b) a second set consisting of approximately 80,283 services, treatments, interventions, and/or actions provided to the patient during the episode of illness.

Processing Statements

Once the narrative statements were collected, the research team had the task of processing and coding the two sets of statements. Because none of the existing coding strategies available at the time (1980s) were based on live research data, none were useful or found to be appropriate. As a result, the Georgetown research team determined there was a gap and a need to develop two new sets of vocabularies that could be used to code the concepts derived from the narrative statements. Hundreds of narrative statements were keyboarded using permuted **keyword sorts** that were processed, evaluated, and statistically analyzed to determine and develop the concepts needed to code the two sets of narrative statements. Narrative statements with similar meanings stated in different words with the same meaning were clustered together for analysis.

Example: Narrative Nursing Diagnosis/Problem Statements:
Many statements used different words to mean the same nursing condition or problem and were merged to form a single concept. For example, *difficult breathing, inhalation problem, and breathing problem* and were merged to form the concept "**Breathing Pattern Impairment**."

Example: Narrative Nursing Service/Intervention Statements:
Many statements used different words to mean the same nursing service or intervention and were merged to form a single concept. For example, *control of urinary drainage, care for bladder drainage, and control of urinary seepage* were merged to form the concept "**Bladder Care.**"

The concepts for the two sets of narrative statements—(a) patient problems/nursing diagnoses and (b) nursing services/interventions—were sorted together, separately, and matched together by patient. By using this technique, the research team empirically developed a tentative vocabulary list of approximately 200 discrete nursing diagnoses/problems and 800 discrete nursing services/interventions.

Development of Nursing Action Types

The research team further noted that each of the 800 discrete nursing services/interventions consisted of two separate parts: (a) a single service or intervention (core concept) and (b) an action type (specific concept). The specific services or interventions were repeated over and over using different actions such as (a) Assess Urinary Catheter Care, (b) Perform Urinary Catheter Care, (c) Teach/Instruct family on Urinary Catheter Care, or (d) Manage/Contact/ call physician regarding Urinary Catheter Care. The core concept (atomic, granular level) was **Urinary Catheter Care**, and the Action Types varied and focused on four different types of actions, each of which required different expertise and different nursing content/knowledge and took different lengths of time.

1. **Assess Urinary Catheter Care:** Addressed the assessment status or observation/monitor of the urinary catheter's condition.
2. **Perform Urinary Catheter Care:** Addressed the actual hands-on care of the urinary catheter.
3. **Teach Urinary Catheter Care:** Addressed the instruction or education of the patient and/or caregiver on how to take care of the urinary catheter.
4. **Manage Urinary Catheter Care:** Addressed the communication with the physician/ provider regarding the condition of the urinary catheter (e.g., blocked, bloody).

As a result, the 800 nursing services/interventions were separated into two levels (sets): (a) core concept (atomic, granular) intervention and (b) four Action Types. The latter includes (a) assess or monitor, (b) perform or provide direct care, (c) teach or educate, and/or (d) manage or refer. This strategy provided a unique, flexible, coding scheme and reduced the number to 160 core interventions concepts with the four Action Types, totaling the original 640 HHCC System Nursing Interventions/Actions.

Care Components

The two sets of concepts—(a) nursing diagnoses/problems and (b) nursing services/interventions—once coded and validated, had to be grouped and/or classified for ease of use and analytic purposes. The purpose of the analyses was to develop categories/groups for classifying the nursing diagnosis and nursing intervention sets. Because none of the existing classification schemes linked the nursing diagnoses to the nursing interventions and to the nursing outcomes, the HHCC Care Components were developed and used for the classification of the two nursing terminologies (classifications/vocabularies).

The above rationale was used to ensure the linkage of each concept between nursing diagnoses, nursing interventions, and nursing outcomes. By conducting statistical empirical analyses on the two sets of coded vocabularies, the frequencies of the study concepts resulted in 20 logical, consistent, statistically grouped categories called *Care Components* (Saba, 1995). The analyses results were tested and retested to ensure that the care components were reliable and could classify the two vocabulary lists of concepts. Thus, the original HHCC System was developed with two vocabularies (lists of concepts arranged in a hierarchal format), making it possible to document, code, and classify the nursing diagnoses/problems and nursing services/interventions as well as map the two terminologies together and use them in the continuum of care. The Care Component analyses found reliable, logical, and clinically significant care component classes.

Nursing Diagnoses

The initial terminology set of approximately 40,361 patient problems, conditions, and/or nursing diagnoses consisted of assessed signs and symptoms for the entire episode of care that required nursing and other allied providers of healthcare services. The original classification of 145 nursing diagnoses consisted of nursing diagnoses collected from the research findings and noun phrases were empirically developed from processing the key words from the narrative statements such as "**medication risk**," "**polypharmacy**," or "**dying process**" (see Figure 2.4).

Nursing Outcomes

The original 145 Nursing Diagnoses were used to derive 435 Nursing Outcomes. The outcomes were used for the Expected Outcomes/Goals of care as well as for the results of care or the Actual Outcomes of the patient's problems/nursing diagnoses that required nursing interventions/services to resolve. The patients' nursing diagnoses were evaluated on admission and discharge and assigned outcomes using one of three qualifiers: (a) **Improve(d)** or resolve(d) (condition changed), (b) **Stabilize(d)** or maintain(ed) (condition did not change), and (c) **Deteriorate(d)** or die(d) (condition worsened). These three qualifiers were used for two steps in the nursing process: (a) Expected Outcome (Outcome Identification/Goal) and (b) Evaluation (Actual Outcome/met or not met condition).

Nursing Interventions

The initial research study obtained over 80,283 narrative statements of nursing interventions, services, and/or actions performed for the entire episode of care. The narrative statements formed the foundation for the empirical development of the original 160 HHCC Nursing Intervention. The 160 Nursing Interventions included: (a) 28 HCFA Skilled Treatment Codes (Health Care Financing Administration, 1977) required by the government; (b) a core set of concepts (major categories and subcategories) based on logical groupings and permuted key word sort; and (c) four Action Type qualifiers (Assess, Care, Teach, and Manage) designed to expand and enhance the list of 160 Nursing Interventions to 640 Nursing Interventions with four Action Types. See Figure 2.5.

Coding Structure

The research team reviewed available code/data sets (government and private) and determined there was a gap in code sets designed for computer processing. The team determined

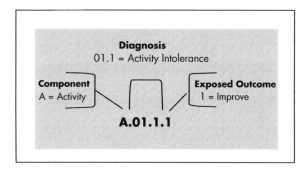

FIGURE 2.4 ■ CCC System Diagnoses codes.

FIGURE 2.5 ■ CCC System
Intervention codes.

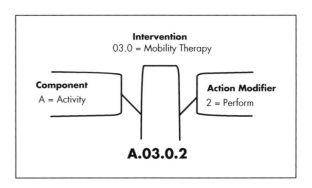

the requirements for the coding of the original classifications/terminologies. The essential requirement was that the coding structure be designed for computer processing. Each concept in the two terminologies had to have a unique code so the concepts could be linked to each other and mapped to other classification systems. Furthermore, each concept had to be coded in a hierarchical structure as well as defined and classified in a standardized manner. Finally, the codes had to be designed so that the concepts could be processed, retrieved, and aggregated for analysis purposes. As a result, the research team developed a coding strategy and framework based on the coding structure and classification format of the Tenth Revision of the *International Statistical Classification of Diseases and Related Health Problems (ICD-10*; World Health Organization, 1992), which was specifically designed for computer processing.

The ICD-10 consists of a five-character alphanumeric code and was used to code all concepts in the CCC classifications/terminologies. The first alphabetic character represents the care components used to classify and link nursing diagnoses, interventions, and outcomes together; the next three characters are digits representing the diagnosis and intervention core concepts (major and subcategories), and the last and fifth character is a digit representing the three outcome qualifiers or the four Action Type qualifiers.

> **Example: Activity Care Component (A) Links Diagnosis, Intervention, and Outcome Together**
>
> * *Nursing Diagnosis:* **Physical Mobility Impairment: A01.5**
>
> * *Expected Outcome (Goal):* **Improve Physical Mobility Impairment***:* **A01.5.1**
>
> * *Core Nursing Intervention:* **Mobility Therapy: A03.0**
>
> * *Nursing Intervention/Action:* **Perform Mobility Therapy: A03.0.2**
>
> * *Actual Outcome (Goal Met):* **Physical Mobility Impairment Improved: A01.5.1**

● Applied Uses

General Uses

The CCC System is in general use in diverse areas of nursing practice and in different EHR and HIT systems applications. The CCC System provides a coded standardized nursing terminology, framework, and information model following the nursing process for nursing and allied health professionals. The CCC System is being used in all clinical settings for documenting nursing practice, including the administration and management of nursing departments. The CCC System is also being used in nursing education for teaching and educating nursing students as well as supporting nursing educational programs. In addition, the CCC System is being used to conduct nursing research.

Nursing Practice

The CCC System's two interrelated terminologies, CCC of Nursing Diagnoses and Outcomes and the CCC of Nursing Interventions/Actions, facilitate the capture (**input**) of standardized coded concepts (data/elements) for the electronic documentation of patient care at the point of care and facilitates the processing of the care data for documenting care as well as for generating **output** for the analysis of nursing practices. The CCC concepts are standardized—defined, classified, and coded—making it possible to link the care process: nursing diagnoses to nursing interventions and nursing outcomes. Based on the CCC System information model and framework for documenting nursing practice, software applications follow the six steps/standards of the nursing process in the EHR and HIT systems.

Nursing Practice Uses

The CCC System facilitates using the EHR system's clinical pathways, plans of care, care protocols for specific disease conditions, population groups, or care staff. The CCC System can also be used to develop decision-support and expert systems. The CCC System makes it possible to evaluate nursing practices, develop guidelines, develop evidence-based practices, and advance nursing knowledge though the data analysis of actual nursing care for which the nurse is accountable.

Nursing Practice Applications

The CCC System is being used in EHRs for the documentation of nursing practice and nursing plans of care regardless of healthcare setting. The CCC System is being implemented into existing EHR systems primarily following the three strategies below:

1. Healthcare facilities (hospitals, ambulatory clinics, or nursing practice programs) obtain CCC System permission (sign a permission form) to integrate the CCC concepts (data/elements) into the facility's data dictionary. The healthcare facility uses the CCC System to develop and code its own plans of care.
2. An EHR/HIT vendor/consulting firm obtains CCC System permission (signs a permission form) and uses the CCC System to develop a proprietary standardized set of plans of care, which is marketed commercially to healthcare facilities.
3. An EHR/HIT vendor/consulting firm obtains CCC System permission (signs a permission form) and inputs the CCC System's concepts into their proprietary data dictionaries for use by customers/clients to adapt and/or develop care plans.

Applied Uses in Nursing Practice

The applied uses of the CCC System in nursing practice include numerous hospitals implementing plans of care and nursing documentation in EHR or HIT systems. The implementation of the CCC System is technology neutral, allowing any EHR or HIT system to integrate the CCC System terminologies. A few examples of CCC System implementation in nursing practice are the following:

- Southcoast Hospitals Group, Fall River, MA (3 hospitals)
- Claxton–Hepburn Medical Center, Ogdensburg, NY
- Hospital Corporation of American, Nashville, TN (163 hospitals)
- Rush Medical Center, Chicago, IL
- Vanderbilt University Medical Center, Nashville, TN

Siemens Medical Solutions integrated the CCC System terminologies in the Siemens vocabulary manager of Sorian©. In Sorian, the CCC System terminologies are now available to clients worldwide for the documentation of nursing practice.

The CCC System is also being used in many countries outside the United States. Finland has adapted the CCC System and called it the Finnish Care Classification (FinCC). In 2005, FinCC was named the national nursing classification standard for documenting nursing practice in *all* Finnish hospitals. The FinCC is currently being translated into Swedish. The CCC System has been translated into German and Norwegian. In Norway, the CCC System has been implemented as SabaKlass. In South Korea for example, the CCC System is used in the Seoul National University Hospital EHR. In South Australia, the Central Adelaide Health Service, Adelaide, SA, has developed an application using the CCC System for the nursing and midwifery programs to document nursing practice following the nursing process. See Chapter 4 for examples of applied CCC System uses from several of these applications, with screen prints.

Nursing Education

The CCC System is being taught as part of every nursing informatics (NI) course that addresses nursing terminologies recognized by the American Nurses Association (ANA). The CCC System offers educators *free* CCC System software and the CCC System terminologies to teach nursing students how to electronically document nursing practice following the nursing process using a standardized nursing terminology. Chapter 7 is included to provide information to educators about how to teach the documentation of a nursing POC using the CCC System information model. Several educators have successfully tested and used the CCC System software on a personal digital assistant device and other handheld devices, such as the iPad, to support the documentation of student clinical practice.

Educational Technologies

Today, nursing educators are using many new technologies and strategies for teaching and learning. The rapidly evolving technology offers online learning, distance learning, and web applications for nontraditional nursing educational programs. These programs provide student instruction separate from the classroom and faculty.

Second Life is a three-dimensional virtual world for engaging students with course content. It creates a virtual laboratory for real or simulated environments and/or a platform for interactive experiences, bringing new dimensions to teaching best practices (Warren, Connors, & Trangenstein, 2011). Simulation laboratories are another unique technology being used to teach students core clinical techniques and safe patient care practices. The CCC System supports nursing student documentation with coding for the nursing diagnoses, interventions, and actions.

Nursing Research

The CCC System is useful in all nursing research methods: quantitative, qualitative, and mixed method. Nursing Research designed to develop decision-support systems and evidence-based systems and evaluate best practices requires a standardized nursing language and unified nursing process framework. The CCC System is the first national nursing terminology standard and framework that includes all six standards of the nursing process, the standard of professional nursing practice (American Nurses Association, 2010). Any nursing research that requires a nursing terminology, coded nursing data, or standardized nursing practices can use the CCC System as a base vocabulary. Doctoral students have used, and continue to use and study, the CCC System to conduct dissertation research. Nursing informatics researchers use the CCC System to document patient care in an EHR to aggregate and analyze the coded data to develop disease management protocols, measure outcomes, and determine workload measures, resources, and costs. The NI researchers also conduct meta-analyses using nursing ontology literature and bibliographic materials to evaluate the advantages of using standardized terminologies in practice and to promote the adoption of EHR/HIT systems for nursing.

Research Studies

The CCC System has been evaluated by several informatics theorists and researchers who conducted ontology research, evaluation studies, and other analyses with the CCC System. The major NI experts who have studied the CCC System have evaluated various aspects of the terminology as well as compared the CCC System to several of the ANA-recognized classifications. In these articles, the NI experts identified the major features and the important characteristics of the CCC System that are described in Chapter 3.

Several research studies have been conducted using the original CCC System (HHCC, Version 1.0) and, more recently, the CCC System, Version 2.0. The NI research on the CCC System regardless of ontology focus, healthcare setting, and time period, have all resulted in similar positive findings on the importance of the CCC System for documenting the **essence of care**. The NI researchers unanimously concluded that the CCC System meets the essential criteria for a terminology as defined by the International Organization for Standardization (2003) and the "Desiderata" by Cimino (1998). The references to the major research and evaluation studies are listed in the Chapter 4 References.

Nursing Administration

The CCC System is used as an innovative tool in nursing administration to measure nursing workload, provide administrative outcome information, and determine the cost of nursing care and resources. Other CCC System uses for nursing management are possible when nursing care data are coded and aggregated for the analysis of different disease conditions, population groups, and healthcare settings. The CCC System can be also be used for data mining

---

EXHIBIT 2.1 ■ Summary of the Clinical Care Classification System

Nursing Practice Applications:

- Capture patient care data using a standardized coded nursing terminology.
- Code electronic clinical encounters: diagnoses, interventions, and outcomes.
- Track nurses' contribution to patient care and care outcomes.
- Provide standardized concepts (data/elements) for clinical pathways and decision support.
- Enable evidence-based practice protocols to process and analyze patient care data and to evaluate the effects of nursing care on patient outcomes.

Nursing Education Applications:

- Teach students how to electronically document and code POCs based on the nursing process.
- Track student assignments: procedures and protocols.
- Test and evaluate online the clinical documentation of students' patient care.
- Teach and evaluate student use of simulations.
- Use Second Life to enhance educational experiences.
- Use the CCC System application to enhance nursing educational experiences.

Nursing Research Applications:

- Search online nursing literature for nursing ontology and the CCC System.
- Research the use of relative value units and the CCC of Nursing Interventions/Action Types.
- Analyze and interpret nursing output in the EHR.
- Support research to advance NI science and knowledge.

Nursing Administration Applications:

- Capture standardized quality indicators and measures.
- Capture and measure the impact of care on outcomes.
- Determine and measure nursing workload, resources, and cost.
- Support the prediction of patient acuity and care needs.

and to demonstrate that the nursing care of patients does improve healthcare quality, ensure patient safety, and improve care outcomes. A summary of the CCC applied uses and applications is shown in Exhibit 2.1.

● References

American Nurses Association. (2010). *Nursing: Scope and standards of practice.* Silver Spring, MD: ANA.

Cimino, J. J. (1998). Desiderata for controlled medical vocabularies in the twenty-first century. *Methods of Information in Medicine,* 37, 304–403.

Department of Health and Human Services (HHS). (2007). January 12 Letter of Secretary of Michael O. Leavitt. Retrieved from http://www.hhs.gov/healthit/documents/m20070123/012207letter.html

Health Care Financing Administration. (1997). *Medicare home health agency manual.* Washington, DC: HCFA, DHHS.

International Organization for Standardization. (2003). Nursing language: Terminology models for nurses. *ISO Bulletin,* 16–18.

Saba, V. K. (1991). *Home healthcare classification project.* Washington, DC: Georgetown University (NTIS Pub # PB92-177013/AS).

Saba, V. K. (1995). A new paradigm for computer-based nursing information systems: Twenty care components. In R. A. Greenes, H. E. Peterson, & D. J. Proti (Eds.), *Medinfo '95 Proceedings* (pp. 1404–1406). Edmonton, Canada: IMIA.

Saba, V. K., Moss, J., & Whittenburg, L. (2011). Overview of the Clinical Care Classification: A national nursing standard coded terminology. In V. K. Saba & K. A. McCormick (Eds.), *Essentials of Nursing Informatics* (5th ed., pp. 217–229). New York, NY: McGraw–Hill.

Taylor, S. (2007). Moving past theory: Use of a standardized coded nursing terminology to enhance nursing visibility. *CIN, Computers, Informatics, Nursing,* 25(6), 324–331.

Warren, J. J., Connors, H. R., & Trangenstein, P. (2011). A paradigm shift in simulation: Experiential learning in Second Life. In V. K. Saba & K. A. McCormick (Eds.), *Essentials of Nursing Informatics* (5th ed., pp. 691–631). New York, NY: McGraw–Hill.

World Health Organization. (1992). *ICD-10: International statistical classification of diseases and related health problems: Tenth revision: Volume 1.* Geneva, Switzerland: WHO.

Features, Standards, and Policies 3

This chapter focuses on the Clinical Care Classification (CCC) System© definitions, features, standards, and policies in Version 2.5: (a) **Definitions** explain the technical differences between the overlapping terms used in the field of languages and ontologies; (b) **Features** address the attributes of the terminology as identified by the theorists in the field; (c) **Standards** highlight the basis for the CCC System as a national nursing standard; and (d) **Policies** describe how the CCC System is administered by SabaCare Inc.

● Definitions

The CCC System's two interrelated terminologies, the CCC of Nursing Diagnoses and Outcomes and the CCC of Nursing Interventions/Actions, have been described as a data set, code set, terminology, dictionary, classification, taxonomy, and nomenclature (Coenen et al., 2001). The CCC System's terminologies have also been defined by the International Organization for Standardization (ISO) as follows:

1. **terminologies** because the CCC System represents a system of concepts (ISO, 1087; ISO, 1990),

2. **classifications** because of the CCC System's hierarchical structure (ISO, 11179-1; ISO, 1999),

3. **taxonomies** because of the relationships between concept levels (major categories and subcategories, (ISO, 11179-1; ISO, 1999) and

4. **nomenclatures** because the CCC terminologies follow a set of preestablished rules officially (ISO 1087; ISO, 1990, 2003).

● Features

The CCC System has several features that are unique and characteristic of a terminology that meets the criteria for a controlled vocabulary proposed by Cimino (1998) in his article "Desiderata for Controlled Medical Vocabularies in the Twenty-first Century." The CCC concepts in the CCC System's two terminologies, the CCC of Nursing Diagnoses and Outcomes and the CCC of Nursing Interventions/Actions, are **granular** or **atomic** and are formally **defined** to ensure **nonambiguity** and **nonredundancy**. The terms in the CCC System have concept permanence and unique concept **identifying codes** that are used **only once** and remain forever unchanged (retired or deleted codes are never reused), and therefore, the CCC System is **context-free**. The CCC System is also polyhierarchical, having multiple levels of granularity.

The CCC of Nursing Diagnoses terminology uses three qualifiers for combining **Expected Outcomes** and/or **Actual Outcomes**, whereas the CCC of Nursing Interventions/Actions uses four qualifiers for identifying types of actions, making the interventions **multiaxial**, multihierarchical, and **combinatorial**. The CCC System has a **structured framework** with **coded concept**s that are classified, consistent, and usable for electronic processing **input** and **retrievable** as output for **analyses**. The **atomic-level concepts** (data) are coded and can be used for multiple purposes. The CCC System can be used to document nursing care process and therefore provides a **legal record** of patient care. The CCC System supports clinical decision-making and captures **data/concepts** that can be retrieved, aggregated, and used for analysis and research (Zielstorff et al., 1998; Cimino, 1998, 2006; Henry & Mead, 1997).

Additionally, several other criteria are met by the CCC System such as (a) being specifically designed for **computer processing** and computer-based systems, (b) **requiring no licensing**

EXHIBIT 3.1 ■ Major Features of the Clinical Care Classification System

---

- Consists of discrete atomic-level concepts using qualifiers to enhance and expand the concepts.
- Data are collected once and used many times for many purposes including efficient aggregation.
- Copyrighted and in the public domain; available with permission without any cost or license.
- Specifically designed for electronic health records (EHRs) and healthcare information technology (HIT) systems as well as other electronic information processing systems.
- Tested and applicable in ALL healthcare settings.
- Conforms to Cimino (1998) criteria for a standardized healthcare terminology.
- Coded standardized framework for electronic documentation, retrieval, and analysis.
- Codes based on ICD-10 (WHO, 1992) structure for information exchange promoting interoperability.
    - * Uses a coding structure of five alphanumeric digits to link the two CCC System terminologies to each other and to map to other EHR/HIT systems.
- Designed for determining workload (productivity), resources (needs), outcomes (quality), and care costs.
- Concept terminology with online source files so public and private organizations may harmonize nursing information formats for cross-organizational sharing of information.
- Facilitates the electronic documentation of patient care at the point of care.
- Uses a framework of care components to classify the two CCC System terminologies and represent 4 healthcare patterns focusing on a holistic approach to patient care.
- Consists of flexible, adaptable, and expandable concepts/data elements.

Sources: Saba, 2011; Saba, Moss, & Whittenburg, 2011; Saba, & Taylor, 2007.

fees, (c) being in the **public domain**, and (d) being responsive to terminology constituents. The major features of the CCC System are listed in Exhibit 3.1.

These features are characteristic of a terminology that can be used in all healthcare settings for the documentation of nursing plans of care and nursing practice. However, any nursing terminology must comply with the healthcare standards that have been determined essential for today's information exchange and interoperability in and between healthcare systems.

● Standards

The major Standards Development Organizations (SDOs) that have integrated the CCC System into their respective standards are briefly described below and listed in Exhibit 3.3. The need for a terminology to be integrated into such SDOs reflects the sound and unified structure of the CCC System for use in EHR systems.

American Nurses Association

In 1991, the original CCC System was initially recognized by the American Nurses Association (ANA) Steering Committee on Databases to Support Clinical Nursing Practice and approved by the ANA Congress on Nursing Practice in 1992 (McCormick et al., 1994). For the core criteria for ANA recognition of nursing databases, classifications, and nomenclatures, see Exhibit 3.2. The ANA Database Committee recognized the CCC System as being a valid and useful approach to naming and classifying nursing practices as well as a comprehensive coded nursing terminology standard meeting nursing data and clinical practice standards requirements for computer-based HIT systems (ANA Steering Committee on Databases to Support Clinical Nursing Practice, 1992). The ANA's recognition of the CCC System led to the approval and integration of the CCC System in other healthcare standards organizations and electronic nursing database resources. (See Appendix B: Clinical Care Classification [CCC] System Milestones:

EXHIBIT 3.2 ■ American Nurses Association Criteria for Recognition of Terminology Supporting Nursing Practice

The following criteria provide the framework for the evaluation for recognition of a terminology supporting nursing practice (September 22, 2008):

1. The terminology supports one or more components of the nursing process.
2. The rationale for development supports this terminology as a new terminology itself or with a unique contribution to nursing/healthcare.
3. Characteristics of the terminology include:
   - Support of one or more of the nursing domains
   - Description of the data elements
   - Internal consistency
   - Testing of reliability, validity, sensitivity, and specificity
   - Utility in practice showing scope of use and user population
   - Coding using context-free unique identifier
4. Characteristics of the terminology development and maintenance process include:
   - The intended use of the terminology
   - The centricity of the content (patient, community, etc.)
   - Research-based framework used for development
   - Open call for participation in initial and ongoing development
   - Systematic, defined, ongoing process for development
   - Relevance to nursing care and nursing science
   - Collaborative partnerships
   - Documentation of history of decisions
   - Defined revision and version control mechanisms
   - Defined maintenance program
   - Long-term plan for sustainability
5. Access and distribution mechanisms are defined.
6. Plans and strategies for future development are defined.

From: American Nurses Association (2008, September). Criteria for Recognition of Terminology Supporting Nursing Practice. Unpublished Document. Reprinted with permission.

2011–1988.) The major SDOs, part of the American National Standards Institute (ANSI), are of interest because these ANSI organizations validated the CCC System information structure and extended their organizational credentials to support the evolution of nursing informatics.

Unified Medical Language System

In 1993, once recognized by the ANA, the National Library of Medicine (NLM) selected the CCC System (previously known as the Home Health Care Classification HHCC) as one of four nursing languages to be integrated into the Metathesaurus of the Unified Medical Language System (UMLS). The terminologies that were selected met the ANA Database Steering Committee criteria for documenting nursing practice in emerging technologies (http://www.nlm.nih.gov?research/umls/support.html).

Cumulative Index of Nursing and Allied Health Literature

In 1993, the next crucial integration event was the submission for indexing into the Cumulative Index of Nursing and Allied Health Literature (CINAHL) which is considered to be the most complete index of all nursing and allied health literature. Today, CINAHL is primarily used by nurses to access information found in the nursing literature: books, journals, proceedings, and other primary literature sources (CINAHL, 2005).

ABC Codes

In 1998, the ABC codes for complementary and alternative medicine (Alternative Link Inc., 2001; 2006) adapted selected CCC Nursing Interventions. The ABC codes were developed and designed to accurately communicate medical and nursing procedures and services to health insurance companies and/or to monitor the charges for patient services by individual medical practitioners/providers. The ABC codes were designed by Alternative Link Inc., to meet the business requirements of providers who use codes (data concepts) to determine the fees for patient encounters.

Health Level Seven

In 1999, the CCC System was registered in Health Level Seven (HL7) as a standard language. Health Level Seven is involved in the development of international healthcare informatics interoperability standards. Through a consensus process, HL7 develops health information management and technology standards for the exchange, sharing, integration, and retrieval of electronic healthcare information. The HL7 standards support information exchanges in clinical practice as well as the management and evaluation of healthcare services for most information technology and terminologies used in the world. Therefore, the CCC System is an interoperable terminology standard for the communication of codes from one system to another (http://www.HL7.org).

Logical Observation Identifiers Names and Codes

In 1999, the CCC of Nursing Diagnoses and Outcomes was integrated into the Logical Observation Identifiers Names and Codes (LOINC®) standard. The LOINC® standard is a universal code system for laboratory and clinical observations developed by the Regenstrief Institute, Inc., Indianapolis, Indiana. As a healthcare standard for the exchange of data from different healthcare information systems, LOINC® is used for research, management, clinical care, outcomes, and other clinical documentation purposes (http://LOINC.org).

American National Standards Institute (ANSI)–Healthcare Informatics Standards Board

In 1998/1999, the CCC System was recognized as a nursing standard and published by the ANSI–Healthcare Informatics Standards Board (ANSI-HISB) in the *Inventory of Clinical Information Standards* (1998/1999). Furthermore, the CCC System was presented to the National Committee on Vital and Health Statistics (NCVHS) Developers of Coding and Classification Panel, Subcommittee on Healthcare Data Needs, Standards, and Security, for the implementation of the Health Insurance Portability and Accountability Act of 1966 (www.ncvhs.dhhs.gov).

National Committee on Vital and Health Statistics

During the 1990s, the CCC was submitted as a recognized nursing standard to several federal agencies including several NCVHS subcommittees which investigated and prepared recommendations to Department of Health and Human Services (HHS) on how to implement the new legislation using electronic standards. Several standards-related healthcare information organizations reviewed the CCC System as a nursing terminology standard since being recognized by the ANA. The historical milestones are listed, and as the HHCC was updated and renamed to the CCC System, each version was submitted to appropriate SDOs.

Systematized Nomenclature of Medicine Clinical Terms

In 2000, the original CCC System (HHCC, Version 1.0) was submitted and integrated into the Systematized Nomenclature of Medicine Clinical Terms (SNOMED CT). The SNOMED CT is a comprehensive clinical terminology, originally created by the College of American Pathologists. The CCC System, Versions 1.0 and 2.0, are mapped by SNOMED CT and are available to anyone with permission. See the SNOMED CT description in relationship to the CCC System in Chapter 5 (http://www.nlm.nih.gov/research/umls/Snomed/snomed_main.html).

International Organization for Standardization Technical Committee: Health Informatics (ISO/TC215: ISO Standard 18104)

In 2003, the CCC System was recognized, confirmed, and approved as a terminology meeting the two reference terminology model structures, nursing diagnoses and nursing actions, that comprise the "Integration of a Reference Terminology Model for Nursing," the international standard passed by the ISO Technical Committee: Health Informatics (ISO/TC215). The "Integration of a Reference Terminology Model for Nursing" was designed to accommodate various nursing terminologies and classifications in use at the time (ISO, 2003). The nursing reference terminology standard was essential as an information model for creating comparable nursing data across settings and countries.

Patient Medical Record Information

In 2003, the federal government, via the NCVHS committees, focused on the implementation of the Health Insurance Portability and Accountability Act of 1996, Part II, Patient Medical Record Information (PMRI). The CCC System was recognized in the PMRI as a nursing terminology standard and included in the recommendation to the secretary of HHS for the PMRI implementation.

Office of the National Coordinator for Health Information Technology

In 2004, the Secretary of HHS implemented the President's Executive Order (13335) recognizing the importance of HIT systems and established the Office of the National Coordinator for Health Information Technology (ONC) with the goal "to support the adoption of HIT and the promotion of nationwide health information exchange to improve healthcare (http://healthit.hhs.gov/portal/server.pt/community/healthit_hhs_gov_onc/1200).

Healthcare Information Technology Standards Panel

In 2005, the Office of the National Coordinator for Health Information Technology (ONC) established a public/private partnership and volunteer Healthcare Information Technology Standards Panel (HITSP). The panel's objectives were to identify, determine, and select the electronic standards, code sets, classifications, and terminologies to implement the president's mandate that everyone in the United States have an EHR by 2014/2015. The CCC System was recognized and accepted January 23, 2007, by HHS secretary Michael Leavitt as a named standard within the HITSP Interoperability Specification for electronic health records, biosurveillance, and community empowerment. The CCC System was named by HHS as the first national nursing terminology for health information exchange and interoperability (http://www.hhs.gov/healthit/community/meetings/m20061031.html).

Health Information Technology for Economic and Clinical Health Act of 2009

In 2009, the Obama administration passed the American Recovery and Reinvestment Act (ARRA) of 2009, which included the Health Information Technology for Economic and Clinical Health (HITECH) Act of 2009 to facilitate the nationwide adoption of EHRs with incentive support for healthcare providers. The HITECH Act mandated that ONC offer online support to the healthcare providers in the United States to encourage the adoption of EHRs by 2014/2015. The ARRA of 2009 funded the HITECH program to provide incentives for all hospitals, healthcare facilities, and physicians/providers to improve patient care through technology. Also in 2009, HHS created two new national committees: (a) the Health Information Technology Policy Committee and (b) the Health Information Technology Standards Committee. The HHS Policy Committee was charged with making recommendations to the ONC for the adoption of a nationwide health information infrastructure, whereas the Standards

Committee was charged with determining the standards, implementation, and certification criteria for the electronic exchange and use of health information.

Meaningful Use

After one year of HHS committee planning, "meaningful use" emerged, which was designed to improve patient care by having better access to more complete patient information, including consumer information, through EHRs. Meaningful use was designed for implementation in three stages. The main focus of Stage 1 is on computerized provider order entry systems designed to electronically capture and share information as well as develop a list of reconciled patient problems. Stage 1 measures were finalized in 2011. The focus of Stage 2

EXHIBIT 3.3 ▦ CCC System in Standards and Other Health Care Information Technology Organizations

- **HITSP** (Healthcare Information Technology Standards Panel): In 2007/2008, the CCC System was recognized as the first named national nursing standard interoperable within the specifications developed for EHR systems.

- **ISO** (International Organization for Standardization): In 2003, the CCC System was tested, proven, and accepted as an international nursing standard based on the ISO "Integration of a Reference Terminology Model for Nursing" (ISO 18104).

- **SNOMED CT** (Systematized Nomenclature of Medicine Clinical Terms; owned by the International Health Terminology Standards Development Organization): In 2000, SNOMED RT (Reference Terminology) and, later, SNOMED CT integrated and mapped the CCC System of Nursing Diagnoses and Outcomes and Nursing Interventions/Actions as a nursing terminology standard in the SNOMED CT database. (See SNOMED CT in Chapter 5.)

- **ICNP** (International Classification for Nursing Practice): In 1999, the CCC System was one of the nursing terminologies contributed for use as the basis for the original alpha version of the ICNP and integrated into the ICNP developed by the International Council of Nurses.

- **ANSI** (American National Standards Institute): In 1998/1999, ANSI, as a national SDO, approved the CCC System as an interoperable terminology.

- **LOINC®** (Logical Observation Identifiers Names and Codes): In 1999, LOINC® integrated the CCC of Nursing Diagnoses and Outcomes into Clinical LOINC® System nomenclature for documenting outcomes.

- **HL7** (Health Level Seven): In 1999, HL7 registered the CCC System as a language standard for the electronic transmission of healthcare data and approved it as an interoperable terminology

- **ABC codes**: In 1998, the ABC codes (Alternative Link Inc.) integrated several adapted CCC Nursing Interventions and Actions into the ABC codes for complementary and alternative medicine to communicate medical and nursing procedures to healthcare providers.

- **ANA**: In 1996, the ANA recognized the CCC System as an appropriate terminology for information technology vendors applying for approval from the Nursing Information and Data Set Evaluation Center to use for their nursing documentation.

- **CINAHL** (Cumulative Index to Nursing and Allied Health Literature®): In 1993, CINAHL integrated the CCC System into its nursing index.

- **UMLS** (Unified Medical Language System): In 1993, the NLM integrated the CCC System into the their Metathesaurus of the UMLS.

- **ANA** (American Nurses Association): In 1991, the ANA recognized the CCC System, and in 1992, the ANA Congress on Nursing Practice recognized it as a nursing standard appropriate for supporting clinical nursing practice in the EHR.

is on electronic quality indicators, to be available by 2013, and the main focus of Stage 3 is the electronic outcomes of patient care, to be achieved by 2015. The CCC System is meets meaningful-use criteria with the implementation of patient plans of care (PPOCs) resulting from computerized provider order entry. The use of the CCC System as a nursing terminology for PPOCs supports Stage 2 quality indicators as well as the Stage 3 patient care outcomes.

The SDOs have identified the CCC System for use in documenting nursing practice within the EHR and/or HIT systems and for the exchange of health information across and between health information systems for nursing practice, education, and research. With the HITECH legislation and meaningful use initiatives, the CCC System is being applied as a nursing terminology meeting the documentation requirements for PPOCs.

Translations

The CCC System, Version 2.0 has been translated into several languages: Dutch, Finnish, Norwegian, Chinese, Portuguese, Spanish, German, Korean, Turkish, Slovene, and Taiwanese. The CCC in Finland is called the Finnish Care Classification, and in Norway, the CCC is called SabaKlass. The CCC System continues to be translated into many languages.

● Maintenance Policy

The CCC is administered by SabaCo, which is incorporated in the State of Virginia. The office is located in Arlington, Virginia. Dr. Virginia K. Saba, EdD, RN, FAAN, FACMI, is the current president and CEO of SabaCo. SabaCo has an advisory board called the National CCC Scientific Advisory Board, which consists of at least five permanent members, ad hoc members, and consultants to the group. The active members have changed with each of the updates but are all nursing terminologists and/or experts in the field of nursing taxonomies, classifications, nomenclatures, and/or terminologies.

- The CCC National Scientific Advisory Board meets each spring to review suggested concepts, terms, or labels that are proposed by CCC Clients for consideration. If there are sufficient concepts, terms, or labels to warrant a formal update, the evaluation process is set in motion as listed in the following revision policy.
- The CCC has had four releases, including the CCC System, Version 2.5, Fall 2011. The CCC System, Version 2.5, changes from Version 2.0 are listed in Appendix A. The changes are:
  1. Care Components: 1 renamed and 2 revised definitions
  2. CCC Nursing Diagnoses: 4 new diagnoses, 10 retired diagnoses, and 16 revised definitions
  3. CCC Nursing Interventions: 14 new interventions, 11 retired interventions, and 25 revised definitions
- CCC System, Version 2.5, News Release (Exhibit 3.5)
- CCC System permission form review (Exhibit 3.6)
- Website (www.sabacare.com and www.clinicalcareclassification.com) contains CCC Version 2.5 content and tables, including the revisions shown in the Appendices.

● Revision Policy

The detailed policy steps for revising the CCC System have been developed by the CCC System National Scientific Advisory Board as follows:

- Convene an annual face-to-face meeting in the spring.
- Review all submitted concepts, terms, or labels.
  * Identify the source of each submission.
  * Review the rationale for the submission change request/justification.

- Review and approve or disapprove new concepts, terms, or labels/definitions.
- Prepare new definitions and codes for the new concepts, terms, or labels.
- Review the existing version to determine whether there needs to be changes in any of the codes and/or concepts, terms, and/or definitions:
  * Retire/Delete: May have a new term;
  * Revise definition: Language may be more appropriate;
  * Revise code: Change from major to a subcategory.
- If the number of codes and/or concepts, terms, or labels are sufficient to warrant preparing a new revision, the developer or copyright holder is required to:
  * Solicit Board assistance to review and assist with coding and defining of the revised concepts, terms, or labels
  * Request that the SabaCare webmaster upload the revised version to www.sabacare. com
  * Prepare and distribute a news release regarding a new version
  * Prepare a new brochure describing the new version
  * Distribute the new version to appropriate organizations where the CCC System is integrated
  * Notify all known individual clients/users of revisions
  * Distribute the new version to all foreign translators of any CCC Version

● **Copyright and Trademark**

The CCC (Version 2.5) is copyrighted by Dr. Virginia K. Saba, EdD, RN, FAAN, FACMI.

- CCC System, Version 2.5, received a Library of Congress award and copyright awards by the United States Copyright Office.
  * CCC System, Version 1.0, copyright 1994
  * CCC System, Version 2.0, updated copyright 2004
  * CCC System, Version 2.5, updated copyright 2011
- The CCC System has been placed in the public domain and requires a signed permission form from a user/customer requesting use. (See Sample Permission Letter in Exhibit 3.5, page XX.)
- Anyone attempting to reproduce the CCC System must have developer/copyright holder permission and must include a disclaimer indicating that the CCC cannot be copyrighted by any other person or publisher.
- The CCC System received a certificate of registration for its logo from the U.S. Patent and Trademark Office on November 25, 2005, reissued in 2011 (required every 5 years). (See Exhibit 3.6, page XX.)

The CCC system continues to expand as the new concepts, terms, and labels are recommended by the different nursing specialty groups and users. The information model and structure of the CCC System readily accommodates expansion as new concepts emerge.

EXHIBIT 3.4 ▥ Service Mark Principal Register (Logo)

Int. Cl.: 35
Prior U.S. Classes: 100, 101, and 102   Reg. No. 3,019.288
U.S. Patent and Trademark Office   Registered November 2005

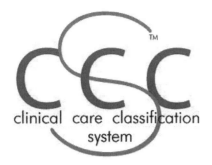

SABA, VIRGINIA K. (UNITED STATES INDIVIDUAL)
Email: **vsaba@att.net**
Website: **http://www.Sabacare.com**

FOR PROVIDING INFORMATION IN THE FIELD OF CLINICAL DATA STANDARDS
FOR CODING PATIENT AND NURSING CARE DIAGNOSES, INTERVENTIONS, AND
OUTCOMES, IN CLASS 35 (U.S. CLASSES 100, 101, AND 102)

FIRST USE: 2-0-2004; IN COMMERCE: 2-0-2004
NO CLAIM IS MADE TO THE EXCLUSIVE RIGHT TO USE "CLINICAL CARE
   CLASSIFICATION
SYSTEM" APART FRPOM THE MARK AS SHOWN.
SERIES NO.: 76-595,572; FILED: 6-4-2004
ELIZABETH PIGNATELLO, EXAMINING ATTORNEY

● **News Release for CCC System Version 2.5**

EXHIBIT 3.5 ▥ Clinical Care Classification (CCC) System News Release

For information, contact Dr. Virginia K. Saba at vsaba@att.net.
For immediate release
SABACARE Announces Clinical Care Classification (CCC) System, Version 2.5
Washington, DC—2011—SabaCare is proud to announce the release of the Clinical Care
   Classification (CCC) System, Version 2.5.
The **Clinical Care Classification (CCC) System**, Version 2.5, refines the purpose of the
   terminology/classification—the documentation of nursing and patient care in any
   healthcare environment where nurses practice such as ambulatory care, outpatient clinics,
   and hospital settings from medical and surgical to critical care units. The CCC is designed
   for use by multidisciplinary integrated care teams and by other healthcare providers.
The update from CCC System, Version 2.0, to **Version 2.5** has new nursing diagnoses and new
   intervention concepts approved by the National CCC Scientific Advisory Board, who meet
   annually to review the terminology. Version 2.5 follows the coding guidelines of the UMLS
   of the NLM.
The **CCC System, Version 2.5,** contains

   1. REVISED Care Component: from Coping Component (D) to **Coping/Neuro Compo-
      nent (D)**
   2. 4 NEW Nursing Diagnoses, 10 RETIRED (deleted) Diagnoses, and 16 REVISED Nurs-
      ing Diagnosis definitions
   3. 10 NEW Nursing Interventions, 11 RETIRED (deleted) Interventions, and 25 REVISED
      Nursing Intervention definitions

(continued)

EXHIBIT 3.5 ■ (*Continued*)

A MAJOR CHANGE was the retirement of six age groups for the nursing diagnoses and the nursing interventions. Age groups were determined to be a demographic axis and not a true nursing diagnosis or nursing intervention concept.

Specific elements of the Clinical Care Classification (CCC) System, Version 2.5, include:

CCC Care Components: 21 Care Components to classify and code the terminologies.

CCC of Nursing Diagnoses: 176 Nursing Diagnoses (59 major and 123 subcategories).

CCC of Nursing Outcomes: derived from the Nursing Diagnoses CCC of Nursing Diagnoses, contains 546 Nursing Diagnoses Outcomes using three modifiers (Improved, Stabilized, or Deteriorated) to label and code Expected and/or Actual Outcomes.

CCC of Nursing Interventions: 804 Nursing Interventions/Actions (201: 77 major and 124 subcategories of core interventions), each using one of four Action Type modifiers (Assess, Perform, Teach, or Manage) to label and code the 804 **unique Nursing Interventions.**

All CCC System changes from Version 2.0 to 2.5 are available at www.sabacare.com and in **APPENDICES A1, A2, and A3.**

CCC System Contact Information
For additional information, visit: **www.sabacare.com or www.clinicalcareclassification.com**.
Virginia K. Saba, EdD, RN, FAAN, FACMI
Developer of the Clinical Care Classification (CCC) System
CEO and President, SabaCare Inc.
Consultant: Nursing Informatics; CCC System
Adjunct Professor, Uniformed Services University, Bethesda, MD
Nursing Advisory Board, George Mason University, Fairfax, VA
Tel: 703-521-6132
Fax: 703-521-3866
Email: vsaba@.att.net

● **CCC System Version 2.5 Permission Form**

EXHIBIT 3.6 ■ CCC System Permission Form

SabaCare Inc.
Tel: 703-521-6132/Fax: 703-521-3866/email: vsaba@att.net
Clinical Care Classification (CCC) System Permission Form

To: Dr. Virginia K. Saba, CEO SabaCare Inc.

_____ [name of entity] ("the Company") requests permission to have nonexclusive, royalty-free, worldwide rights in all languages and in all editions and formats—printed hardcopy and/or electronic version—to the Clinical Care Classification (CCC) System terminologies for use (through distribution, reproduction, incorporation, etc.) in its products and related services. The CCC System (formerly known as the HHCC System) consists of two terminologies, (a) the CCC of Nursing Diagnoses and Outcomes and (b) the CCC of Nursing Interventions and Actions, both of which are classified by 21 care components. The CCC System is copyrighted as TX 6-100-481.

OBLIGATIONS OF THE COMPANY:

1. The CCC System will be used only in any one or both of the following ways: (a) in any dictionary, vocabulary server product/application, or other compilation of terminology, printed or electronic, provided that such use consists of **ONLY** the CCC System and no other nursing system terminology, language, vocabulary, or classification system, and/or (b) in any clinical applications, primarily for use by nurses, as developed by the Company.
2. The CCC System, if used as stated above in 1(a), will not be sold or otherwise provided for any monetary charge, although reasonable charges for associated costs (copying, distribution,

(continued)

EXHIBIT 3.6 ▨ (*Continued*)

etc.) may be made. The CCC System, if used as stated above in 1(b), may be sold as part of the Company's clinical applications.

3. The CCC System will not be separately copyrighted by the Company.
4. The Company will give full credit to SabaCare Inc. for use of the CCC System in the Company's product collateral and in any copyright registration based on the CCC System as a preexisting work.
5. The Company will share with SabaCare Inc. any new concepts (nursing diagnoses/outcomes or interventions/actions) identified while using the CCC System.
6. The CCC System when updated will be provided in an electronic format to the Company.

Company Name:_____

Address: _____

City:_____

State:_____ **Zip:**_____

Signature: _____
  (**Authorized Representative of the Company**)
Title:_____ **Date:** _____

APPROVAL OF REQUEST:

The foregoing permission is hereby granted:

Approved By: _____ **Date of Approval:** _____

Title: _____

© V. K. Saba—Revised 8/20/2009

References

Alternative Link Systems, Inc. (2001; 2006). *ABC Coding Manual for Integrative Healthcare.* Albuquerque, NM: ABC Coding Solutions-Alternative Link Systems, Inc.

American National Standards Institute–Health Informatics Standards Board (ANSI–HISB). (1998/1999). *Inventory of clinical information standards.* Washington, DC: ANSI.

ANA Steering Committee on Databases to Support Clinical Nursing Practice. (1992). *Database activities to support the effectiveness initiatives: Report.* Washington, DC: ANA.

Cimino, J. J. (1998). Desiderata for controlled medical vocabularies in the twenty-first century. *Methods of Information in Medicine, 37,* 304–403.

Cimino, J. J. (2006). In defense of the Desiderata. *Journal of Biomedical Informatics, 39*(3), 299–306.

CINAHL Information Systems. (2005). *Cumulative index for nursing and allied health literature.* Glendale, CA: CINAHL.

Coenen, A., McNeil, B., Bakken, S., Bickford, C., & Warren, J. J. (2001). Toward comparable nursing data: American Nursing Association criteria for data sets, classification systems, and nomenclatures. *Computers in Nursing, 19*(6), 240–246.

Henry, S. H., & Mead, C. N. (1997). Nursing classifications systems; Necessary but not sufficient for representing "what nurses do" for inclusion in computer-based patient record systems. *Journal of the American Medical Informatics Association, 4*(3), 222–232.

International Organization for Standardization. (ISO) (1990). *International standards ISO 1087: Terminology—Vocabulary.* Geneva, Switzerland: ISO.

International Organization for Standardization (ISO) (1999). *International Standards ISO 1179: Metadata Registry* (MDR). Geneva, Switzerland: ISO.

International Organization for Standardization (ISO). (2003, September). Nursing language: Terminology models for nurses. *ISO bulletin* (pp. 16–18).

McCormick, K. A., Lang, N., Zielstorff, R., Milholland, D. K., Saba, V. K., & Jacox, A., (1994). Toward standard classification schemes for nursing languages: Recommendations of the American Nurses Association Steering Committee on Databases to Support Clinical Nursing Practice. *Journal of the American Medical Informatics Association, 1*(6), 421–427.

Saba, V. K. (2011). *Clinical care classification (CCC) of nursing interventions.* Retrieved from http://www.sabacare.com

Saba, V. K., Moss, J., & Whittenburg, L. (2011). Overview of the Clinical Care Classification System: A national nursing coded terminology. In V. K. Saba & K. A. McCormick (Eds.), *Essentials of nursing informatics* (5th ed., pp. 217–229). New York, NY: McGraw–Hill.

Saba, V. K. & Taylor, S. (2007). Moving past theory: Use of a standardized coding nursing terminology to enhance nursing visibility. *CIN: Computers, Informatics, Nursing, 25*(6), 324–331.

World Health Organization (1992). ICD-10 *International Statistical Classification of Diseases and Related Health Problems: Tenth Revision* (Vol. 1) Geneva, Switzerland: WHO.

Zielstorff, R. D., Tronni, C., Basque, J., Griffin, L. R., & Welebob, E. M. (1998). Mapping nursing diagnosis nomenclatures for coordinated care. *Journal of Nursing Scholarship, 30*(4), 369–373.

CCC System© Collaboration With SNOMED CT© and ICNP®

4

This chapter highlights the use of the Clinical Care Classification (CCC) System within two reference terminologies: (a) Systematized Nomenclature of Medicine Clinical Terms (SNOMED CT) and (b) International Classification for Nursing Practice (ICNP)®. Each of the terminologies, SNOMED CT and ICNP, has integrated the CCC System nursing terminologies, the CCC of Nursing Diagnoses and the CCC of Nursing Interventions/Actions into its reference data files. The CCC System is a point-of-care terminology used to document nursing practice. A reference terminology such as SNOMED CT and ICNP, is used in meaningful use requirements for data exchange, transmission, and interoperability. The following section is a presentation of the integration of the CCC System within SNOMED CT, followed by a presentation of the CCC System within ICNP.

CCC System© and SNOMED CT©

Cynthia B. Lundberg and Debra Konicek

SNOMED CT is a comprehensive clinical terminology that provides clinical content and expressivity for clinical documentation and reporting. The use of SNOMED CT ensures consistency in exchanging and understanding clinical information. It can be used to code, retrieve, and analyze clinical data. SNOMED CT resulted from the merger of SNOMED Reference Terminology (SNOMED RT), developed by The College of American Pathologists (CAP), and Clinical Terms, Version 3, developed by the National Health Service of the United Kingdom.

In 2007, the CAP, the originator of SNOMED CT for the past 40 years, transferred the intellectual property to the International Health Terminology Standards Development Organization (IHTSDO). The purpose of the transfer was to obtain a global terminology standard that supports interoperability. SNOMED CT provides the core general terminology for the electronic health record (EHR) and contains more than 311,000 active concepts with unique meanings and formal logic-based definitions organized into hierarchies. The IHTSDO is responsible for editorial governance and international distribution of SNOMED CT.

The Office of the National Coordinator for Health Information Technology (ONC) recognizes SNOMED CT as a standard terminology in the United States and has adopted SNOMED CT as a standard for the entry of structured data in certified EHR technology. To meet the American Recovery and Reinvestment Act of 2009 (ARRA) "meaningful use" objective to "maintain an up-to-date problem list of current and active diagnoses" for the Medicare and Medicaid EHR Incentive Programs, eligible professionals, hospitals, and critical access hospitals will need to maintain an up-to-date problem list of current and active diagnoses using SNOMED CT (Center for Disease for Medicare and Medicaid Services, 2011).

SNOMED CT terminology is composed of concepts, terms, and relationships with the objective of precisely representing clinical information across the scope of healthcare. Content coverage is divided into 19 hierarchies that include:

Clinical finding	Physical force
Procedure	Events
Observable entity	Environment/geographical location
Body structure	Social context
Organism	Situation with explicit context
Substance	Staging and scales
Pharmaceutical/biological product	Linkage concept
Specimen	Qualifier value
Special concept	Record artifact
Physical object	

● SNOMED CT Uses

Healthcare software applications focus on collection of clinical data, linking to clinical knowledge bases, information retrieval, as well as data aggregation and exchange. Data encoded using SNOMED CT may be recorded in different ways at different times and across sites of care. Knowledge bases for nursing link nursing problems/diagnoses to interventions and outcomes based on research and evidence-based practice. SNOMED CT is a reference terminology that supports the infrastructure of the knowledge bases developed by the nursing classification systems, such as the CCC. SNOMED CT contains the concepts necessary to support the electronic description and sharing of knowledge bases.

Standardized information improves analysis. SNOMED CT provides a standard for clinical information, with software applications that can use the concepts, hierarchies, and relationships as a common reference point for data analysis. SNOMED CT serves as a foundation upon which healthcare organizations can develop effective analysis applications to conduct outcomes research, evaluate the quality and cost of care, and design effective treatment guidelines and clinical decision support systems that can be used to improve the quality of patient care.

Standardized terminology provides several benefits, especially to clinicians, patients, researchers, administrators, software developers, and payers. A clinical terminology aids in providing healthcare providers with easily accessible and complete information pertaining to the healthcare process (medical history, illnesses, treatments, laboratory results, etc.), resulting in improved patient outcomes. Clinical terminology also allows a healthcare provider to identify patients based on certain coded information in their records, facilitating follow-up and treatment (IHTSDO, 2011).

● Integration/Convergence of Standardized Nursing Languages within SNOMED CT

The SNOMED CT structure allows for the convergence of nursing content from a variety of standardized nursing language sources currently recognized by the American Nurses Association. Nursing concepts with similar meaning are placed within the same hierarchies. Nursing diagnoses are located within clinical findings, nursing interventions are found within procedures, and nursing outcomes concepts are modeled within the observable entity hierarchy. Frequently, nursing concepts become synonyms of existing SNOMED CT concepts. It is important to understand how nursing concepts from a variety of existing classification systems converge and interrelate to one another within SNOMED CT.

Nursing Content Integration/Convergence Process

The basic underlying principles for the addition of nursing concepts are described below. Nursing concepts are integrated into SNOMED CT via several mechanisms:

1. A nursing concept may be identical to an existing SNOMED CT concept (exact match).

2. A nursing concept may be a synonym of an existing SNOMED CT concept and is added as such.

3. A nursing concept may be new (not currently contained within the SNOMED CT terminology). These concepts are added as new, given a SNOMED CT code, modeled using current attributes, and assigned a specific **IsA** (parent–child) relationship, placing it within the appropriate hierarchy

In each of the above scenarios, the concept is also assigned an internal (not released) identifier representing the source nursing terminology. This "marker" then allows for these concepts to be uniquely identified in order to populate the mapping tables that will be generated. These mapping tables, which can be acquired from the CAP SNOMED Terminology Solutions, provide the linkages between the specific nursing terminologies and SNOMED CT. For example, the CCC mapping table identifies the relationship links between the CCC source terminology and SNOMED CT.

● CCC Nursing Map

The CCC map to SNOMED CT contains nursing diagnoses, outcome qualifiers, and intervention concepts that can be used to document patient care in any healthcare setting. This content provides a rich variety of nursing concepts that will enhance and expand the SNOMED CT efforts toward being a "healthcare" terminology. Future nursing content efforts will be focused on assessing end-user nursing documentation needs. We look to the users and developers of EHR systems within the United States and internationally to provide guidance in terms of possible sources of additional nursing content (IHTSDO, 2011).

Examples of Mappings between CCC System and SNOMED CT

Examples of mappings of the CCC System with SNOMED CT can be obtained directly from The College of American Pathologists - SNOMED Terminology Solutions (CAP-STS); some are shown in Tables 4.1.1 and 4.1.2.

1. CCC of Nursing Diagnoses: All concepts have been mapped directly to the SNOMED CT Clinical Finding hierarchy.

2. CCC of Nursing Interventions/Actions: All concepts have been mapped directly to the SNOMED CT procedure hierarchy. The concepts consist of SNOMED codes for the interventions with each of the four action types (assess, perform, teach, and manage).

TABLE 4.1.1 ■ SNOMED CT/CCC of Nursing Diagnoses Integration Examples

SNOMED CT© Finding (Diagnosis)	CCC Diagnosis
77427003 Activity intolerance	A01.1 Activity Intolerance
399122003 Swallowing problem	J24.5 Swallowing Impairment
50177009 Body temperature above reference range	K25.2 Hyperthermia
32000005 Difficulty using verbal communication	M28.1 Verbal Impairment
7058009 Noncompliance with treatment	G20.0 Noncompliance
161838002 Infant feeding problem	J54.0 Infant Feeding Pattern Impairment
78648007 At risk for infection	K25.5 Infection Risk
20573003 Ineffective breathing pattern	L26.2 Breathing Pattern Impairment
373191003 Self-toileting deficit	O39.0 Toileting Deficit

Note. CCC = Clinical Care Classification System; SNOMED CT = Systematized Nomenclature of Medicine, Clinical Terms.

TABLE 4.1.2 ■ SNOMED CT/CCC of Nursing Interventions/Actions, Version 2.0, Integration Examples

SNOMED CT Procedure	CCC Interventions/Actions
385884006 Bed rest care	A61.0.2 Bed-bound Care
370871008 Ambulation therapy	A03.1.2 Ambulation Therapy
37799002 Urinary bladder training	T58.2.2 Bladder Training
408885009 Breast-feeding support education	J66.0.3 Breast-feeding Support (Teach)
50723001 Blood pressure-taking education	K33.1.3 Blood Pressure (Teach)
385980003 Cardiac rehabilitation management	C08.1.4 Cardiac Rehabilitation (Manage)
408957008 Chronic pain control management	Q47.2.4 Chronic Pain Control (Manage)
385725001 Emotional support assessment	E13.0.1 Emotional Support (Assess)
410223002 Mental healthcare assessment	P45.0.1 Mental Healthcare (Assess)

Note. CCC = Clinical Care Classification System; SNOMED CT = Systematized Nomenclature of Medicine, Clinical Terms.

3. CCC Of Nursing Outcomes: A SNOMED CT code consists of each of the three qualifiers for the expected outcomes and/or actual outcomes (improve[d], stabilize[d], and deteriorate[d]). The outcome relationships within CCC can be represented in the EHR by combining a CCC nursing diagnosis with a qualifier.

● Summary

The power of the SNOMED CT standardized terminology is its ability to support interoperability. Combining the CCC System for documentation of nursing practice at the point of care with the power of SNOMED CT terminology within the electronic healthcare record enhances the ability of all clinicians to share data with CCC users.

● References

Centers for Medicaid and Medicare Services (CMS). (2011). *EHR incentive program.* Retrieved from https://questions.cms.hhs.gov/app/answers/detail/a_id/10150/~/%4Behr-incentive-program%5D-to-meet-the-meaningful-use-objective-%E2%80%9Cmaintain-an

International Health Terminology Standards Development Organization (IHTSDO). (2011). *About SNOMED CT.* Retrieved from http://www.ihtsdo.org/index.php?id=snomed-ct0

International Health Terminology Standards Development Organization (IHTSDO). (2011). *SNOMED Clinical Terms User Guide January 2011 release.* Retrieved from http://www.ihtsdo.org/fileadmin/user_upload/Docs_01/Publications/doc_UserGuide_Current-en-US_INT_20100131.pdf

ADDENDUM 4.1.1

Mapping CCC Nursing Concepts/Terms Using SNOMED CT©

Patricia C. Dykes

A direct concept mapping exists for most Clinical Care Classification (CCC) System concepts to SNOMED CT concepts. However, for some SNOMED CT core intervention concepts, the CCC Action Type is embedded within the SNOMED CT concept. In this scenario, the CCC concept must be postcoordinated with a CCC Action Type to complete a direct

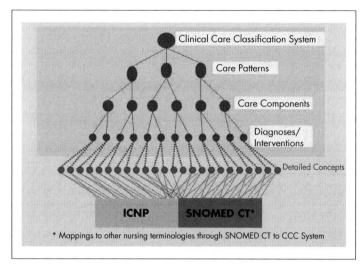

FIGURE 4.1.1 ▦ Integrated Terminology Framework for Nursing.
Note. CCC = Clinical Care Classification; ICNP = International Classification for Nursing Practice; SNOMED CT = Systematized Nomenclature of Medicine Clinical Terms.

mapping. For example, by postcoordinating the CCC concept "Transfer Care" with the CCC action type "Perform/Care/Provide/Assist" (A03.3.2), there is a direct mapping to the SNOMED CT concept "Patient Transfer" (C0030704). A key advantage of mappings between the CCC System concepts and the SNOMED CT concepts is that the benefits of both terminology systems can be leveraged within the EHR and support interoperability.

The CCC System provides an information model that supports documentation of the plan of care and linkages between nursing diagnoses, interventions, and patient outcomes. This classification linkage is known as a knowledge base. The granular concepts in SNOMED CT provide a means to document a detailed set of clinical interventions. The mapping between CCC System concepts and SNOMED CT concepts provides a framework for leveraging the CCC plan of care information model at a higher level while inheriting the more specific clinical concepts that exist in SNOMED CT. Because many of the American Nurses Association-approved nursing terminologies, including the CCC System, are integrated within SNOMED CT, this framework provides a means to utilize nursing terminologies from across multiple domains of nursing practice. As illustrated in Figure 4.1.1, a concept from any nursing classification system that can be converged into SNOMED CT can potentially be leveraged for documentation using the CCC information model (or knowledge base) in an EHR or health information technology system.

ADDENDUM 4.1.2

Plan of Care Using CCC System© and SNOMED CT©

Luann Whittenburg

A patient plan of care (PPOC) meets the meaningful use problem list requirement of computerized provider order entry as well as other interoperability data requirements. In meaningful use, Stages 2 and 3, the PPOC will be applicable for the collection of quality indicators and outcome measures. In addition, the PPOC can collect data for the Centers for Medicare and Medicaid Services "no-pay" diagnoses that prevent the reimbursement of facilities for "reasonable preventable" patient care conditions, such as injuries from patient falls, pressure sores, urinary tract infections, and other conditions for which nurses have care responsibilities.

In Table 4.3.1, the PPOC case study of a patient with pneumonia is coded using the CCC System. The PPOC provides two sets of codes: (a) CCC codes and (b) CCC codes mapped to SNOMED CT. The PPOC follows the six steps/standards of the nursing process (American

Nurses Association, 2010): (a) assessment (care components), (b) diagnosis (nursing diagnosis), (c) outcome identification (expected outcome), (d) planning (nursing interventions), (e) implementation (Action Types), and (f) evaluation (actual outcomes) for the electronic documentation of nursing practice supported by the CCC framework.

An inpatient PPOC may have a minimal number of nursing diagnoses that highlight the medical condition of the patient, which may require multiple nursing interventions/actions during an episode of care. When a patient is transferred to another inpatient unit in the same facility, the PPOC remains active, with revisions and updates to the PPOC about nursing care processes for continuity of care. When a patient is transferred to another health care facility (e.g., rehabilitation hospital), the PPOC accompanies the patient at the time of transfer. The PPOC, if electronically transferred to the receiving facility as SNOMED CT codes, transforms into the CCC System for use at the point of care by nursing and allied health professionals. This PPOC process makes the interoperability of mapped CCC System codes to SNOMED CT manageable for transfer.

CCC System SNOMED CT PPOC Scenario

A 70-year-old man is admitted to a hospital unit after presenting to the emergency department with productive cough, acute rib pain with coughing, increased work of breathing, pulse oximetry saturation of 88%, temperature of 102.2 °F, heart rate of 108, and blood pressure of 156/88. Chest X-ray done in the emergency department showed bilateral lower lobe and right middle lobe infiltrates. Medical diagnosis is pneumonia.

The step-by-step process of creating a PPOC for a patient with pneumonia is coded using the CCC System and SNOMED CT as shown in Table 4.1.3. A patient is admitted to a hospital with pneumonia requiring nursing care. The admitting nurse reviews the physician/provider orders and develops an individualized PPOC based on the nursing process. The PPOC becomes the framework for documenting patient care during the inpatient stay. The nurse reviews the PPOC shift by shift and, at a minimum, daily to ensure that patient progress and care quality are maintained and that nursing interventions are evaluated. The CCC System framework allows patient-centric care evaluation incorporating nurse and allied health professional feedback when updating the PPOC. The individualized PPOC with nursing diagnoses, interventions/actions, and outcomes is specified in the example.

● Reference

American Nurses Association. (2010). Nursing: Scope and Standard of Practice. Silver Springs, MD: ANA

TABLE 4.1.3 ■ Coded Pneumonia Plan of Care Using CCC and SNOMED CT

Nursing Plan of Care	Care Component/ Signs and Symptoms (Assessment)	Nursing Diagnoses (Diagnoses)	Expected Outcomes (Outcomes Identification)	Nursing Interventions (Planning)	Nursing Action Types (Implementation)	Actual Outcomes (Evaluation)	Evidence
CCC Codes	Respiratory: L	Respiratory Alteration: L26.0	L26.0.2: Stabilized	Pneumonia Care: L36.0 Positioning Therapy: A61.1	L36.0.2 A61.1.2	L26.0.2: Stabilized	Ribs splinted for coughing; bed elevated 30° (not coughing, able to get out of bed)
SNOMED Codes		Respiratory Alteration: 129893005	409052007 129893005	Respiratory Care Adjustment: 129893005 Positioning Patient: 22982408		409052007 129893005	
CCC Codes	Respiratory: L	Breathing Pattern Impairment: L26.2	L26.2.1: Improve	Breathing Exercises: L36.1	L36.1.3	L26.2.1: Improved	Taught use of breathing inhaler (able to breathe normally)
SNOMED Codes		Ineffective Breathing Pattern: 20573003	390771008 20573003	Breathing Exercise Education: 385849007		390771008 20573003	
CCC Codes	Respiratory: L	Gas Exchange: L26.3	L26.3.1: Improve	Oxygen Therapy Care: L35.0	L35.0.2	L26.3.1: Improved	Regulated humidified oxygen (O2) per nasal cannula and titrated to keep oxygen saturation at 92% on room air (oxygen no longer needed)

(continued)

TABLE 4.1.3 ■ Coded Pneumonia Plan of Care Using CCC and SNOMED CT (*Continued*)

Nursing Plan of Care	Care Component/ Signs and Symptoms (Assessment)	Nursing Diagnoses (Diagnoses)	Expected Outcomes (Outcomes Identification)	Nursing Interventions (Planning)	Nursing Action Types (Implementation)	Actual Outcomes (Evaluation)	Evidence
SNOMED Codes		Impaired Gas Exchange: 70944005	390771008 70944005	Oxygen Therapy: 57485005		390771008 70944005	
CCC Codes	Sensory: Q	Acute pain: Q63.1	Q63.1.1: Improve	Acute Pain Control: Q47.1 Medication Treatment: H24.4	Q47.0.2 H24.4.2	Q63.1.1: Improved	Pain scale score less than 3 and medicated with morphine (rib pain ceased)
SNOMED Codes		Acute Pain: 274663001	390771008 274663001	Pain Control: 225782006 Administration Medication: 18629005		390771008 274663001	
CCC Codes	Physical Regulation: K	Physical Regulation Alteration: K25.0	K25.0.1: Improve	Vital Signs: K33.0.2 Medication Treatment: H24.4	K33.0.2 H24.4.2	K25.0.1: Improved	Vital signs taken every 4 hours (vital signs normal); gave antibiotics (PCN 1GM IM; temperature normal, PCN discontinued)
SNOMED Codes		Physical Regulation Alteration: 129856004	390771008 129856004	Vital Signs: 61746007 Administration Medication: 18629005		390771008 129856004	

Note. CCC = Clinical Care Classification System; SNOMED CT = Systematized Nomenclature of Medicine, Clinical Terms.
* PCN, Penicillin; 1 GM, 1 Gram; IM, Intramuscular Injection

Harmonizing Nursing Terminologies: CCC System© and ICNP®

Amy Coenen

In the 1990s, the ICNP was developed by the International Council of Nursing (ICN). It included Home Health Care Classification (HHCC) (Version 1.0) concepts in its original Alpha release of 1996. Since then, the ICNP has been tested and revised into its latest ICNP, Version 1.0 (2005). It is a classification of nursing phenomena, actions, and outcomes, and serves as a unifying framework into which existing classifications can be cross-mapped to compare nursing data. The ICNP is being mapped to the CCC enabling nursing classification implementers to use both interchangeably.

The ICNP is a major component of the ICN eHealth Programme (http://www.icn.ch/pillarsprograms/ehealth). The ICNP is a formal terminology for nursing practice and is used to represent nursing diagnoses, outcomes, and interventions. Since its inception in 1989, many nurses and terminology experts have contributed research and development projects, translations, critical reviews, and evaluations to advance the ICNP. The ICNP 2011 Release reflects more than 20 years of ongoing research and development.

The primary motivation for an international nursing terminology involves sharing and comparing nursing data across settings, countries, and languages. These data can be used to support clinical decision-making, evaluate nursing care and patient outcomes, develop health policy, and generate knowledge through research. In addition to promoting comparable nursing data, the ICNP is intended to facilitate use of nursing data in analyses using interdisciplinary and administrative data sets.

As a formal terminology, ICNP can be used to cross-map among local, regional, national, and international classifications. The ability to cross-map ICNP with other classification systems means that the important contributions of existing classifications can continue to advance by informing ICNP and being informed by ICNP development.

Because ICNP is a large and complex terminology (3,290 concepts in ICNP 2011), there are strategies and representations that facilitate the use of ICNP in point-of-care health information systems. One approach has been the development of ICNP catalogs or subsets of nursing diagnoses, outcomes, and interventions for a select specialty or focus of nursing practice (e.g., palliative care, community health nursing). Concepts in the ICNP subset can be mapped to an encoded in other nursing and healthcare classifications or terminologies.

Using a formal ontological approach, ICNP can complement existing nursing classification, such as the CCC System. The ICN and the developer of the CCC System have initiated

TABLE 4.2.1 ■ Example of Mapping Concepts from CCC to ICNP

CCC Nursing Diagnosis (Code)	ICNP 2011 Nursing Diagnosis (Code)
Tissue Perfusion Alteration (S48.0)	Ineffective Tissue Perfusion (10001344)
Acute Pain (Q45.1)	Acute Pain (10000454)
Sleep Pattern Disturbance (A01.6)	Impaired Sleep (10001300)

CCC Nursing Intervention (Code)	ICNP 2011 Nursing Intervention (Code)
Perform Transfer Care (A03.3.2)	Transferring Patient (10033188)
Teach Wound Care (R55.0.3)	Teaching about Wound Care (10034961)
Perform Bereavement Support (E14.1.2)	Supporting the Mourning Process (10026489)

collaboration through cross-mapping projects (Matney et al., 2008). A resulting map identifies how CCC System concepts are represented using ICNP (Table 4.2.1). This work will facilitate evaluation and ongoing development of both terminologies and allow users to compare data using CCC System codes with data from other standard classifications or terminologies mapped to ICNP. In addition to providing an interface terminology for users, a CCC System cross-mapping to ICNP would allow users to apply a conceptual model (CCC Care Component classes) to organize content delivered at the interface of EHR systems.

The ICN and the makers of the CCC System, along with researchers and other experts, can work together in health information systems development to support clinical practice and advance nursing science. These two distinct terminologies serve different but complementary purposes. Ongoing collaboration among nursing and other healthcare terminology developers will advance the capability to describe, compare, and evaluate nursing practice regionally, nationally, and internationally.

● Reference

Matney, S., DaDamio, R., Couderc, C., Dlugos, M., Evans, J., Gianonne, G., Haskell, R., Hardiker, N., Coenen, A., Saba, V. (2008). Translation and integration of CCC nursing diagnoses into ICNP®. *Journal of the American Medical Informatics Association, 15*(6), 791–793.

Current CCC Applications 5

The only nursing terminology that makes sense—useful at the point of care, reflects nursing practice, and makes sense to the entire clinical team—is the CCC. —Debbie Raposo, RN, BSN

This chapter describes samples of current applications of the Clinical Care Classification (CCC) System in electronic health record (EHR) and health information technology (HIT) systems by healthcare vendors, software developers, hospitals, universities, clinics, and other healthcare facilities involved in healthcare terminology and standards efforts. The sample applications have been developed by actual implementers of the CCC System in clinical practice and education.

Current samples of the CCC System in working applications were selected from a large number of submissions from CCC clients. The implementers of EHR systems have designed plan of care (POC) systems using the CCC for documenting nursing practice. Other EHR developers have designed unique applications using the CCC for a specific purpose or program or for an entire country (Finland)!

Each of the applications described below have implemented the CCC System using different approaches and design strategies. The first group uses the CCC System for the documentation of nursing practice in inpatient hospitals: (a) Southcoast Hospitals Group, Fall River, MA; (b) Claxton Hepburn Medical Center, Ogdensburg, NY; (c) Vanderbilt University Medical Center, Nashville, TN; and (d) Healthcare Corporation of America, Nashville, TN. Medicomp Systems, Chantilly, VA, developed a CCC System nursing POC and documentation application for the MEDCIN® engine and knowledgebase for ambulatory care and inpatient facilities. A sample school health record from the cumulative school record health module in a multi-school district in Colorado is also included. Two other sample applications are from international clients: FinCC is used in most hospitals and serves as a national nursing system for ALL hospitals in Finland, and another application developed for the nurses and midwives of South Australia, Adelaide, South Australia, are included for your use. Each selected application has included screen print samples to further illustrate the various design strategies for using the CCC System. The sample applications include:

Part 5.1: Southcoast Hospitals Group, Fall River, MA

Part 5.2: Claxton Hepburn Medical Center, Ogdensburg, NY

Part 5.3: Vanderbilt University Medical Center, Nashville, TN

Part 5.4: Healthcare Corporation of America, Nashville, TN

Part 5.5: Medicomp Systems, Chantilly, VA

Part 5.6: Cumulative School Record in multischool district in Colorado

Part 5.7: Finnish Care Classification Kuopio, Finland (FinCC)

Part 5.8: Nurses and Midwives of South Australia, Adelaide, South Australia

Each of the individual parts is presented as, and focuses on, selected applications of the CCC System to demonstrate the wide range of its use and implementations in the healthcare industry—EHRs and HIT systems.

Using CCC with Meditech and IATRIC Visual Flowsheet

Debbie Raposo

On March 23, 2009, Southcoast Hospitals Group became the first site to "go live" with the Clinical Care Classification (CCC) System electronically using our vendor product, Meditech, and Iatric Visual Flowsheet. This methodology can easily be used by all patient care partners. It truly allows for interdisciplinary plans of care and education records. Care plans have become a useful and meaningful part of the everyday job of our healthcare professionals. They are easy to read and easy to follow and make sense to the patient and all other participants in our patient's care.

As problems and/or interventions are identified or modified by any care partner, so is the plan of care. It can be modified by any licensed discipline care provider who is working with this patient. It is a truly interdisciplinary plan of care.

Maximizing Meditech's functionality also helped with the process of building care plans. Twenty-one customer-defined screens accounted for the 21 care components within the CCC System. We capture the CCC coding behind the scenes based on the partner-in-care documentation in assessments and education records.

The plan of care for the patient is as fluid as the patient. As other partners in care identify a new problem or meet an outcome of a current problem, they can add to or modify the care plan to meet the patient's changing needs. Partners in care can also easily add or remove interventions as needed for the patient.

We are all speaking the same language with CCC. Every partner in care (rehab, dietary, care coordination, speech, respiratory, pharmacy, social work) is using the same problems, outcomes, and interventions. We are all using the same methodology to care for our patient. No more isolation of care by disciplines. We are all on the same page and speaking the same language.

The CCC System provides for a **realistic** and **achievable** plan of care for patients. We all know that potentials exist. We assess for them all the time. It is what we **DO.** Until a potential becomes a problem, we do not **NEED** it as part of our patient's plan of care. We know it as a potential because we are experienced, licensed professionals.

Shown below to illustrate the system are a series of five screens and one exhibit with some system findings.

EXHIBIT 5.1.1 ■ Admission Assessment for Fall Risk

```
                        **** Fall Risk Assessment ****
     Recent History of Falls (+7) ? Y    Fall Risk Score   Intervention Class
         Altered Elimination (+3) ? N          0 - 2            Normal Risk
      Confusion/Disorientation (+4) ? N         3 - 7            Moderate
                  Medication (+3) ? Y          8 - 15            High
            Dizziness/Vertigo (+3) ? N         16 or more        Severe
                Poor Mobility (+2) ? Y
          Sensory Impairment (+3) ? N    * High and Severe Class Requires Ruby Slipper Program
         Age Greater Than 75 (+1) ? N
                   Total Score: 12
  Fall Risk Intervention Class: High
            Safety Comment:
```

This is our version of a fall risk assessment that is done upon admission and at least one time every shift. Based on this nursing assessment of "high risk for falls," a trigger for the safety component of care and safety education record is evoked, sending the nursing order to the Meditech order entry system provider order entry (POM). The nurse must then opt out of the component of care and education records that are not a high priority for the patient.

EXHIBIT 5.1.2 ▨ POM (Provider Order Entry) Meditech Order Entry System

-	Category	Orders	Pri	Date/Time	Status	Stop	My
	Education: Safety (NUR)			02/15 1118	Active		
			PRN				
	Component: Safety (NUR)			02/15 1118	Active		
			PRN				

This is an "**OPT OUT**" functionality in our order entry system. The nurse must use his/her clinical judgment and professional experience to decide which identified problems to focus on and which ones, while identified, are not the main focus for this admission. The care components and education records are nurse orderable interventions via Meditech. The care components can be added or completed as the patients progress through their hospital stay.

EXHIBIT 5.1.3 ▨ Customer-Defined Screen Created in Meditech to Document the Plan of Care Using the CCC Care Components, Outcomes

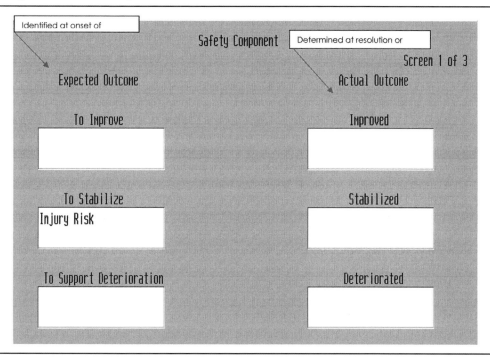

On screen 1, we identify the expected outcome. We later return to this screen to close out the component of care by documenting the actual outcome when the goal is achieved or the patient is discharged from the hospital.

EXHIBIT 5.1.4 ■ Customer-Defined Screen Created in Meditech to Document the Plan of Care Using the CCC Care Components, Interventions

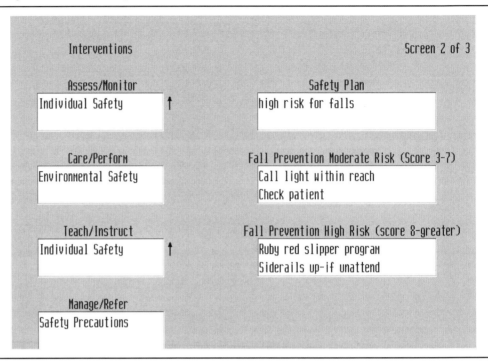

Screen 2 of the customer-defined screen is the interventions screen. Here we determine the interventions we are going to assess/monitor, perform/care, teach/instruct, or manage/refer. Partners in care (rehab, dietary, respiratory, pharmacists, discharge planners, care coordinators, and social workers) all contribute to the outcomes and interventions as they identify changes in the patient plan of care.

EXHIBIT 5.1.5 ■ IATRIC Visual Flowsheet Viewable by All Patient Care Providers

	06/29/11 13:49 - 14:48
Care Plan Reviewed	
Care Plan Reviewed	
Safety Component	
Name/Discipline	RAPOSO, DEBBIE CIS MIS
To Stabilize	Injury Risk
Assess/Monitor	Environmental Safety Individual Safety
Care/Perform	Environmental Safety
Teach/Instruct	Environmental Safety Individual Safety
Manage/Refer	Safety Precautions
Safety Plan	high risk for falls
Fall Prev. Moderate Risk (Score 3-7)	Call light within reach Check patient
Fall Prev. High Risk (Score 8-greater)	Ruby red slipper program Siderails up-if unattend

This "view" of the plan of care is attached to all providers. We all can easily see what the plan is for the patient. All partners in care can see that the expected outcome is to stabilize injury risk. We are going to reach that outcome by providing interventions to assess/monitor environmental safety and individual safety, perform/care environmental safety, and teach/instruct environmental safety and individual safety. Our patient has been identified based on assessment for a high risk of falls, and in addition to the CCC interventions, we are going to place the patient on a Ruby Red Slipper Program (we place red rubber-soled slippers for each patient at high risk as well as a picture of red slippers on the head wall) and ensure that the side rails are up if no one is with the patient. Any care provider who opens this screen can quickly see the plan of care for the patient and is aware of the interventions that have been put in place to keep this patient safe.

EXHIBIT 5.1.6 ■ Fall Risk Data Summary: Preliminary Results of Data on Falls Based on Implementation of CCC as the Standard Language for All Care Providers and Other Fall Reduction Strategies

---

Pre-CCC, February 2008– February 2009 Fall Data (Preautomation)
Site 1 = 0.58%
Site 2 = 0.58%
Site 3 = 0.57%
Post- and in-process CCC, February 2009–February 2010 Data (Postautomation)
Site 1 = 0.31%   Implemented CCC March 2009 and online documentation
Site 2 = 0.56%   Implemented CCC Sep 2009 and online documentation
Site 3 = 0.85%   Implemented CCC Jan 2010 and online documentation
Postimplementation of CCC, May 2009–May 2010 Data (Postautomation)
Site 1 = 0.03%
Site 2 = 0.31%
Site 3 = 0.35%

Other important factors occurring in tandem with this result are hourly rounding, patient care observer role, therapeutic assistant role, "falls rooms, safety zones, and reeducation of staff."

The implementation of the CCC System has allowed us to collect coded and standardized data on falls. Utilizing CCC as our standardized language and other fall prevention strategies has reduced our incidence of falls dramatically. We have maintained this reduction for this current year.

PART 5.2

Meditech's Process Intervention Screen Using CCC Structure

Amber Greer

Claxton–Hepburn Medical Center is a 130-bed community hospital located in Northern New York State on the Canadian border. A project to revise the Meditech Magic inpatient Nursing Module using Clinical Care Classification (CCC) structure began in 2007. An interdisciplinary team with representation from medical–surgical, obstetrics, intensive care unit, clinical nutrition, respiratory, occupational physical therapy, and education collaborated in the redesign of 75 electronic documentation screens using CCC structure. This project has been successfully live since 2009 for inpatient documentation in all the represented departments.

The first screen—process intervention in Meditech (Figure 5.2.1)—depicts the starting point for the documentation. On this screen, the nurse can see all the interventions on the patient's record. The nurse chooses the intervention set that is most closely related to the patient's problem. From here, the nurse can add additional problems and interventions from a pick list based on CCC language. Once the nurse chooses the interventions/problems, she/he can then document the problems. The second screen (Figure 5.2.2) shows documentation related to the respiratory problem. The last screen (Figure 5.2.3) is the respiratory general care interventions. This is where the nurse documents the patient's assessment, care teaching, and any referrals/notifications that have been made regarding this patient.

FIGURE 5.2.1 ■ Process intervention in Meditech.

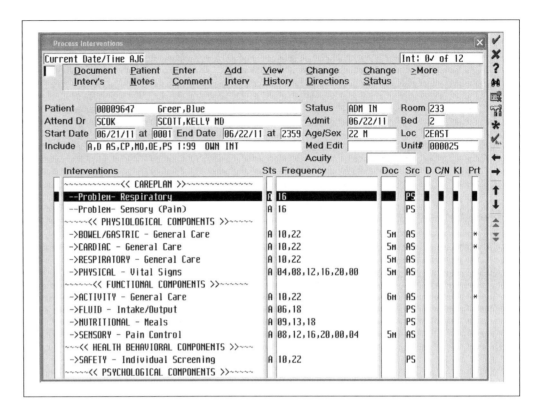

FIGURE 5.2.2 ■ Respiratory problem/diagnosis screen. This screen shot represents the respiratory problem or diagnosis component. Included in the screen structure of all 21 problems are a problem or diagnosis, expected outcome, actual outcome, and the interventions used. The "problem" screens represent the "care plan" pieces of the documentation.

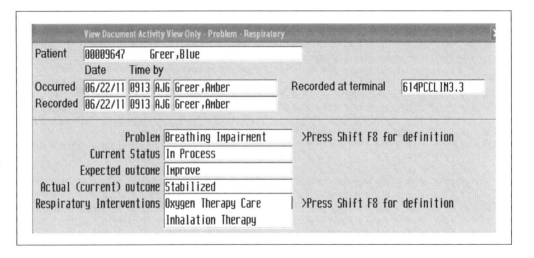

View Document Activity View Only - RESPIRATORY - General Care

Patient	00009647	Greer,Blue		
	Date	Time by		
Occurred	06/22/11	0914	AJG	Greer,Amber
Recorded	06/22/11	0929	AJG	Greer,Amber

Recorded at terminal   614PCCLIN3.3

ASSESS Y Respiratory WNL N ~ Unimpaired respirations; Symetrical chest expansion
Breath sounds clear; No cough or secretions;
No oxygen necessary.

Document abnormals only

Rhythm	Tachypnea
Effort	Deep / Dyspnea on exertion
Assymetrical chest expansion	
RUL Breath Sounds	Crackles (Rales)
LUL Breath Sounds	Crackles (Rales)
RLL Breath Sounds	Crackles (Rales) / Diminished
LLL Breath Sounds	Crackles (Rales) / Diminished
Cough	Non-productive / Ineffective
Secretions	
O2 Usage	Dependent
Other	

CARE Y

Action	Inhalation therapy / Oxygen therapy care
Oxygen Setting	2 liter
Oxygen Device	Nasal cannula
Incentive Spiromter encouraged	Y
IS Vital capacity (mL)	1000
Times capacity reached	2
Performance barriers	Pain
Comment	

TEACH Y

Topic	Incentive spirometer / Plan of care
Details	
Learner	Patient / Spouse
Method	Discussion / Demonstration
Response	Demonstrates Ability

NOTIFY N

Notified	
Content	

FIGURE 5.2.3 ■ Respiratory general care intervention. This screen is used for documenting the intervention for "general respiratory care." Each screen is divided into the four CCC Action Types: "assess," "perform/care," "teach," and "manage/notify." The "normal" assessment of the component type is defined on the screen. The nurse then documents the assessment of the "abnormals only" and then follows with documentation of the care, teaching, and notification pertaining to each particular component for the patient.

Implementing a Nursing Documentation Framework Using the Clinical Care Classification© Terminology

Deborah Ariosto

Our decision to use the Clinical Care Classification (CCC) System© Vanderbilt University Medical Center (VUMC) was based on its accessibility; its cross-continuum applicability; the simplicity of the outcomes (improve, stabilize, support decline) and intervention action types (assess, perform/care, teach, manage); as well as the linkages to multidisciplinary Systematized Nomenclature of Medicine Clinical Terms (SNOMED CT©). As you will see below, having a coded terminology in the background, invisible to the users, gave us enormous flexibility in creating a variety of different displays for different workflows. We have really appreciated the foundational work of Dr. Virginia K. Saba and her colleagues and encourage others to put it to good use.

● Nursing Priority Problem Documentation and Visualization

Implementing a terminology structure yielded more benefit than we imagined when we started organizing nursing care planning around the CCC nursing diagnoses. Like most large academic medical centers, we have a high energy around local innovation that challenges standardization efforts designed to share/reuse data across the continuum. The CCC offered us a balance by providing a high-level organizing framework upon which to hang unit or entity based documentation to visualize nursing care across the enterprise.

What that means operationally is that we ask that nursing documentation requests be framed using CCC. When accreditation and standards asked for better restraint documentation, we captured it under the "safety" category. In a recent study on delirium, researchers successfully reorganized their study assessments (medication risk, etc.) and interventions (sleep pattern control, etc.) using the CCC without compromising their study integrity. This was a win–win by embedding the study data collection into the usual electronic workflow (instead of having to use an additional paper collection tool), resulting in timely collection and reporting of study data to the research team.

The CCC shows great promise in helping with our efforts to build towards an interoperable, multidisciplinary care plan. The CCCs have matching SNOMED CT© codes that will enable future work across all disciplines and capture the spirit of meaningful use. Currently, 85% to 95% of our inpatients have coded nursing problems. In addition, CCC nutrition categories work hand-in-glove with the American Dietary Association (ADA)-specific terminology, such as *body nutrition deficit* or *knowledge deficit of dietary regimen*. We have also built a patient education and engagement record that uses the CCC coded concepts of knowledge deficit, self-care, and health behavior that is being piloted by pharmacists, dietitians, and nurses. The patient education and engagement record is getting much attention as we look through the long-range lens of accountable care to achieve better patient outcomes.

We have developed several other electronic views of what we call our "nursing priority problem" (nursing diagnosis) list. By organizing data collected by nursing under the CCC categories, we were able to create a graphical view to quickly see priority problems by patient, by nurse assignment, or at the unit level. Exhibit 5.3.1 shows a rendered view of the VUMC developed electronic health record (EHR) StarPanel™ priority problem dashboard. Each letter represents a corresponding CCC diagnosis in each care category. Colors and shading represent the timeliness of the documentation. Nurse managers use this for focused rounding and educators for teaching how to improve plans of care. Exhibit 5.3.2 shows a drill-down from the **"Plan"** column on the dashboard to display more detail on interventions and goals. We are also looking at embedding

EXHIBIT 5.3.1 ■ Priority Problems (CCC) on the StarPanel™ Dashboard, Obstetric Unit View

	LOS	Plan	Physiological									Life	Psych		Functional					Behavioral		
			Reg	Pul	Car	Perf	Skin	Met	GI	UR		NCog	PsyS	Flui	Nut	Pain	Act	Self	HBhv	Med	Safe
Patient 1	10 d	*									L					P					S
Patient 2	:23M																				
Patient 4	2d	*									L			F		P					
Patient 5	2d	*									L					P	A				
Patient 6	2d	*	P	C				M			L			F							

■ Patient 6 has current goals for cardiac (M), metabolic (M), and lifecycle (L) problems; older pulmonary (P) and fluid balance (F) problems highlighted. Plan details shown in Exhibit 5.3.2.

Note. CCC = Clinical Care Classification (CCC) System© Vanderbilt University Medical Center. Used with permission. All rights reserved.

decision support for potential priority problems in next releases of the dashboard. For example, if a patient has a high fall risk score, it will light up the "safety" column box for that patient.

Phase I of our implementation introduced CCC nursing diagnoses into the care planning process in June 2010. User-defined screens in our McKesson Horizon Expert Nursing Documentation™ system (HED) enabled us to create a tab with the CCC problem categories and selections. Our plan of care consists of a generic evidence-based pathway (e.g., fx hip, heart failure, antepartum) that is individualized to the patient using the CCC problem list. A sample HED plan of care screen is shown in Exhibit 5.3.3.

We initially pushed out the concept of a "priority problem list" instead of reintroducing "nursing diagnoses," which had too much of an emotional connection with the failed terminology attempts of long ago. Interviews with nurses have shown an extremely positive response regarding the priority problem list's usability. While the terminology was a little awkward initially, nurses were generally pleased with the succinct visualization of their assessments. This view is now embedded in the physician team summary as well (Exhibit 5.3.2). At the beginning of each shift, nurses identify the top 2 to 4 CCC problems (Exhibit 5.3.3) that are a priority and set short-term goals for each one (Exhibit 5.3.4). These priorities are based on (a) asking patients what their priority is (i.e., pain), (b) identifying high-risk, actual or potential problems (i.e., skin integrity), and (c) determining what is keeping patients from moving to the next phase in their care (i.e., activity intolerance). Later in their shift, nurses indicate whether the short-term goals were met and if plan changes are needed. Day and night-shifts nurses may have different goals (ambulation vs. sleep), so current priority goals are visualized in real time (green) on the unit-based StarPanel™ priority problem dashboard (Exhibit 5.3.1).

EXHIBIT 5.3.2 ■ Patient 6 Drill-Down from Dashboard to Plan (*) Detail

Pathway Name: Antepartum; **Phase:** HD#12, 29.5 wks. **(07/05 5:26) Shift Summary:** No S&S of labor, good fetal movement, bg within paramter, vss, pain 2/10. **Plan summary (07/05 5:26)** Continue monitoring vss, bg, s/s of labor, fetal movement. Pt has ob u/s in the morning

Priority Problems	Short-Term Goal
(06/25/11 21:04) Gestational risk r/t risk for preterm delivery	(07/04/11 19:55) Pt will not have any s/s of labor
(06/26/11 19:30) Glucose alt r/t type 1 diabetes	(07/05/11 07:57) Pt BG will remain <200
(06/28/11 13:40) BP alteration r/t HTN	(07/05/11 07:57) Maintain BP <160/100 this shift
(07/01/11 21:04) Fluid excess r/t pregnancy	(07/03/11 20:41) Fluid balance/edema monitoring
(07/02/11 20:00) Fluid excess r/t magnesium admin	(07/02/11 20:00) Min 30cc/hr urinary output while on magnesium therapy
(07/02/11 20:00) Gas exchange r/t potential/ RT incr fluid	(07/02/11 20:00) Maintain clear lung sounds on mag
(07/05/11 08:11) Labor risk r/t PTL	(07/05/11 07:57) No s/sx labor this shift

EXHIBIT 5.3.3 ■ Horizon Expert Documentation™ Build for Priority Nursing Problems

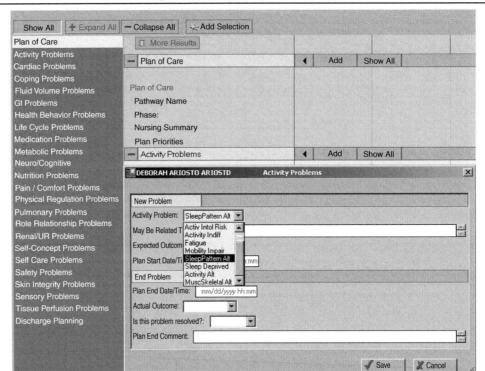

EXHIBIT 5.3.4 ■ Obstetric Priority Problems (CCC) and Trended Plan of Care in the Mckesson Horizon Expert Nursing Documentation™ View

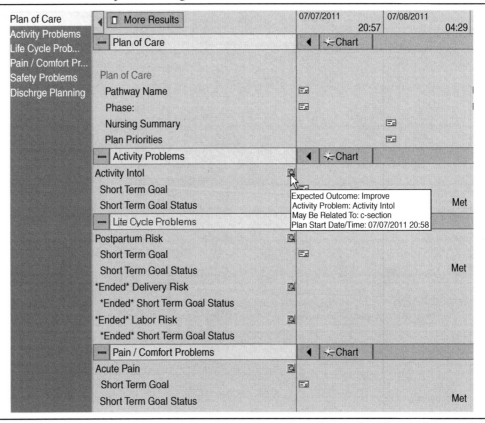

EXHIBIT 5.3.5 ■ Vanderbilt University Medical Center (VUMC) StarPanel™ Priority Problems (CCC), Longitudinal View

Key: Each line is a CCC Diagnosis/Problem. Hovering over the colored nodes along the line displays short-term goals (yellow [outline]) and whether these goals were met (green [medium gray] or not met (red [black]).

Note. CCC = Clinical Care Classification (CCC) System© Vanderbilt University Medical Center. Used with permission. All rights reserved.

With the initiation and resolution of each problem, the desired outcomes are determined (improve, stabilize, support decline), and actual outcomes are evaluated (improved, stabilized, decline supported). The presence of explicit outcomes relating to supporting patient deterioration has been powerful in sparking renewed discussions on the types of interventions needed to best achieve this in our palliative care settings. Our longitudinal view of patient problems (Exhibit 5.3.5) has been helpful for identifying ongoing problems for patients who are frequently readmitted. This view has been a helpful addition in recalling the "patient story" during retrospective chart review.

Nursing diagnosis has widespread adoption. We are currently looking at the best approaches to map our current interventions with the CCC interventions, which will be challenging. The diagnosis model has proven to work well across our adult, pediatrics, and obstetric settings. We will be testing it soon in our psychiatric hospital to help with care transition between medical, surgical, and psychiatric settings.

PART 5.4

Healthcare Corporation of America Implements Clinical Care Classification Data Elements in Meditech 6.0 Functionality

Jane Englebright, Kelly Aldrich, and George Grayson

● Hospital Corporation of America

The Hospital Corporation of America (HCA) is one of the largest healthcare providers in the United States, operating 166 hospitals; 112 surgery and endoscopy centers; and over 600 physician practices, oncology centers, and imaging facilities in 23 states and England. HCA-affiliated facilities include general community, suburban, and rural hospitals as well as academic health centers and tertiary referral hospitals. These facilities provide approximately 5% of the major hospital services in the United States.

● Implementing CCC

The HCA has a long history of using computerized documentation in nursing practice, including 10 years of experience with bar-coded medication administration. The Clinical Care Classification (CCC) System was identified as a mechanism for improving clinical practice and clinical documentation in a new clinical information system implementation. The HCA used CCC to define

TABLE 5.4.1 ■ Where HCA Embedded CCC Elements in Meditech 6.0 Functionality

CCC Elements	MediTech 6.0 Functionality
CCC problems	Problem/diagnosis dictionary
CCC expected outcomes	Outcome dictionary and query
CCC interventions	Intervention dictionary or query
CCC actual outcomes	Outcome dictionary and query
	Care plan dictionary not used

and to code the essence of care at the clinical intervention level to meet a variety of quality improvement strategies. While CCC coding is not visible to the end users, the framework is easily recognized by the clinical team, and the coding is embedded and available for reporting and analysis.

Two examples of the HCA implementation of the CCC System follow:

● **Streamlining Clinical Documentation**

Computerized documentation accumulates vast amounts of data very rapidly. The **"essence of care"** can be obscured in the sheer volume of data available. A critical component of using the CCC taxonomy in computerized documentation entails separating essential information from nonessential information and determining the level of detail required in the medical record.

The first step in this process is defining guiding principles about what must be in the patient record. The HCA Chief Nursing Officer Council defined the following priorities:

1. Needed for patient care
2. Needed for regulatory requirements
3. Needed for billing compliance

Every element of documentation was evaluated against these criteria. Data were deemed to be needed for patient care if it was sent to a display panel, a report, or a notification. Data were deemed to be needed for regulatory requirements when a specific standard from the Joint Commission or condition from Center for Medicare and Medicaid (CMS) could be cited. Data was deemed to be needed for billing compliance when a specific billing guideline was cited.

Examples of items eliminated from clinical documentation include the following:

- Inventory of belongings
- Standard safety precautions
- Hand-off communication

An example of abbreviated documentation is hygiene care, except for behavioral health, rehabilitation, and ventilated patients where hygiene care is part of their treatment.

● **Plan of Care**

Constructing a plan of care for a hospitalized patient that focuses on the **essence of care** and meets regulatory requirements is especially challenging when using a computerized system. Computer-assisted care planning enables assessment findings to suggest patient problems for the plan of care. This time-saving decision-support functionality can generate an overly complex plan of care that actually obscures the essence of care if left unchecked.

Maintaining a focus on the **"essence of care"** requires reserving the plan of care for the three to four priority problems that are the focus for the current episode of care. We accomplished this by creating two new categories of nursing interventions, routine care and individual considerations for care, that are standard care elements but not part of the plan of care.

Routine care interventions are those care activities that are required for all patients, regardless of the individual patient problems. These activities are necessary for care, often required by standards, and not directed to specific patient goals. Some examples are admission assessment, activities of daily living, discharge process, and monitoring of vital signs.

Individual considerations for care are patient characteristics and preferences that are important to planning and providing care and to all caregivers. These items are often required by

Assessments

Clinical Risk Reassessment ✓

Apply Clinical Risk Reassessment Values	⦿ All Normal (Editable) ○ All abnormal (Editable) ○ All Normal (Non-Editable)
Orientation and thought processes unchanged from admission	⦿ Yes ○ No
Appropriately engaged in care activities/care planning	⦿ Yes ○ No
Bilateral lung sounds clear & equal	⦿ Yes ○ No
Calves symmetrical without pain with dorsiflexion	⦿ Yes ○ No
Skin on sacrum intact without redness	⦿ Yes ○ No
Skin on heels and elbows firm and intact without redness	⦿ Yes ○ No
Free of pain or burning upon urination	⦿ Yes ○ No
Abdomen soft, non-distended & non-tender	⦿ Yes ○ No
Active bowel sounds all quadrants	⦿ Yes ○ No
Free of feelings of constipation	⦿ Yes ○ No
Last BM date	11/10/10
Days elapsed since last BM	2

Examples of items abbreviated in clinical documentation include the following:

* Hygiene Care (Except behavioral health and rehabilitation patients)
* Clinical Risk Assessment (combines risk assessment from common hazards of hospitalization)

FIGURE 5.4.1 ■ Example of clinical documentation. Clinical reassessment screen designed to identify commonly occurring complications in the hospitalized adult patient.

standards and are not linked to specific patient goals. Some examples of individual considerations for care include learning preferences, language, religious preferences, advanced directives, and dietary preferences. Eliminating routine care interventions and individual considerations for care from the plan of care allows the nurse to focus on the patient problems that are suggested within the computer system based on the patient assessment. The problems present in the CCC framework, and the nurse is asked to select the three to four high-priority problems that are amenable to nursing intervention within the anticipated length of stay for this episode of care. The result is a focused plan of care that communicates priority needs and actions for each patient and a related, but separate, work list of tasks that the nurse needs to accomplish.

EXHIBIT 5.4.1 ■ Worklist: Routine Care Activities

Routine care activities appear on the nursing task list but are not linked to problems or outcomes on the plan of care.

	Care Item			Last Done	Status/ Due	NOW	Today 09:00
A	Comprehensive Assessment	ONCE			-1m		
A	First point of contact	ONCE			-1m		
A	Health History	ONCE	P		-1m		
A	Height & Weight	ONCE			-1m		
A	Vital Signs	BID			3m		
A	Clinical Reassessment	QS					
A	Intake and Output	QS					
A	Intravascular Access	.PRN	A				
A	Manage-Refer-Contact-Notify	.PRN					
A	Pain Assessment	.PRN					
A	Teach	.PRN					

EXHIBIT 5.4.2 ■ Individualized Considerations of Care

Individual considerations for care are shown in the patient list for all care providers to access, as displayed below. Based on the selection, problems for the patient are then added to the plan of care, and all are coded with the CCC.

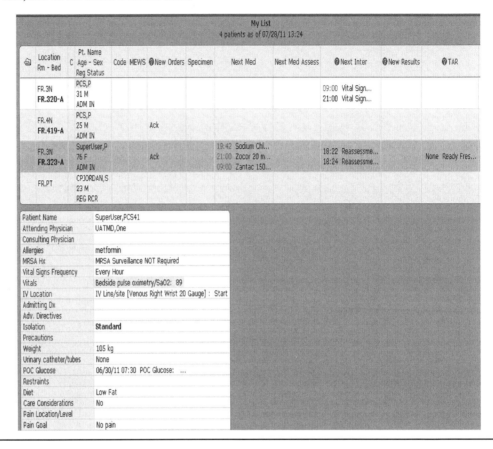

EXHIBIT 5.4.3 ■ Suggested Diagnoses and Interventions for the Plan of Care

Assessment findings generate suggested diagnoses and interventions that the nurse evaluates for inclusion in the plan of care. The nurse is responsible for selecting the priority problems that reflect the essence of care for this patient during this episode.

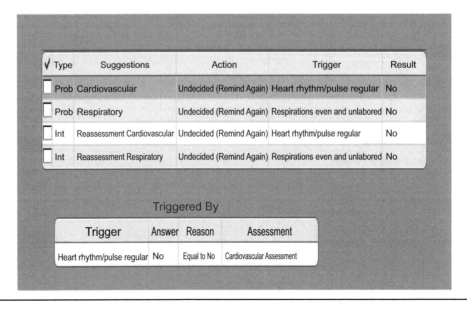

The CCC System© in Medicomp's Point of Care Knowledge Engine (MEDCIN®)

Luann Whittenburg

● MEDCIN® Nurse Module

The Nurse Module was designed for the Clinical Care Classification (CCC) System to support integrated care and the documentation and care planning functions of nurses and allied health professionals. The CCC is directly linked in the Medicomp Nurse Module to clinical terminology that may be found in the patient's electronic health record. Starting with one or more clinical diagnoses, relevant nursing diagnoses are discovered using the Intelligent Prompting™ capabilities of the MEDCIN® engine. A plan of care is dynamically constructed from the data present in one or more of the nursing encounters. The plan of care is presented in a view that illustrates all of the nursing activity related to the patient. The nurse, at any time, views the plan of care by selecting the "Show Plan of Care" menu; this displays the active nursing diagnoses selected in the "Data Entry View" (Figure 5.5.1). The context menus allow access to additional CCC System intervention selections relevant to a diagnosis as well as access to additional intervention Action Type selections relevant to a nursing intervention.

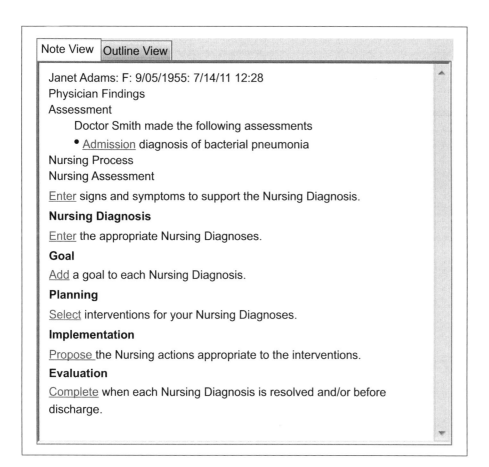

FIGURE 5.5.1 ■ MEDCIN® initial plan of care guided by the American Nurses Association nursing process.

● **Plan of Care Selection**

MEDCIN® selects from the electronic health record history pool of documentation to create a patient plan of care. MEDCIN® is a knowledge engine of standardized clinical terminology and vocabulary cross-mapped to leading codification systems such as the Systemized Nomenclature of Medicine Clinical Terms (SNOMED CT©); Current Procedural Terminology (CPT®); International Classification of Diseases 9th Revision Clinical Modification (ICD9-CM/ICD10-CM); *Diagnostic and Statistical Manual of Mental Disorders (DSM)*; Logical Observation Identifiers, Names and Codes (LOINC®); RxNORM; Current Dental Terminology (CDT®); and the CCC System for nursing and allied health. The MEDCIN® Engine indexes the CCC System to the full array of terminology standards and concepts with intelligent prompting, allowing for the presentation and documentation of relevant clinical symptoms, history, physical findings, and diagnoses to the CCC System concepts from the mapped to leading codification systems such as the SNOMED CT©, CPT®, ICD9-CM/ICD10-CM, DSM, LOINC®, RxNORM and CDT.

MEDCIN® used a diagnostic index to provide method to link signs and symptoms as well as clinical diagnoses to CCC nursing diagnoses, interventions, actions, goals, and outcomes. At the point of care, the diagnostic index focuses on nursing interventions relevant to CCC nursing diagnosis and carries the proper CCC code, allowing for aggregate data analysis. A new systematic methodology was developed to integrate a structured nursing terminology, the CCC System, as a contextual hierarchical tree into a clinical knowledgebase hierarchy: MEDCIN®.

This innovative methodology has populated the MEDCIN® clinical database with the CCC nursing terminology and demonstrates that the contextual hierarchy is the appropriate method for integrating the CCC terminology into the clinical databases (Figure 5.5.2). The contextual hierarchy of the MEDCIN® Engine supports the design of an electronic plan of care following the nursing process. The nursing process is used in an information system to measure the outcomes of nursing care and provide meaningful use information for patient care

FIGURE 5.5.2 ■ MEDCIN® plan of care with nursing diagnosis—actual outcome.

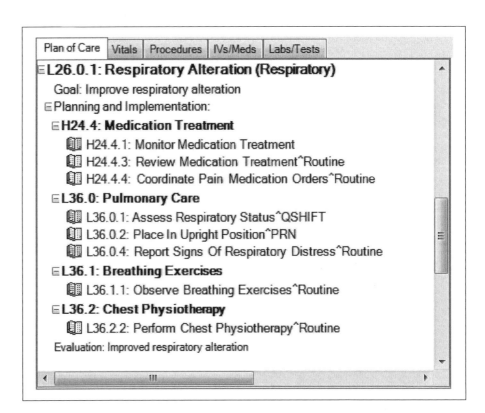

Frequency of Intervention Actions

Interventions	CCC Code	Intervention Actions	Frequency
L35.0 Oxygen Therapy Care	L35.0.1	Monitor Oxygen Saturation	1
	L35.0.2	Provide Oxygen Therapy	1
	L35.0.4	Collaborate With Respiratory Therapist	2
L36.0 Pulmonary Care	L36.0.1	Assess Respiratory Status	1
	L36.0.2	Perform Pulmonary Care	1
	L36.0.3	Explain Pulmonary Care	1
L36.1 Breathing Exercises	L36.1.1	Assess Breathing Status	2
	L36.1.3	Explain Breathing Exercises	1
	L36.1.4	Manage Breathing Exercises	1
L36.2 Chest Physiotherapy	L36.2.1	Assess Sputum Appearance	4
	L36.2.2	Perform Chest Physiotherapy	4
	L36.2.3	Explain Breathing Exercises	1
	L36.2.4	Collaborate With Respiratory Therapist	3

FIGURE 5.5.3 ■ Sample frequency of intervention actions report.

The Medicomp Nurse Module also provides a means to generate reports by aggregating CCC findings for a single patient or multiple patients. The reports include (and are not limited to) "Frequency of Intervention Actions" (Figure 5.5.3). The plan of care can be generated as a report. Each report can be printed or exported to a PDF or an XPS file.

CCC Use in Electronic Cumulative School Record with Health Module

Edith Vick

The nurse's role within public, private, parochial, and charter schools varies widely according to perceived needs. The nurse working in schools may have extensive involvement in direct care of significant student health needs and health program compliance management or may be less involved, working within a consultative model.

As record keeping is done electronically in most schools, school nurses can struggle with implementing a standardized language in daily practice. Here, two barriers exist. One is the nurse's lack of understanding of standardized language and how it facilitates documentation and information capture. The other is the framework of the available technology to support insertion of standardized language for meaningful use.

The Clinical Care Classification (CCC) is a concrete and functional language ideal for use in school nurse practice. The CCC is easily implemented into existing technology even if the framework of the technology has limitations for language insertion, such as limiting characters in text boxes or not allowing use of the decimal point for numerical codes.

Examples of CCC inserted into a cumulative school records program with a health module for a small school district of up to 400 students aged 3 to 21 years are provided. The school nurse attends weekly, increasing frequency according to student/school needs.

FIGURE 5.6.1 ■ CCC Nursing Diagnoses and Interventions for identified student health needs.

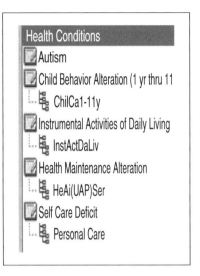

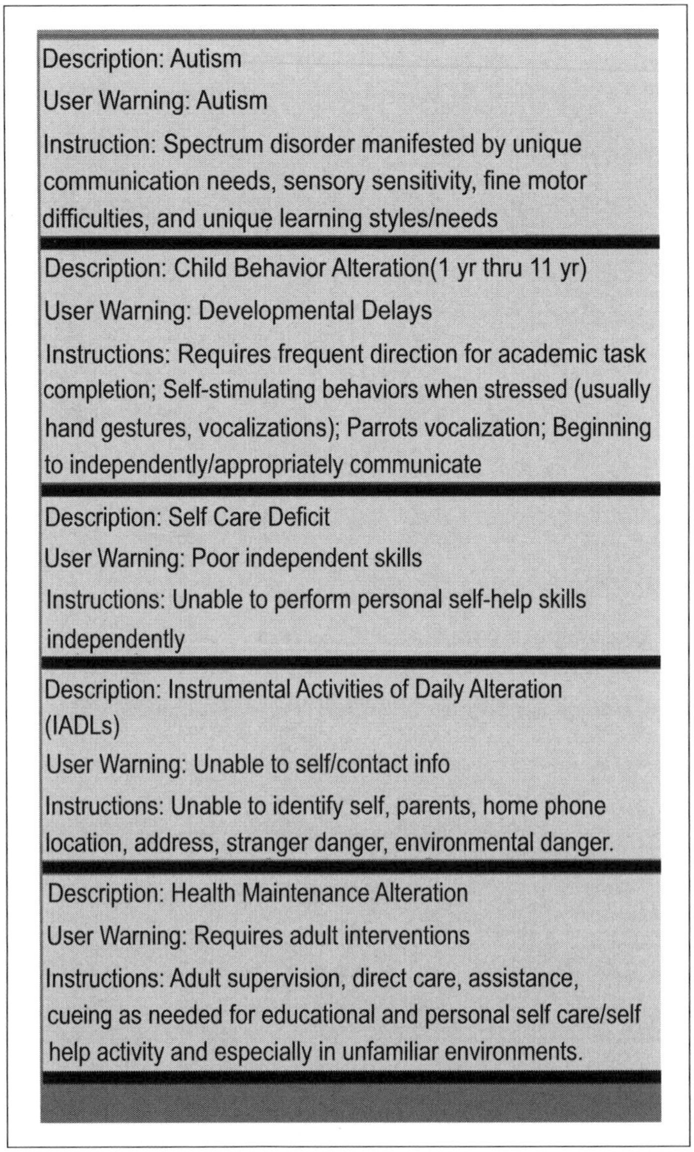

FIGURE 5.6.2 ■ CCC Nursing Diagnoses in identified student health alert (nursing assessment).

Description: Autism

User Warning: Autism

Instruction: Spectrum disorder manifested by unique communication needs, sensory sensitivity, fine motor difficulties, and unique learning styles/needs

Description: Child Behavior Alteration(1 yr thru 11 yr)

User Warning: Developmental Delays

Instructions: Requires frequent direction for academic task completion; Self-stimulating behaviors when stressed (usually hand gestures, vocalizations); Parrots vocalization; Beginning to independently/appropriately communicate

Description: Self Care Deficit

User Warning: Poor independent skills

Instructions: Unable to perform personal self-help skills independently

Description: Instrumental Activities of Daily Alteration (IADLs)

User Warning: Unable to self/contact info

Instructions: Unable to identify self, parents, home phone location, address, stranger danger, environmental danger.

Description: Health Maintenance Alteration

User Warning: Requires adult interventions

Instructions: Adult supervision, direct care, assistance, cueing as needed for educational and personal self care/self help activity and especially in unfamiliar environments.

Condition	Treatment
299.0 Autism Start/End Date: 08/18/2010-12/31/2021 Status: Life Long	
U61.3 Child Behavior Alteration (1 yr thru 11 yr) Start/End Date: 08/18/2010-12/31/2021 Status: To Improve	**763 ChilCa1-11y** Start/End Date: 08/18/2010-12/31/2020 Status: MRCN
O38.2 Instrumental Activities of Daily Living Alteration (IADLs) Start/End Date: 08/18/2010-12/31/2020 Status: To Improve Comments: Parents advised to attach personal information to child in some way	**432 InstActDaLiv** Start/End Date: 08/18/2010-12/31/2020 Status: CPPA Comments: Do not leave unsupervised; Personal ID/contact info on child for out of school building activity
G17.0 Health Maintenance Alteration Start/End Date: 08/18/2010-12/31/2020 Status: To Stabilize	**211 HeAi(UAP)Ser** Start/End Date: 08/18/2010-12/31/2020 Status: MRCN Comments: UAPs delegated to provide personal care
O38.0 Self Care Deficit Start/End Date: 08/18/2010-05/31/2019 Status: To Improve	**43 Personal Care** Start/End Date: 08/18/2010-05/31/2019 Status: CPPA Comments: Requires direct care/assistance/supervision/cueing with personal skills/self-help activity

FIGURE 5.6.3 ■ CCC Nursing Diagnoses, Expected Outcomes, and Interventions in identified student healthcare plan.

The cumulative records program is an online program accessed by password from any computer. Each school district purchases the online program through a vendor, who provides technology support as needed. The records program technology framework is extensive and requires administrative permissions to access insertion of the CCC language into the program. Exploring the technology framework to determine where to appropriately insert the CCC was a time-intensive task and continues to evolve as familiarity of the program grows.

The program technology allows development of a plan of care for students with identified health problems requiring intervention during the school day. Medical diagnoses are provided by the online technology for the nurse to select and associate with the student, if desired. After assessing the student, the school nurse selects the appropriate CCC nursing diagnosis or diagnoses. The technology framework allows the association of the CCC Interventions with the CCC Nursing Diagnoses, which are selected by the school nurse (Figure 5.6.1).

The program technology provides a method of communication to teachers. The school nurse may choose to select the alert, which serves to document assessment of the student and communicate to teachers the student's abilities, limitations, and health needs (Figure 5.6.2).

The technology does not allow for the CCC Interventions decimal points and limits text; therefore, an adjustment was made and documented for consistency in use. The school nurse may print a student condition/treatment (diagnosis/intervention) and add a parent/guardian signature to a student plan of care, as needed (Figure 5.6.3).

The technology framework of the daily log requires the CCC actual outcome and Action Type codes and text to be inserted together and abbreviated owing to text limitations, for example, "CP AO-1. Improved" (care plan actual outcome was improved) and "RN-4.MRCN" (RN provided service of: manage, refer, contact, notify; Figure 5.6.4).

The program technology does provide reporting ability. A report of all school nurse-identified student health conditions (Figure 5.6.5) and/or a report of student health conditions associated with a student name can be generated. Additional reporting capability exists

Student Name	HCP Identified Needs	CPOther - Identified Needs RN - 3. TEIS	HeAi(UAP)Ser
Recorded By: School Nurse	Date/Time: 09/23/2010 11:41 AM	Comments: Reviewed wih UAP staff regarding personal care needs and Medicaid billing documentation/submission	
Student Name	HCP Identified Needs	CPOther - Identified Needs RN - 4. MRCN	HeAi(UAP)Ser
Recorded By: School Nurse	Date/Time: 11/04/2010 11:49 AM	Comments: UAPs compliant with personal care plan/documentation; Documentation submitted for medicaid billing	
Student Name	Staff Referral	CPOther - Identified Needs RN - 4. MRCN	ChilCa1-11y
Recorded By: School Nurse	Date/Time: 01/06/2011 01:00 PM	Comments: IEP meeting; discussion with parent regarding personal ID/contact info on child, and care plan	
Student Name	HCP Identified Needs	CPOther - Identified Needs RN - 4. MRCN	HeAi(UAP)Ser
Recorded By: School Nurse	Date/Time: 03/03/2011 12:01 PM	Comments: UAPs compliant with personal care plan; Medicaid billing submitted	
Student Name	HCP Identified Needs	CP AO - 1. Improved RN - 4. MRCN	ChilCa1-11y
Recorded By: School Nurse	Date/Time: 05/26/2011 12:02 PM	Comments: Lessened self stim behaviors at school	
Student Name	HCP Identified Needs	CP AO - 1. Improved RN - 4. MRCN	HeAi(UAP)Ser
Recorded By: School Nurse	Date/Time: 05/26/2011 12:05 PM	Comments: UAPs compliant with plan	
Student Name	HCP Identified Needs	CP AO -1. Improved RN - 4. MRCN	InstActDaLiv
Recorded By: School Nurse	Date/Time: 05/26/2011 12:07 PM	Comments: School staff complaint with supervision and ID on child for out of school building activity; Parent has not provided personal ID/contact for child to wear on person	
Student Name	HCP Identified Needs	CP AO - 1. Improved RN - 4. MRCN	Personal Care
Recorded By: School Nurse	Date/Time: 05/26/2011 12:10 PM	Comments: Child beginning to initiate personal self help skills	

FIGURE 5.6.4 ▨ CCC Actual Outcomes and Action Types in health office visit log.

within this electronic records program; however, at this time, technology assistance is needed by this user to access it.

This is a small sample of CCC implementation for student healthcare plan development and documentation within an online electronic school records program. Implementing the CCC provides a clear, succinct, and functional means of identifying and communicating student health-related needs relevant to Individual Education Plan (IEP) as mandated by Individuals with Disabilities Education Act plan development, 504 (Americans with Disabilities Act) plan development, transition planning into adulthood, and school Medicaid billing. Utilizing the CCC in electronic school records for student healthcare plans captures the depth of professional school nursing work and provides a means of efficient, targeted management of large populations.

Health Conditions (non-grouped)

Code	Description	Total	Alerts
314.00	ADD/Attention deficit disorder	1	1
314.01	ADHD/Attention deficit disorder with hyperactivity	1	1
477.90	Allergic Rhinitis, cause unspecified	1	1
995.30	Allergy, unspecified	2	2
704.00	Alopecia	1	1
995.00	Anaphylaxis, allergic shock	1	1
493.90	Asthma, unspecified	3	3
299.0	Autism	1	1
749.00	Cleft palate, cleft lip	1	1
759.83	Fragile X syndrome	1	1
333.10	Tremor, essential and other	1	1
Grand Total		**14**	**14**

ND Health Behavioral

Code	Description	Total	Alerts
G17.0	Health Maintenance Alteration	3	3
Grand Total		**3**	**3**

ND Physiologic

Code	Description	Total	Alerts
U61.3	Child Behavior Alteration (1 yr thru 11 yr)	3	2
Grand Total		**3**	**2**

ND Health Behavioral

FIGURE 5.6.5 ■ CCC Nursing Diagnoses in grades PS–5 student report.

FIGURE 5.6.5
(cont'd) ▨ CCC Nursing
Diagnoses in grades PS–5
student report.

Code	Description	Total	Alerts
H21.0	Medication Risk	2	2
Grand Total		2	2

ND Health Behavioral

Code	Description	Total	Alerts
N33.0	Injury Risk	2	2
Grand Total		2	2

ND Functional

Code	Description	Total	Alerts
038.2	Instrumental Activities of Daily Living Alteration (IADLs)	1	1
038.0	Self Care Deficit	1	1
Grand Total		2	2

ND Functional

Code	Description	Total	Alerts
Q44.1	Auditory Alteration	2	2
Q44.7	Visual Alteration	18	18
Grand Total		20	20

PART 5.7

Finnish Care Classification for Nursing Documentation

Anneli Ensio, Ulla-Mari Kinnunen and Minna Mykkanen

● Introduction

In Finland, the target of national nursing documentation has been to unify and standardize nursing documentation and to connect it with the interdisciplinary core documentation of patient care. These core elements of a patient record have been defined for the national code server and will be used when electronic patient records are stored in a national patient record archive by 2014. One reform in the new HealthCare Act (active as of January 5, 2011) is the improvement of the mobility of patient records. Every electronic patient register and patient record archive in different health centers and hospitals in a hospital district forms a joint register of patient records. In the beginning of 2000, the terminology chosen—the Home Health-Care Classification (HHCC)—was translated and modified as the Finnish Care Classification (FinCC). The structure of the FinCC is equal to the HHCC/Clinical Care Classification (CCC). The changes in content of the FinCC have followed the cultural validation in 2001 and feedback of users in 2007 and 2010.

The National Nursing Documentation Project (2005–2008) has had significant meaning for nurses in Finland. During that project, the nationally unified and standardized nursing documentation model has been developed and piloted. The structure of the Finnish nursing documentation model is based on the decision-making process and a standardized nursing terminology. Nursing diagnosis, interventions, and outcomes are documented in a structured way using the FinCC. Later, these databases enable also evaluation, analysis, and utilizations for meaningful use of information for different purposes. Most important is that with these tools, we make nursing visible.

● Finnish Care Classification, Version 2.01

The structure of the FinCC follows the structure of the CCC, and it is based on a three-level hierarchical format. FinCC includes three separate classifications: the Classification of Nursing Diagnoses (FiCND), Nursing Interventions (FiCNI), and Nursing Outcomes (FiCNO) Version.2.0.1. The development work started in the late 1990s by defining nursing interventions and diagnoses at the University Hospital of Kuopio in Finland and expanded considerably in 1995 when the Ministry of Social Affairs and Health launched the (above presented) broad project within public healthcare organizations. In the next 4 years, the common model for the nursing documentation grew and was implemented in different electronic patient record systems. Much emphasis has been focused on education and training when the documentation model has been implemented. The structured form of care plans gives several possibilities for meaningful use of the nursing documentation.

The latest FiCND and FiCNI, Version 2.0.1, contain 19 components (Table 5.7.1), which are divided into a number of main categories and further into subcategories. The FiCNO includes three qualifiers: improved, stabilized, and deteriorated. The development and maintenance of the FinCC has been organized at the University of Eastern Finland (former Kuopio University), at the department of Health and Social Management. The 10-member terminology expert group, comprising members from different healthcare organizations in Finland, supervises the terminology development, networks with the users and researchers, and is responsible for the continuing evaluation of the FinCC. Also, the translation to Swedish has just been completed.

Feedback from the users of the FinCC was collected in 2007 and 2010. In Spring 2010, an electronic questionnaire was sent to the FinCC contact persons in Finnish hospitals and health care centers where the FinCC was in use. The aim of the study was to find out the experiences of FinCC users, especially how usable the 19 components of FiCND and FiCNI are and how the terminology could further be evolved. The research looked for answers by the aid of following questions:

1. Is the component useful at your unit?
2. Is the component unambiguous to nurses at your unit?
3. Is the component unambiguous in your multiprofessional care group?
4. Is the content of the component comprehensive?
5. Is the component concrete enough?

TABLE 5.7.1 ■ FINCC Components, Version 2.01

Activity	Health Services	Metabolic	Sensory
Elimination	Medication	Role Relationship	Skin Integrity
Coping	Nutrition	Safety	Continuity of Care
Fluid Volume	Respiration	Activities of Daily Living (ADL)	Life Cycle
Health Behavior	Cardiac	Psychological Regulation	

The answers (n = 148) were given by a group of nurses or by one nurse at a time. The medication, elimination and skin integrity components reached the best agreement. On the other hand, coping, role relationship, and life cycle needed revision and further development. Based on the study results, valuable user feedback, and the work of the expert group, FinCC, Version 3.0, and a User Guidebook available in 2012. The user guidebook is currently also in process.

Documentation of Wound Care as an Example of Using the FinCC

In the FinCC, wound care is documented using the skin integrity component. The FiCND has such main categories as acute wounds, chronic wounds, and information necessity of skin integrity. The FiCNI includes main categories like wound monitoring, wound care, wound care guidance, monitoring burn, burn care, burn care guidance, pressure ulcer prevention and care, and pressure ulcer guidance.

Patient: Mr. X

Case history: The patient had a huge abscess on the back of his right hand. He could not remember what has happened to his arm. His friends brought him to the hospital. Now the abscess has been evacuated and totally removed 3 days ago. There are still two open wounds. He has diabetes mellitus and no medication.

The example of the standardized nursing documentation in the electronic patient record system in use at Kuopio University Hospital in Finland can be seen in Figure 5.7.1. Even if it shows a limited picture of nursing care plan, it gives an overview of 1-day documentation of wound care. The nursing process becomes visible when nursing diagnoses, interventions, and outcomes are documented using the FinCC. In addition to components and main and subcategories, there is always a possibility to describe patient condition with narrative text.

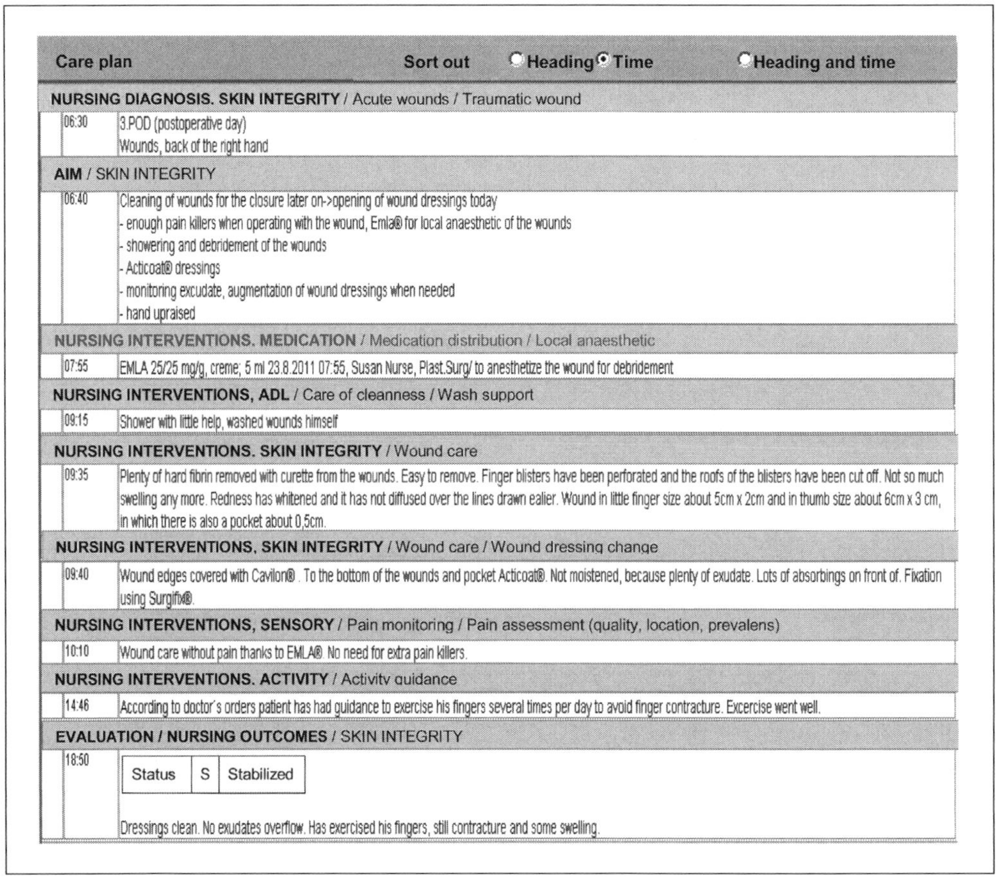

Care plan   Sort out   Heading   Time   Heading and time

NURSING DIAGNOSIS. SKIN INTEGRITY / Acute wounds / Traumatic wound
06:30 3.POD (postoperative day)
Wounds, back of the right hand

AIM / SKIN INTEGRITY
06:40 Cleaning of wounds for the closure later on->opening of wound dressings today
- enough pain killers when operating with the wound, Emla® for local anaesthetic of the wounds
- showering and debridement of the wounds
- Acticoat® dressings
- monitoring excudate, augmentation of wound dressings when needed
- hand upraised

NURSING INTERVENTIONS. MEDICATION / Medication distribution / Local anaesthetic
07:55 EMLA 25/25 mg/g, creme; 5 ml 23.8.2011 07:55, Susan Nurse, Plast.Surg/ to anesthetize the wound for debridement

NURSING INTERVENTIONS, ADL / Care of cleanness / Wash support
09:15 Shower with little help, washed wounds himself

NURSING INTERVENTIONS. SKIN INTEGRITY / Wound care
09:35 Plenty of hard fibrin removed with curette from the wounds. Easy to remove. Finger blisters have been perforated and the roofs of the blisters have been cut off. Not so much swelling any more. Redness has whitened and it has not diffused over the lines drawn ealier. Wound in little finger size about 5cm x 2cm and in thumb size about 6cm x 3 cm, in which there is also a pocket about 0,5cm.

NURSING INTERVENTIONS, SKIN INTEGRITY / Wound care / Wound dressing change
09:40 Wound edges covered with Cavilon® . To the bottom of the wounds and pocket Acticoat®. Not moistened, because plenty of exudate. Lots of absorbings on front of. Fixation using Surgifix®.

NURSING INTERVENTIONS, SENSORY / Pain monitoring / Pain assessment (quality, location, prevalens)
10:10 Wound care without pain thanks to EMLA®. No need for extra pain killers.

NURSING INTERVENTIONS. ACTIVITY / Activity guidance
14:46 According to doctor's orders patient has had guidance to exercise his fingers several times per day to avoid finger contracture. Excercise went well.

EVALUATION / NURSING OUTCOMES / SKIN INTEGRITY
18:50

Status	S	Stabilized

Dressings clean. No exudates overflow. Has exercised his fingers, still contracture and some swelling.

FIGURE 5.7.1 ■ Example of nursing documentation using the FinCC.

In organizations where standardized documentation is in use, nursing databases expand and give several possibilities to reuse the information for different purposes in the fields of care, education, and management. This is a considerable benefit, which enables also cooperation and teamwork at an international level, with the global aims of nursing documentation to improve the quality of patient care and increase patient safety.

● Bibliography

Ensio, A., Saranto, K., Ikonen, H., & Iivari, A. K. (2006). The national evaluation of standardized terminology. In H. A. Park, P. Murray, & C. Delaney (Eds.), *Consumer-centered computer-supported care for healthy people. Proceedings of NI2006, Seoul* (pp. 749–752). Amsterdam: IOS Press.

Jylhä, V., Kinnunen, U. M., & Saranto, K. (2008). The use of structured documentation in electronic patient records: Case diabetics. In H. Karsten, B. Back, T. Salakoski, S. Salanterä, & H. Suominen (Eds.), *Proceedings of Louhi ´08. The First Conference on Text and Data Mining of Clinical Documents, Turku, Finland, September 3rd–4th, 2008* (pp. 83–88). Turku, Turun yliopisto: TUCS General Publication 52. Retrieved from https://www.doria.fi/bitstream/handle/10024/41995/proc2008louhi.pdf?sequence=2

KanTa. (2009). National Archive of Health Information. Electronic archive of patient records. 9.10.2009. Retrieved from https://www.kanta.fi/en/electronic-archive-of-patient-records

Kinnunen, U. M., Ensio, A., & Liljamo, P. (2011). Finnish care classification for nursing documentation: Users' voice. In F. Sheerin, W. Sermeus, K. Saranto, & E. H. Jesus (Eds.), *ACENDIO 2011. E-health and nursing. The Proceedings of the 8th Conference of ACENDIO, Madeira, 25/26 March* [DVD] (pp. 250–257). Madeira, Portugal: ACENDIO.

Kinnunen, U. M., Saranto, K., & Miettinen, M. (2009). Effects of terminology-based documentation on nursing. In K. Saranto, P. F. Brennan, H. A. Park, M. Tallberg, & A. Ensio (Eds.), *Connecting health and humans, proceedings of NI 2009 Helsinki, the 10th International Nursing Informatics Congress.* Helsinki, Finland: Amsterdam, IOS Press.

MSAH, Ministry of Social Affairs and Health. (2011, May 3). Patients have access to health services according to care plan even outside their home municipality. Press release 108/2011. Retrieved from http://www.stm.fi/en/pressreleases/pressrelease/view/1560084#en

Saba V. K. (2006). Clinical Care Classification (CCC) System manual: A guide to nursing documentation. New York: Springer Publishing Company.

Saranto K., & Kinnunen, U. M. (2009). Evaluating nursing documentation—research designs and methods—systematic review. *Journal of Advanced Nursing, 65*(3), 464–475.

Tanttu, K. & Rusi, R. (2007). Nursing documentation project in Finland: Developing a nationally standardized electronic nursing documentation model by 2007. In N. Oud, F. Sheerin, M. Ehnfors, & W. Sermeus. *Nursing communication in multidisciplinary Practice. Proceedings of the 6th ACENDIO Conference in Amsterdam in the Netherlands* (pp. 213–217). Amsterdam: ACENDIO.

PART 5.8

Clinical Practice Support (CPS) for Nurses and Midwives in South Australia

Livio Ciacciarelli

● Careconnect.sa Clinical Practice

Careconnect.sa clinical practice support (CPS) assists nurses, midwives, and other healthcare professionals in making prompt, informed decisions about patient care through the following:

1. streamlining assessments
2. interventions and care planning processes

3. minimizing duplicated data entry

4. enabling continuous monitoring of the patient's journey

5. providing the ability to identify and manage risk and monitor patient outcomes by promoting quality patient care based on available best practice.

In 2008, South Australian nursing and midwifery leads identified the need to adopt a standardized language and structure for nursing and midwifery care. The CCC System was explored and determined to be the preferred practice framework to achieve these goals and be used with the careconnect.sa CPS, the enterprise-wide nursing & midwifery clinical information system.

As CPS is an enterprise-wide standards database. It aims to support patients/clients and nurses/midwives in their decision-making with evidence-based best practice using the six steps of the nursing process as outlined in the CCC System framework and illustrated below.

Step 1, Assessment

In Figure 5.8.1: CPS Assessment, the nursing and midwifery assessment becomes the basis for many parts of identify and managing patients' needs. From these data, CPS will begin to formulate and identify the care planning requirements based upon evidence-based pathways.

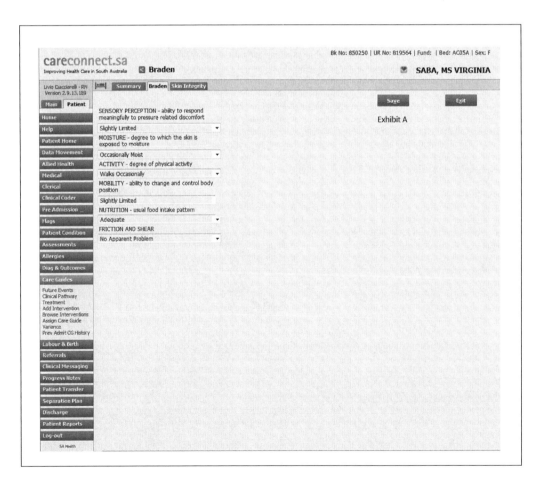

FIGURE 5.8.1 ▦ Clinical practice support assessment. Copyright 1998 by Barbara Braden and Nancy Bergstrom.

Step 2, Diagnosis

In Figure 5.8.2: CPS Assessment Summary, CPS will begin to formulate the following based upon the assessment data entered:

1. Assessment score (e.g., Braden score)
2. Clinical pathway (nursing interventions contained within the care guide)
3. Clinical flags (e.g., pressure ulcer risk)
4. Nursing/midwifery diagnosis
5. Expected outcomes

Step 3, Outcome Identification

In Figure 5.8.2: CPS Assessment Summary, the nurse/midwife is presented with an automated nursing diagnosis based upon data entered from the assessment. The expected outcome is entered prior to the assessment being allowed to be completed.

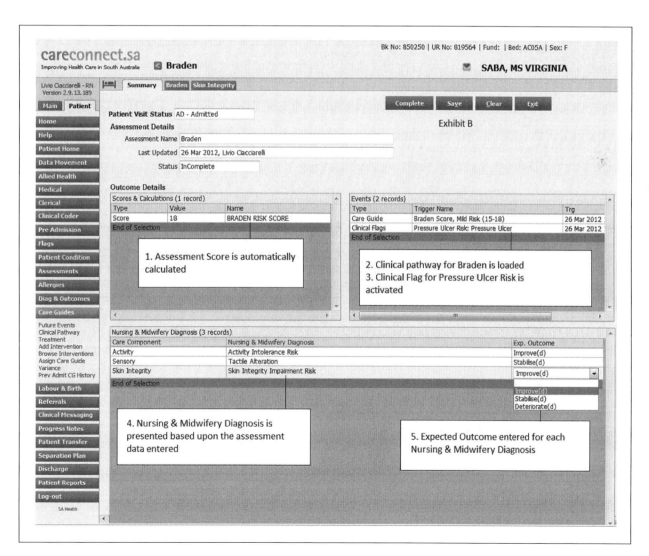

FIGURE 5.8.2 ■ Clinical practice support assessment summary.

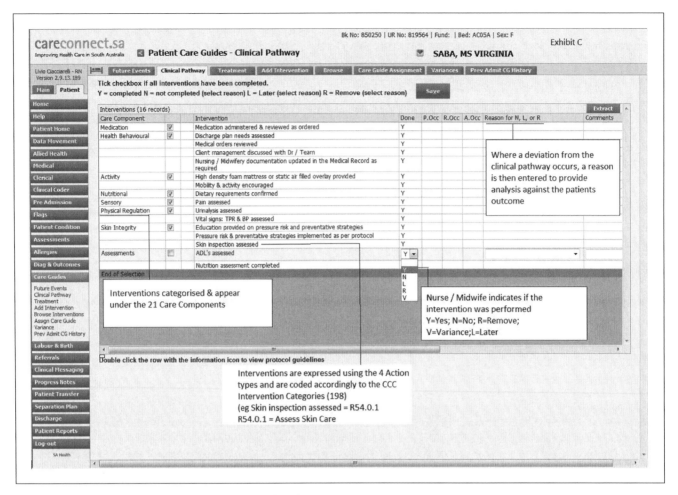

FIGURE 5.8.3 ■ Clinical practice support clinical pathway.

Step 4, Planning, and Step 5, Implementation

In Figure 5.8.3: CPS Clinical Pathway, the clinical pathway is generated from the assessment and contains nursing/midwifery interventions categorized under the 21 care components. The interventions and phrased are coded accordingly to the CCC system intervention categories and the 4 Action Types.

The clinical pathways are based on the statewide review of practice, with a strong link to best-practice and evidence-based guidelines. The nurse/midwife is able to adjust the clinical pathway/nursing interventions according to the patient's requirements, adding or removing interventions as required. Where there is deviation from best-practice care, the clinician is required to document the impact that this variance has on the person's outcome. Information is then used to assist and support changes in monitoring nursing/midwifery practice, work environment, patient acuity, and resource calculation.

Step 6, Evaluation

In Figure 5.8.4: CPS Diagnosis and Outcomes, prior to the patients' discharge, actual nursing/midwifery diagnoses are required to be entered.

Both the expected and actual nursing diagnosis outcomes can then later be compared to the outcome achieved within the clinical pathway, which provides supporting evidence for changes in care provision (work practice, work process, work environment).

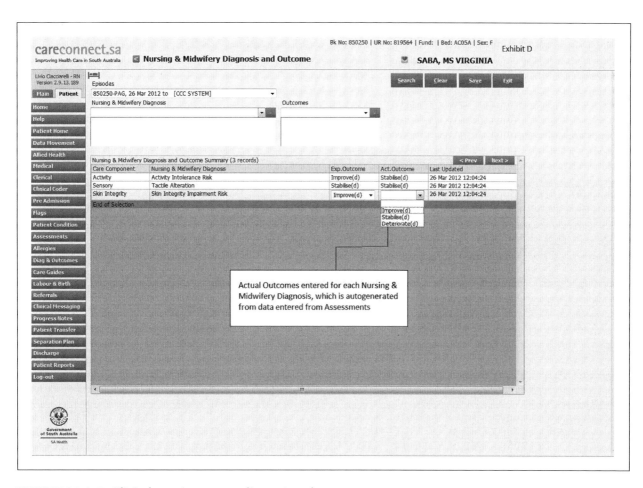

FIGURE 5.8.4 ▦ Clinical practice support diagnosis and outcomes.

6 Nursing Education Application of the Clinical Care Classification Using the Personal Computer

Jennifer E. Mannino and Veronica D. Feeg

As the healthcare system rapidly evolves and the use of the electronic health record (EHR) broadens, nurse educators are confronted with the need for ways to expand an already dense curriculum to teach the knowledge and skills of electronic documentation to students that adequately prepares them for the workforce. The personal computer Clinical Care Classification (PC-CCC) system is a Microsoft Access® version of the Sabacare Clinical Care Classification (CCC) System© terminology. The goal of this chapter is to present the PC-CCC as a useful tool in introducing students to health information technology (HIT) and teaching students EHR documentation using the CCC coded nursing terminology.

● Introduction

Nurse educators face the academic challenge of teaching students—future clinicians—a mountain of continuously changing knowledge and skills that will serve them in practice. As the health system changes, students need to develop learning strategies that help them keep current on the frequent recommendations that emerge from evidence to guide their maturity into professionals. The foundation of the nursing profession is the nursing process. It is necessary to teach nursing students skill in using the nursing process so that they can turn nursing knowledge and theory into practice (Craven & Hirnle, 2009). With mastery, nursing students can refine their systematic approach to solving problems with current information. The nursing process uses cognitive skills and leads students to identify problems that nursing interventions can address, plan a course of action, implement those actions, and evaluate outcomes (Wang, Kao Lo, & Ku, 2004; Yura & Walsh, 1988). In a retrospective study, researchers have concluded that theory and practice of using the nursing process should be introduced early and reinforced throughout remaining courses to improve care planning (Palese, DeSilvestre, Valoppi, & Tomietto, 2009).

Nursing Process and Planning Care

The nursing process is a systematic problem-solving approach to provide individualized patient care (see Table 6.1), which nurses use in all patient care settings to identify and treat the patient's response to potential or actual health problems (Craven & Hirnle, 2009). The practice setting for clinical experiences provides the place and opportunities where students interact with patients and families to acquire cognitive skills. These settings are currently undergoing transformation with the integration of information technologies including the EHR. Setting-based problem-solving and clinical decision-making opportunities give real experiences for students to apply the knowledge they acquire in the classroom. Planning care for an assigned patient gives students a cognitive and psychomotor experience derived from the clinical setting and translated into the activity of charting. This rich field experience helps students practice in a simulated milieu for learning. The ultimate goal is to develop clinical understanding that connects signs and symptoms with holistic clinical plans that recognize the difference between individualized and standardized care (Benner, Tanner, & Cesla, 1996; Billings & Halstead, 1998; Craven & Hirnle, 2009). In hospitals today, nursing students need to learn the additional psychomotor skill of communicating their plans in writing and documenting care in the EHR.

   The nursing student better learns the process of care planning by doing rather than by reading, such as identifying patient goals and determining ways to reach those goals. As students move through the cognitive steps of formulating short-term and long-term goals for the patient, they begin to articulate those plans in the active mental exercise of writing down the plan in a logical, cohesive manner. This can be done in the long-hand narrative format of

TABLE 6.1 ▦ Steps and Definitions of the Nursing Process. (http://www.sabacare.com/
Framework/NursingProcess.html)

Nursing Care Process Steps—Documentation System
The steps of the nursing process include the following: **Assessment** **Diagnosis** **Outcome identification (expected outcome)** **Intervention (planning)** **Type of Action—implementation (monitor/perform/teach/refer)** **Evaluation (actual outcome)**
Care Components: Assessment
Care components provide a standardized framework to document and track care with each patient contact/encounter. Care components link and map the six steps of the care process and provide the analysis and measures for evidence-based practice.
Nursing Diagnoses: Diagnosis
Nursing diagnoses are used to identify the specific atomic-level diagnostic conditions based on the signs and symptoms, assessed care components, and/or patient problems that require care.
Expected Outcome: Outcome Identification
Each nursing diagnosis requires an *expected outcome* as the goal of the care. The three qualifiers used for the outcome identification are to *improve* patient condition, to *stabilize* the patient condition, or to *support* the patient's deteriorating condition.
Nursing Interventions: Planning
The *nursing interventions* are atomic-level services identified to plan and implement patient care. They are needed to satisfy each care component, diagnostic condition, or patient problem assessed as requiring nursing care.
Type of Intervention Action: Implementation
Each nursing intervention requires a *Type of Action* as the major focus of the core nursing intervention. It provides the evidence used to measure care and determine resources. The four qualifiers used to provide the Type of Action are the following: **1. Assess/monitor/evaluate/observe** = Action evaluating patient condition. **2. Care/perform//provide/assist** = Action performing actual patient care. **3. Teach/educate/instruct/supervise** = Action educating patient or caregiver. **4. Manage/refer/contact/notify** = Action managing care on behalf of the patient or caregiver.
Actual Outcome: Evaluation
Each nursing diagnosis requires an *actual outcome* as an evaluation of the outcome of the care process—interventions and Action Types. The same three qualifiers are used to predict the care goals and to evaluate whether they were met or not met.
Patient's condition **improved, stabilized,** or **deteriorated**.

writing care plans on paper, or they can be prompted by computer-based logic in a software program that structures the nursing process steps and guides the student through the logic. The educator can create these assignments to accomplish learning in terms of domains of educational activities described by Bloom, including (a) the *cognitive domain*—using the knowledge and skills of recall, identification, and synthesis; (b) the *psychomotor domain*—using the computer to document the care planning process that emulates an electronic documentation system of care planning; and (c) the *affective domain*—using the experience to develop a sense of confidence in the learner (Chitty & Black, 2007).

Electronic Health Record

As we move into the electronic age of healthcare documentation, institutions of nursing education are urged to prepare students to use HIT. In a 2005 study conducted by Jha, Ferris, et al, a systematic review of EHR adoption, about one fourth of physicians used some form of electronic systems, and approximately 5% of hospitals used HIT (Jha, Ferris, Donelan, DesRoches, Shields, Rosenbaum, & Blumenthal, 2006). However, with recent federal policy stimulus support, including the American Recovery and Reinvestment Act (ARRA), and with the Institute of Medicine calling for the growth of HIT as promising tools to improve quality, numerous recommendations have been issued for health educators in all disciplines to include information technology in curricula (IOM, 2003). The Office of the National Coordinator for Health Information Technology oversees the Health Information Technology for Economic and Clinical Health (HITECH) Act, which provides US Department of Health and Human Services (HHS) with the authority to establish programs to improve healthcare quality, safety, and efficiency through the promotion of HIT, including EHRs and private and secure electronic health information exchange. The HITECH regulations include the expectation that systems meet criteria, including "meaningful use" objectives, defined in stages by the federal government (ONCHIT, 2011).

Nurses in the workplace with expertise in computers are more likely to fully adopt hospital information technology systems and maximize the designed features that enhance patient safety (Moody, Slocumb, Berg, & Jackson, 2004). Renewed efforts to train and implement systems across settings have been ongoing for professionals in hospitals. Given the many systems available, there is no single approach to teaching and/or learning EHR documentation. Gloe (2010) identified the difficulty of new nurses learning to use an EHR with concomitant barriers of moving from novice to expert with limited experiential opportunities. She describes the challenge of selecting an academic EHR to prepare students to enter the modern workplace and acknowledges the need for committee-based selection criteria to choose a vendor in a marketplace of high-cost systems—particularly for the education setting. She concludes that the biggest challenge may be funding the chosen software but supports the need to provide the EHR in the learning environment to produce competent graduates who are ready to work in computerized environments.

● Personal Computer Approach

The personal computer (PC) is ubiquitous in industry and homes today. Students from kindergarten to college use computers for academic and social activities in all aspects of life. The PC offers the nursing student a familiar tool with which assignments can be completed at home or school. Schools have developed innovative ways to integrate information literacy and computer skills through the curriculum (Flood, Gasiewicz, & Delpier, 2010). Planning care via computer is a vehicle to combine knowledge and skills in the student clinical learning experience. A class-based assignment can use practice-setting experiences to apply knowledge that integrates the use of technology with the cognitive skills of the nursing process. The student's learning is enhanced through simulated documentation on the computer. Electronic care planning provides a teacher-guided learning activity.

The PC-CCC was developed by Feeg, Saba, and Feeg (2008) and tested in a randomized clinical trial. It was subsequently field tested (Mannino & Feeg, 2011) with baccalaureate nursing students, yielding positive usability results and improved care planning skills. It creates an unintimidating opportunity for nurse educators to embrace and bring the EHR into the classroom.

The Sabacare CCC© system is a standardized, coded nursing terminology that identifies the discrete elements of nursing practice. Designed to follow the nursing process, it provides a coherent framework to guide use by nursing students when documenting and describing their care. Its unique coding system allows for the documentation and aggregation of nursing care. The system electronically classifies and links coded nursing diagnoses directly with coded nursing interventions. Sample care plans, detailed descriptions, and step-by-step instructions are provided in the instructional materials.

The PC-CCC is a PC version that allows nursing educators to bring the Sabacare CCC into the classroom. Designed for use with Microsoft Access®, the PC-CCC is an evidenced-based electronic care planning database program. The application is available via free download from the Internet. It is easy to install and use on any laptop or desktop computer, PC or Mac, equipped with Microsoft Access®. The database can be stored on a removable storage device (i.e., flash drive, thumb drive, etc.), making it a portable documentation system that electronically records and aggregates nursing interventions.

In addition to learning EHR documentation, The PC-CCC application offers a unique approach to learning the nursing process. The Sabacare data-based system adds more structure and support in identifying patient care. It also provides the educator with the means to monitor, track, and evaluate student experiences at multiple clinical sites over time. The reports generated by the system provide information about the individual student experiences, patient acuity, and clinical experience as a whole.

● Teaching the PC-CCC in the Classroom

The teaching–learning environment for combining the cognitive skills of the nursing process with the psychomotor skills and application of knowledge with documentation needs to be cultivated for optimum learning. The activities should be planned with objective-driven guidance and teacher-directed activities throughout the early learning process. The following describes the classroom and practice-setting activities to use the PC-CCC for planning patient care.

Objectives

The activity is developed around a set of student- and instructor-focused objectives for the activities.

    A. <u>Learning Objectives: Student</u>

- Obtain basic knowledge of HIT
- Provide the novice computer user with a basic set of computer skills
- Empower students with confidence when learning future electronic documentation systems
- Foster the students' understanding of the nursing process and recognize the steps as essential for nurses
- Foster the students' understanding of and ability to prioritize nursing diagnoses and nursing interventions
- Foster the students' understanding of and ability to create nursing care plans
- Encourage critical thinking without memorization

    B. <u>Practice Objectives: Instructor</u>

- Monitor, track, and evaluate student experiences at multiple clinical sites
- Store, analyze, and retrieve documentation prepared by students
- Aggregate and analyze the students' nursing interventions by type and frequency
- Evaluate the students' exposure and experiences at multiple clinical sites meaningfully over time

Planning Instruction

    A. *Students.* The PC-CCC, like any new software application, will take some time to get used to. The best way for educators and students to learn how to use the PC-CCC is

TABLE 6.2 ■ Method of Instruction

Instruction	Objectives *Method*	Time
Electronic health records, PC-CCC	· **Introduce health information technology** · **Obtain basic set of computer skills** *Didactic and demonstration*	30–45 min
Step-by-step guidance (not required for all students)	· **Ensure basic set of computer skills** *Computer laboratory—common patient*	1 hour
Home assignment (clinical experience)	· **Foster understanding of the nursing process** · **Encourage critical thinking** · **Document patient data electronically** *Individual clinical patients*	Submitted

Note. PC-CCC = personal computer Clinical Classification System.

to actually begin using the program. The method of instruction summarized in Table 6.2 is based upon randomized trial procedures developed by Feeg et al. (2008) and actual field testing results reported in the literature (Mannino & Feeg, 2011). Instruction, method, and time may vary according to the level of student understanding, including the following sequence:

1. Begin instruction in the classroom or computer laboratory with an initial 30 to 45 minutes introduction to electronic documentation and the CCC.

2. Follow the initial instruction with a real-time PC-CCC program demonstration highlighting its relationship with the nursing process.

3. Demonstrate how to access, download, and save the program.

4. Finish instruction by providing handouts containing rich patient examples, sample documentation, and step-by-step instructions for the students to take home.

5. Offer time at a later date for follow-up questions and answers.

Once downloaded and saved on a portable flash drive, students can immediately begin documenting patient care electronically using the PC-CCC. Students will first enter the patient data into the database then begin creating care records for each. Once completed, they can print a record or electronically send, as an email attachment, a PDF file or the entire database to their instructor.

B. Teachers. Faculty, including both clinical and classroom teachers, should be actively involved in the monitoring and evaluation process. The information about real situations give the student in the clinical setting a rich source of content to organize relevant to the didactic instruction and the clinical application. The suggested sequence of activities includes the following:

1. Assess each electronic care record for completeness and offer feedback to students about the quality of their care planning documentation.

2. Look for demonstrated use of the nursing process in properly applied, well-stated, and well-supported nursing diagnoses with appropriate nursing interventions and expected outcomes.

3. Be sure that each intervention has a rationale and correct action(s) for providing the intervention.

4. Depending on the intervention and length of time with the patient, an actual outcome may or may not be noted.

5. Be accepting of students' feedback.

6. Ask the students and additional faculty or assistant faculty to complete a PC-CCC evaluation tool (see Tables 6.3A & B).

TABLE 6.3A ▦ Evaluation Tools for PC-CCC (Students)

A. Circle the most appropriate response to the following questions.					
This program aided my ability to understand and prioritize nursing diagnosis.	Strongly agree	Agree	Disagree	Strongly disagree	N/A
This program aided my ability to understand and prioritize nursing interventions.	Strongly agree	Agree	Disagree	Strongly disagree	N/A
Using this program aided my ability to understand nursing care plans.	Strongly agree	Agree	Disagree	Strongly disagree	N/A
Using this program aided my ability to create nursing care plans.	Strongly agree	Agree	Disagree	Strongly disagree	N/A
I would recommend future Nursing 209 students use this program.	Strongly agree	Agree	Disagree	Strongly disagree	N/A
I would like to continue using this program for all nursing courses that require the development of nursing care plans.	Strongly agree	Agree	Disagree	Strongly disagree	N/A

B. Circle the most appropriate response to the following questions related to technical use of the PC-CCC.					
The screen design was organized and clear.	Strongly agree	Agree	Disagree	Strongly disagree	N/A
The format was easy to follow.	Strongly agree	Agree	Disagree	Strongly disagree	N/A
The information was easy to understand.	Strongly agree	Agree	Disagree	Strongly disagree	N/A
The system allowed me to chart my care plan.	Strongly agree	Agree	Disagree	Strongly disagree	N/A
The system was efficient to enter the data.	Strongly agree	Agree	Disagree	Strongly disagree	N/A
I enjoyed the method of entering the data.	Strongly agree	Agree	Disagree	Strongly disagree	N/A
I would recommend using this program at the bedside.	Strongly agree	Agree	Disagree	Strongly disagree	N/A

Note. PC-CCC = personal computer Clinical Classification System.

The feedback results from the evaluation tool can be useful to the teacher. Using a Likert scale, students have the opportunity to report their level of agreement/disagreement in questions pertaining to the application's ease of use and their learning of electronic documentation and the nursing process. The evaluation questionnaire can be helpful in determining the usability of the PC-CCC application for particular assignments and assists the teacher in using feedback to customize and modify procedures and requirements.

● Using the PC-CCC System

Accessing the PC-CCC Database

The application uses a Microsoft Access® database format and requires that the students have this commonly used software on their laptops, home PCs, and/or school-accessible computers. The steps to access the downloadable free application are specific, and students must be connected to the Internet to follow these instructions.

TABLE 6.3B ■ Evaluation Tools for PC-CCC (Faculty)

Directions for faculty: Circle the most appropriate response to the following questions.					
This program aided my students' ability to understand and prioritize nursing diagnosis.	Strongly agree	Agree	Disagree	Strongly disagree	N/A
This program aided my students' ability to understand and prioritize nursing interventions.	Strongly agree	Agree	Disagree	Strongly disagree	N/A
This program aided my students' ability to understand nursing care plans.	Strongly agree	Agree	Disagree	Strongly disagree	N/A
This program aided my students' ability to create nursing care plans.	Strongly agree	Agree	Disagree	Strongly disagree	N/A
I saw a steady progression in the quality of my students' care plans.	Strongly agree	Agree	Disagree	Strongly disagree	N/A
I would recommend future Nursing 209 courses use this program.	Strongly agree	Agree	Disagree	Strongly disagree	N/A

Note. PC-CCC = personal computer Clinical Classification System.

Student Step by Step Instructions

1. Insert a USB storage device (i.e., flash drive, thumb drive, etc.) into the USB port of the PC.
2. Open web browser (Internet Explorer, Netscape, Mozilla, Chrome, etc.).
3. Go to http://faculty.molloy.edu/pcccc
4. Click "download list."
5. Click "class application with sample patient screens."
6. Click "save file" (file information: databases.zip, 1.8 MB, molloy.edu).
7. Once saved, unzip "ClassSample" by double clicking.
8. See "CCC209ClassSample" (file information: Microsoft Access® application size, 4.75 MB).

    Please note: To begin using the application, it must first be moved and renamed.
    Click, hold, and drag the file to the USB storage device (or desktop) AND rename.

9. Rename with term, year, and user's last name (example: spring2010smith).
10. Double click to open the program from the USB drive.

    Please note: To allow the program to open, click on the security "options" and "enable" the program to be opened completely.

11. Review the three example cases contained in this database.
12. Begin preparing the care plan (specific instructions to follow).

Adding a Patient to the PC-CCC Database

Each patient must be added to the PC-CCC database before documenting a care record.

1. To add a patient to the database, click "Patient Data" on Screen A: Switchboard. (All clicks are left clicks unless otherwise noted.) The screen will automatically change from the Switchboard to Screen B: Core Patient Information (see Figure 6.1).
2. Click "add new patient" (see Figure 6.2).
3. Record necessary patient information. (Medical and Nurse ID code can be left blank.)

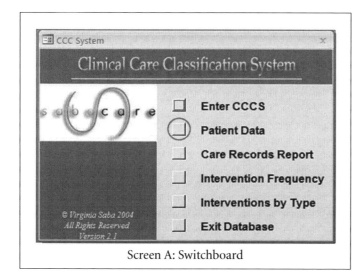

Screen A: Switchboard

FIGURE 6.1 ■ Switchboard leading to core patient information.

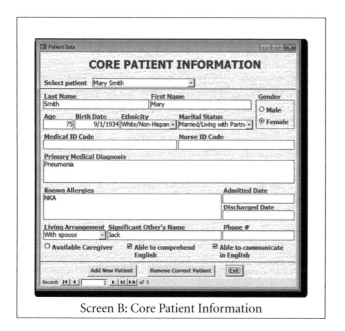

Screen B: Core Patient Information

FIGURE 6.2 ■ Core patient information to add a new patient.

*Please note: This product is PC based and not HIPAA compliant as a stand-alone system; therefore, rules similar to the use and transfer of student-generated paper-documented care plans according to the educational institution must be stressed. Although the program calls for patient names, students are to use fictitious names and no identifying demographic or health data to preserve patient anonymity and maintain HIPPA compliance. Students must be reminded of the American Nurses Association Code of Ethics related to the use of real names.

4. Click "add new patient" a second time. Repeat steps 2 to 4 if adding multiple patients. Patients, including the database sample patients, may be removed by first highlighting the desired patient from the "select patient" drop-down menu then clicking "remove current patient."

5. When complete, click "exit" to return to the Switchboard.

● Creating an Individual Care Record According to the Nursing Process

The CCC System developed by Dr. Virginia K. Saba (http://www.sabacare.com) is consistent with the steps of the nursing process used in practice to assess and document patient care needs. The student will follow the nursing process as a guide in identifying and documenting an individualized care record for each patient. The nursing process is a fundamental problem-solving approach essential to nursing and remains as the foundation for delivering all nursing care. As a result of using the PC-CCC, the student will become more comfortable and confident with their application of the nursing process and the delivery of holistic patient care.

The PC-CCC provides several tracking schemes in developing individual care plans and reviewing them individually, collectively, or aggregately. (a) Individual care planning screens give the user a guided and visually meaningful approach to selecting from check-box and drop-down structures of the nursing process to formulate the problem aspects and the intervention aspects of the plan of care. The terminology is all coded in the background to be linked and populate screens as in the real clinical settings while forcing the user to complete all the steps before the plan can be entered. An individual report can be produced. (b) Collectively, the PC-CCC allows the user to enter each patient's plan of care and produce a collection of all patients that have been recorded on a summary report. (c) Aggregately, the PC-CCC allows the instructor to aggregate information across patients' summaries about the frequency of interventions and portion of total records that include particular actions. These summary aggregated reports can be printed.

1. To begin preparing the care record (a.k.a. nursing plan of care), click "enter CCCS" on the Switchboard.

2. The user has access to all of the PC-CCC functions from the Switchboard. Once clicked, the screen changes to the patient care classification screen (see Figure 6.3).

   Highlight and click on the appropriate patient from the "patient name" drop-down menu (see Figure 6.4).

3. **Assessment**: Through patient assessment, the student identifies a *care component*. Care components provide the standardized framework to document and track the care with each patient contact/encounter. Care components link and map the six steps of the care process and provide the analysis and measures for evidence-based practice.

   Highlight and click on a care component from the drop-down menu (see Figure 6.5).

4. **Diagnosis**: The *nursing diagnosis* is used to identify a patient's problem, its etiology, and presenting signs and symptoms. It is a representation of the nurse's clinical knowledge about the patient and response to an actual or a potential health concern. Nursing diagnoses are used to identify the specific atomic-level diagnostic conditions based on the signs and symptoms, assessed care components, and/or patient problems that require care.

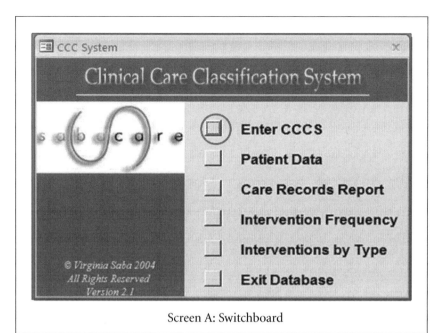

Screen A: Switchboard

FIGURE 6.3 ▥ Switch-board leading to the CCC screen.

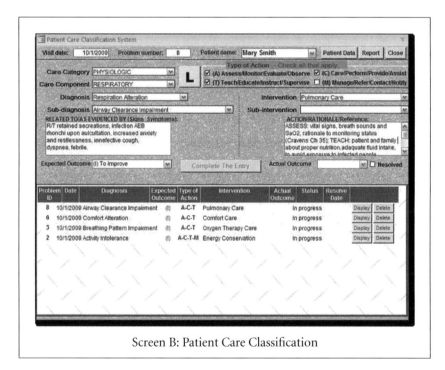

Screen B: Patient Care Classification

Highlight and click on a diagnosis from drop-down menu. Then use free text for the "related to/as evidenced by" data to substantiate the selected diagnosis. The free-text option encourages the student to carefully investigate and consider potential causes for and signs and symptoms of the patient's problem (see Figure 6.6).

5. **Outcome identification**: Each nursing diagnosis requires an *expected outcome* as the goal of the care. The three qualifiers used for the outcome identification are the following: to *improve* the patient's condition; to *stabilize* the patient's condition; or to *support* the patient's deteriorating condition.

Highlight and click on an expected outcome. Students choose what they expect to happen given the patient's condition and the nursing interventions being performed, to improve, stabilize, or support deterioration (see Figure 6.7).

FIGURE 6.4 ■ Patient care classification with "patient name" drop-down menu.

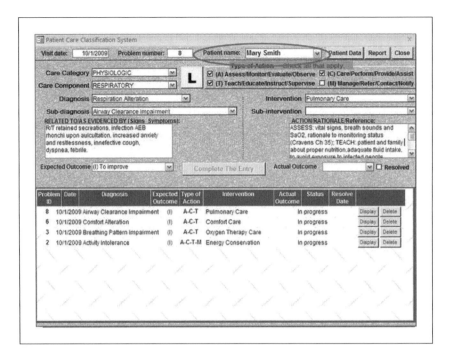

6. **Planning**: The *nursing interventions* are atomic-level services identified to plan and implement patient care. They are needed to satisfy each care component, diagnostic condition, or patient problem assessed as requiring nursing care.

    Highlight and click on "intervention" (and "subintervention" if necessary) from the drop-down menu. Then identify the action(s) and intervention(s) with rationales and references necessary to implement care and achieve the expected outcome. The added free-text option allows the student to customize each plan to meet the patient's specific needs. Having the student type in specifics applicable to the individual encourages critical thinking (see Figure 6.8).

7. **Implementation:** Each nursing intervention requires a *Type of Action* as the major focus of the core nursing intervention. It provides the evidence used to measure care and determine resources.

FIGURE 6.5 ■ Patient care classification with "care component" drop-down menu.

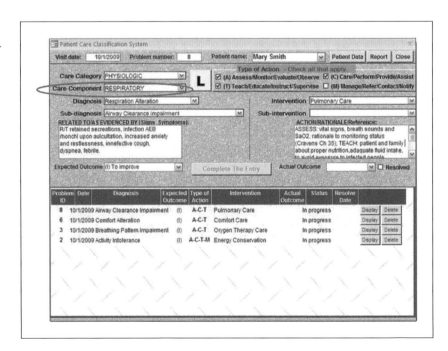

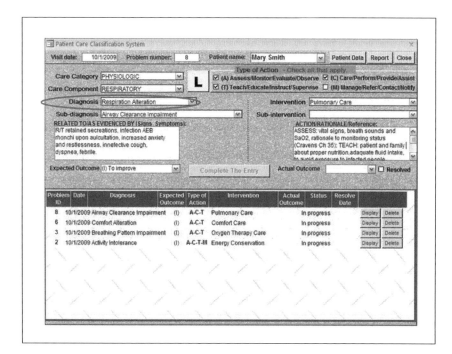

FIGURE 6.6 ▓ Patient care classification with "diagnosis" drop-down menu.

The four qualifiers used to provide the Type of Action are the following:

1. Assess/monitor/evaluate/observe: Action evaluating the patient condition.
2. Perform/care/provide/assist: Action performing actual patient care.
3. Teach/educate/instruct/supervise: Action educating patient or caregiver.
4. Manage/refer/contact/notify: Action managing care on behalf of the patient or caregiver.

Click to check and select appropriate Type of Action(s) to be performed (see Figure 6.9).

"Action" identifies specifically what nursing skills are necessary to carry out the selected nursing intervention and bring about the expected patient outcome. The actions are divided into four main types: assess, care, teach, and manage. These provide data for the type of care needed to produce a specific patient outcome.

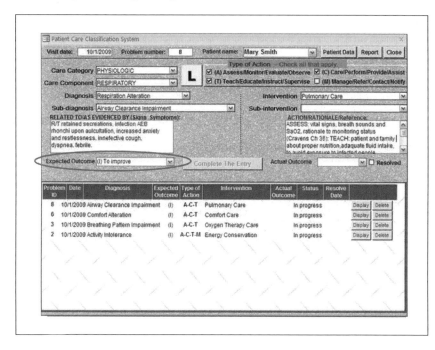

FIGURE 6.7 ▓ Patient care classification with "expected outcome" drop-down menu.

FIGURE 6.8 ▪ Patient care classification with intervention and subintervention.

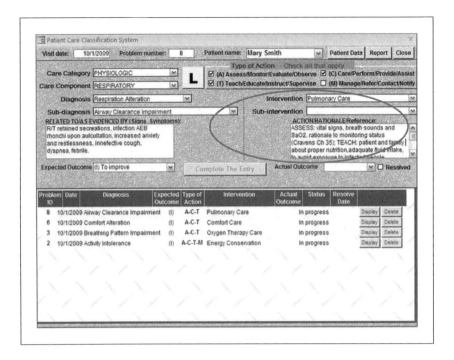

Consider the following example of a nurse administering a medication to a patient to exemplify the many actions necessary to bring about one routine intervention. When nurses administer medication to a patient, they perform at least three separate actions, whereas documentation on a medication administration record notes only one. To begin, the nurse first "assesses, monitors, evaluates, and/or observes" the patient's readiness to receive a medication. This may require a swallowing assessment, auscultation of breath sounds, checking of vital signs, etc. If all results are satisfactory, the nurse will actually "perform, care, provide, and/or assist" with the actual administration of the medication. During this time, the nurse is con-

FIGURE 6.9 ▪ Patient care classification with "type of action(s)" check boxes.

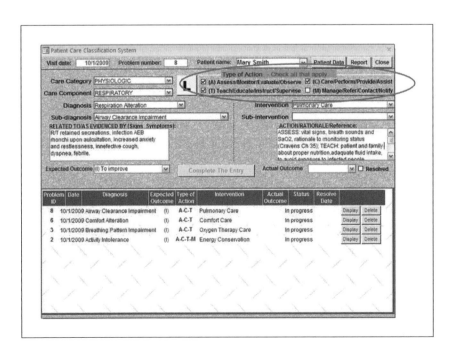

tinuing to assess but also is "teaching, educating, instructing, and or supervising" the patient about medication safety, side effects, therapeutic effects, and so forth.

The four major Action Types capture the **"essence of care."** This is crucial for the student to understand. Nursing care is never static but is dynamic in nature. Emphasis must be placed on care as encompassing the whole patient, not merely a collection of independent skills

Review the plan for accuracy and completeness. Once satisfied, click "record the entry" for a new plan or "complete the entry" for a plan modification. Click "report" to view the individual care record. Click "close" to return to the Switchboard (see Figure 6.10).

8. **Evaluation:** The *actual outcome* demonstrates the evaluation stage of the nursing process. Each nursing diagnosis requires an actual outcome as an evaluation of the outcome of the care process—interventions and Action Types. The same three qualifiers are used to predict the care goals and to evaluate whether they were met or not met.

- Patient's condition **improved**, **stabilized**, or **deteriorated**.

See the sample provided in Figure 6.11, which has four problems listed with an "in progress" status. This represents the four plans of care that are currently being evaluated for this patient. Evaluation of the patient's condition and effectiveness of the nursing care delivered is an ongoing process. To document a condition change, *improved, stabilized,* or *deteriorated,* click on "actual outcome" and highlight the appropriate choice. *Improved, stabilized,* or *deteriorated* will be noted on the problem list in the *actual outcome* column. To close out or "resolve" a plan, after choosing an actual outcome, click "resolved." The status will change from "in progress" to "resolved."

*Please note: Often, owing to time constraints and logistics, a student cannot evaluate the effectiveness of the plan of care. In those instances, the actual outcome is left blank, and the problem remains documented as "in progress."

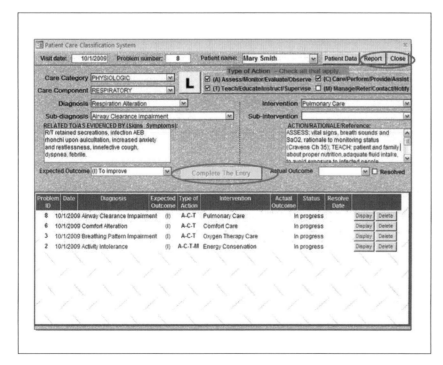

FIGURE 6.10 ■ Patient care classification with "complete the entry," "report," and "close" boxes.

FIGURE 6.11 ▓ Patient care classification with "actual outcome" drop-down menu.

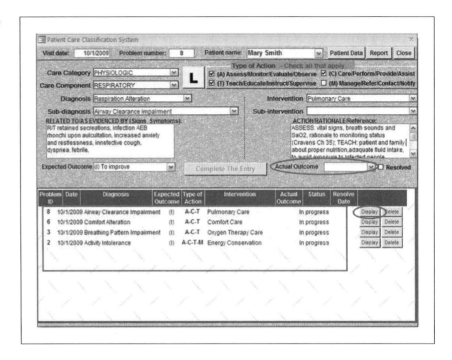

The CCC automatically creates an individual problem list for each patient every time a care record is created. Add additional care records to the patient's problem list as appropriate. *Actual outcomes* can be documented and "in progress" problems can be "resolved" by clicking "display." Problems may be deleted if entered incorrectly.

When complete, click "report" to view individual care records (see Figure 6.12). See the "Printing and Emailing" section for instructions on how to print and email individual care records. See the "Creating Aggregate Reports" section for instructions on how to create database reports. Click "close" to return to the Switchboard.

FIGURE 6.12 ▓ Patient care classification with progress report and "display/delete" options.

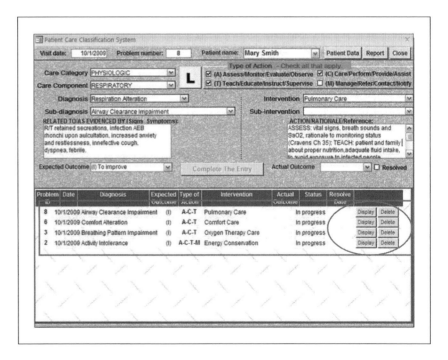

● Individual Care Records

The care record that results from the PC-CCC is a printable, readable form that fills a matrix of headings showing the temporal nature (dates, etc.) of the process and gives the student space to use the cognitive skills of documenting sources of evidence used in diagnosis and rationale for interventions (see Figure 6.13). The richness of the content can be encouraged by developing guidelines that mandate that the student must reference sources of rationale to foster the learned steps of seeking evidence to support nursing actions.

Through the use of the nursing process, the student identified patient Mary Smith (pseudonym) as having the diagnosis of "airway clearance impairment" and requiring a "pulmonary care" intervention. The diagnosis is well supported by the free text describing the patient's condition. In this example, the diagnosis is related to the patient having retained secretions and an infection; Mary Smith presents as being febrile, dyspneic, anxious, and restless; has rhonchi upon auscultation; and has an ineffective cough.

To carry out the "pulmonary care" intervention, the student nurse identifies that this will require three separate nursing actions: (a) to "assess" or evaluate the severity of the condition, noting the patients vital signs, pulse oximetry, and breath sounds; (b) to "care" or perform the actual procedure of assisting with postural drainage, coughing, and deep breathing and providing chest physiotherapy; and (c) to "teach" the patient and family strategies to prevent exacerbation, such as to maintain adequate hydration, avoid infected people, and practice good hygiene, and the importance of getting vaccinated.

● Creating Aggregate Reports

The PC-CCC provides the teacher with several aggregate reports that may be useful at the end of semesters or clinical rotations. These reports can be aggregated by each student by (a) creating a summary of all of the patients who have had plans of care developed or (b) gathering data by types and frequencies of interventions (see Figure 6.14).

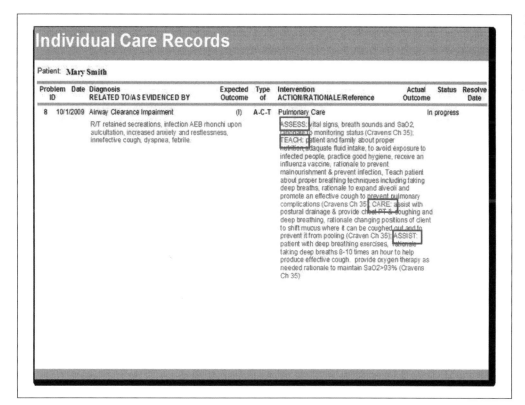

FIGURE 6.13 ▦ Individual care record.

FIGURE 6.14 ■ Switchboard
identifying multiple report options.

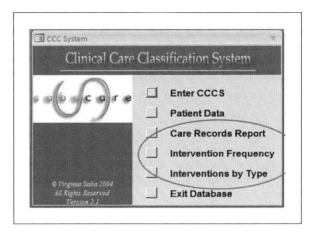

FIGURE 6.15 ■ Care records
report.

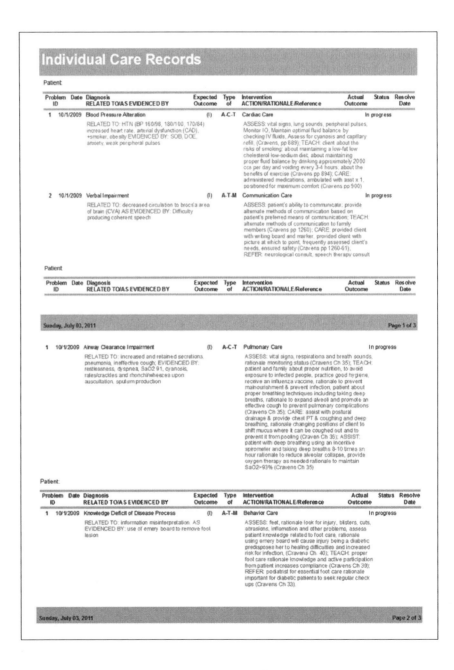

With just one click from the Switchboard screen, the PC-CCC aggregates all data contained within the database. The teacher has the ability to monitor, track, and evaluate the students' learning and experiences at multiple clinical sites over time. The reports can also provide information about an entire clinical group's experience and the partnering institution, such as patient acuity.

a. <u>Care Records Report</u>

The "Care Records" report function generates a cumulative display of the individual care records for all the patients contained in the database (see Figure 6.15). The patients are sorted according to the order in which they were initially entered into the database. At a quick glance, the teacher can evaluate the ongoing quality and completeness of each student's care records without having to store and sort through multiple sheets of paper.

b. <u>Frequency of Interventions</u>

The "Frequency of Interventions" function provides a breakdown of all of the actions that were used to carry out the selected interventions, categorized by care component (see Figure 6.16).

c. <u>Interventions by Type</u>

The "Interventions by Type of Action" displays the frequency and percentage of actions required to carry out the nursing interventions (see Figure 6.17).

FIGURE 6.16 ■ Frequency of interventions report.

Frequency of Interventions

Component	Intervention	Frequency
A ACTIVITY	A01.2.2 Care Energy Conservation	3
	A01.2.4 Manage Energy Conservation	3
	A01.2.4 Teach Energy Conservation	3
	A01.2.1 Assess Energy Conservation	3
C CARDIAC	C08.0.1 Assess Cardiac Care	3
	C08.0.2 Care Cardiac Care	3
	C08.0.4 Manage Cardiac Care	2
	C08.0.3 Teach Cardiac Care	3
D COGNITIVE	D10.0.1 Assess Behavior Care	1
	D10.0.4 Manage Behavior Care	1
	D10.0.3 Teach Behavior Care	1
I METABOLIC	I27.0.1 Assess Diabetic Care	2
	I27.0.2 Care Diabetic Care	2
	I27.0.4 Manage Diabetic Care	2
	I27.0.3 Teach Diabetic Care	2
L RESPIRATORY	L35.0.3 Teach Oxygen Therapy Care	3
	L35.0.1 Assess Oxygen Therapy Care	3
	L35.0.2 Care Oxygen Therapy Care	3
	L35.0.4 Manage Oxygen Therapy Care	2
	L36.0.2 Care Pulmonary Care	2
	L36.0.4 Manage Pulmonary Care	1
	L36.0.3 Teach Pulmonary Care	2
	L36.0.1 Assess Pulmonary Care	2
	L37.0.3 Teach Tracheostomy Care	1
	L37.0.1 Assess Tracheostomy Care	1
	L37.0.2 Care Tracheostomy Care	1
	L37.0.4 Manage Tracheostomy Care	1
Q SENSORY	Q48.0.3 Teach Comfort Care	2
	Q48.0.1 Assess Comfort Care	2
	Q48.0.2 Care Comfort Care	2

FIGURE 6.17 ■ Interventions by type of action.

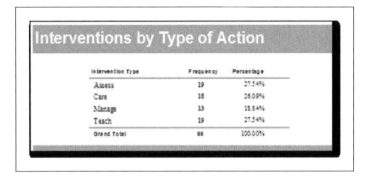

Interventions by Type of Action

Intervention Type	Frequency	Percentage
Assess	19	27.54%
Care	18	26.09%
Manage	13	18.84%
Teach	19	27.54%
Grand Total	69	100.00%

● **Printing and Emailing**

To print a care record or report, click the "file" tab located in the upper left corner of the screen then "print". To email, first save the care record or report as a PDF file then send as an email attachment. Do this by clicking the "PDF" icon tab located in the upper center of the screen.

Please note: This function is available only on computers equipped with Adobe Acrobat Professional. Alternatively, the entire database can be sent as an email attachment.

● **Backing up the PC-CCC Database**

As all electronic system users know and students need to be reminded, information in electronic format should be backed up routinely to prevent data loss. The following steps can be encouraged for students to perform independently over the course of the semester or learning experience.

1. Right click on the PC-CCC icon located on the desktop or in the portable storage device.
2. Select "copy."
3. Move to another directory on the portable storage device or your personal home computer.
4. Right click then select "paste."
5. RENAME the file (example: spring2010smith1).

● **Evaluation Process**

Students and adjunct faculty should be given the opportunity to evaluate using the PC-CCC. The information yielded from ongoing evaluations helps the teacher to modify subsequent uses for classes. Collecting reports from students allows the teacher to also evaluate the student and patient interactions over a period of time to yield important information for modifying clinical placements and/or learning opportunities.

The teacher using the PC-CCC can evaluate a variety of aspects of individual student progress, collective experiences, and aggregated proportions of activities. In addition, the data resulting from these activities can be used for comprehensive reviews of clinical experiences and practice setting opportunities. For example, charts and graphs using Excel can be assembled that yield usable and synthesized information about the semester activities by semester or over time (see Sample Charts 6A and 6B).

Overall, integrating the PC-CCC provides a mechanism for instructing students on electronic charting that is generic and applicable in the multiple hospital and home settings where they may work. At the same time, this coded nursing terminology-based application gives students the real experience of employing a nursing care planning system that documents electronically organized data about patients, resulting in cognitive learning, psychomotor skills, and affective-related confidence-building results.

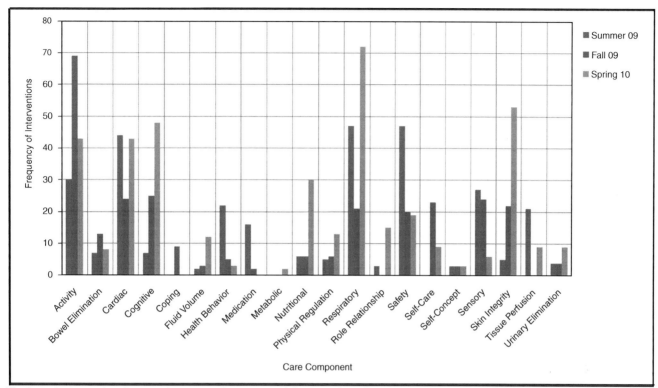

*Each student completed one to three care plans per week for 8 to 10 weeks.

SAMPLE CHART 6A ▦ Interventions (by category) performed by three semesters of sophomore-level nursing students (n = 57).

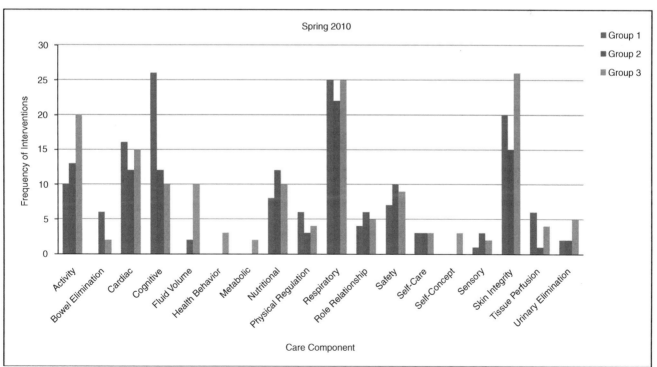

*Each Student completed one to three care plans per week for 10 weeks.

SAMPLE CHART 6B ▦ Interventions (grouped by category) performed by three sophomore-level clinical groups enrolled during the spring 2010 semester (n = 25)

● References

Benner, P., Tanner, C., & Chesla, C. (1996). *Expertise in nursing practice: Caring, a clinical judgment and ethics.* New York, NY: Springer Publishing Company.

Billings, D. & Halstead, J. (1998). *Teaching in nursing: A guide for faculty.* Philadelphia, PA: W.B. Saunders Company.

Craven, R. & Hirnle, C. (2009). *Fundamentals of nursing: Human health and function* (6th ed.). Philadelphia, PA: Lippincott.

Chitty, K. & Black, B. (2007). *Professional nursing: Concepts and challenges.* St. Louis, MO: Saunders, Inc.

Feeg, V., Saba, V., & Feeg, A. (2008). Testing a bedside personal computer clinical care classification system for nursing students using Microsoft Access®. *Computers, Informatics, Nursing, 26*(6), 339–439.

Flood, L, Gasiewicz, N. & Delpier, T. (2010). Integrating information literacy across a BSN curriculum. *Journal of Nursing Education, 49*(2), 101–104.

Gloe, D. (2010). Selecting an academic electronic health record. *Nurse Educator, 35*(4), 156–161.

Institute of Medicine (IOM). (2003). *Health professions education: A bridge to quality.* Washington, DC: National Academies Press.

Jha, A. K., Ferris, T. G., Donelan, K., DesRoches, C., Shields, A., Rosenbaum, S., & Blumenthal, D.(2006). How common are electronic health records in the United States? A summary of the evidence. *Health Affairs, 25*(6), 496–500.

Mannino, J. & Feeg, V. (2011). Field testing a PC electronic documentation system using the Clinical Classification (CCC) system with nursing students. *Journal of Healthcare Engineering, 2*(2), 223–240.

Moody, L., Slocumb, E., Berg, B., & Jackson, D. (2004). Electronic health records (EHR) documentation in nursing: Nurses' attitudes and preferences. *Computers, Informatics, Nursing, 26*(6), 337–344.

Office of the National Coordinator for Health Information Technology (ONCHIT). (2011). Electronic health record and meaningful use. Retrieved from http://healthit.hhs.gov/portal/server.pt?open=512&objID=2996&mode=2

Palese, A., DeSilvestre, D., Valoppi, G., & Tomietto, M. (2009). A 10-year retrospective study of teaching nursing diagnosis to baccalaureate students in Italy. *International Journal of Nursing Terminologies and Classifications, 20*(2), 64–75.

Saba, V. K. (2004). Sabacare Clinical Care Classification System. Retrieved from http://www.sabacare.com

Wang, J., Kao Lo, C., & Ku, Y. (2004). Problem solving strategies integrated into nursing process to promote clinical problem solving abilities of RN–BSN students. *Nurse Educator Today, 24*, 589–595.

Yura, H. & Walsh, M. (1988). *The nursing process: Assessing, planning, implementing, evaluating.* Norwalk, CT: Appleton & Lange.

Documentation Strategies

7

> *Nursing vocabularies emerged as critical to the advancement of the profession. They were created to name nursing phenomena and to document and code clinical nursing practice. The CCC System supports the electronic capture of discrete patient care data for documenting the "**essence of care**" and measuring the relationship of nursing care to patient outcomes.* —Virginia K. Saba

● Getting Started

This chapter provides "**get started**" information about how to implement the Clinical Care Classification (CCC) System into electronic health record (EHR) and healthcare information technology (HIT) systems. Information on the CCC System includes the following: (a) information model, (b) theoretical framework following the nursing process, and (c) coding structure. This chapter also provides an overview of the design strategy for the development of a nursing plan of care (POC), with examples of three unique POCs: standardized, individualized, and interactive.

● CCC System Information Model

The CCC System framework following the nursing process and the CCC Information Model are guides to designing nursing POC documentation. The CCC System framework is a unified approach for the electronic capture and organization of nursing care data in an EHR/HIT system. The CCC information model illustrates the six steps/standards of the nursing process (American Nurses Association, 2010). The CCC information model shown in Figure 7.1 illustrates the dynamic, interrelated, and continuous feedback process performed by nurses for the documentation of a plan of care.

The model represents the interrelationship between the CCC of Nursing Diagnoses and Outcomes and the CCC of Nursing Interventions/Actions. The arrows in the information model are bidirectional, indicating a continual flow of information as well as feedback among three key nursing documentation; variables (diagnoses, interventions, and outcomes) within the six steps/standards of the nursing process. The model also illustrates how the **Assessed signs and symptoms** initiate the **Nursing Diagnoses** with their **Expected Outcomes (goals)**, which leads to the **Nursing Interventions/Action Types** required to achieve the **Actual Outcomes (disposition of the Diagnoses Outcomes)**. The model also illustrates how the evidence of the **Actual Outcomes** is based on **Nursing Interventions/Actions**.

● Nursing Process

The CCC System follows the six steps/standards of professional practice (ANA, 2010) as a theoretical framework. The nursing process steps/standards focus on patient care provided by nurses regardless of where nurses practice or their educational preparation. The nursing process operationalizes and demonstrates the art and science of nursing. The six steps, called *standards*, of the nursing process describe the competent level of nursing care, encompass all significant actions taken by nurses to provide care to patients/clients, and form the basis for clinical decision-making. The standards of practice and the standards of professional performance are addressed in *Nursing: Scope and Standards of Practice* (ANA, 2010), which identifies

FIGURE 7.1 ▩ Clinical Care Classification Information Model.

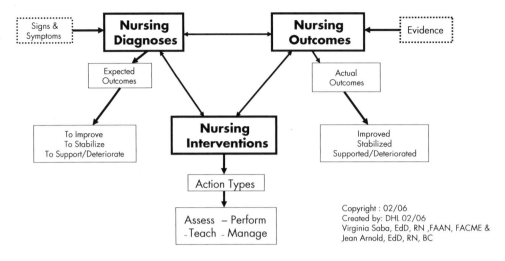

the specific professional responsibilities of nurses engaged in clinical practice. The six steps/standards of the nursing process apply to all nurses in all areas of clinical practice in all nursing environments and settings.

Nursing Process and CCC System

The CCC System framework uses the ANA nursing process as a theoretical framework for documenting nursing care. This framework makes it possible to document, link, and track the six steps/standards of the nursing process in the CCC System for an episode of care and provides a means to measure outcomes and professional clinical decision-making. Each of the six nursing process steps/standards (assessment, diagnosis, outcome identification, planning, implementation, and evaluation) correlates with the CCC System framework presented in detail below (Exhibit 7.1).

● CCC System Coding Structure

The CCC System uses a five-character alphanumeric structure to code the two nursing terminologies—CCC of Nursing Diagnoses and Outcomes and the CCC of Nursing Interventions/Actions. The CCC System coding structure is based on the format of the *Tenth Revision of the International Statistical of Diseases and Related Health Problems: Tenth Revision (ICD-10)* specifically designed for computer processing (World Health Organization, 1992).

The CCC System coding structure supports computer processing in EHR/HIT systems and provides linkages between the two CCC System terminologies and word mappings to other health-related classifications. The CCC System concepts (data/elements) are input once and used multiple times within the application. The concepts are stored in a database and retrieved to evaluate patient care. The data elements can also be aggregated and reused for research purposes. The coding strategy for each CCC System terminology consists of the following:

> First position: One alphabetic character code for Care Component (A to U)
>
> Second and third positions: Two-digit code for a core concept followed by a decimal point
>
> Fourth position: One-digit code for a subcategory, if available, followed by a decimal point
>
> Fifth position: One digit code for
>
> —one of three Expected or Actual Outcomes and/or
>
> —one of four Nursing Intervention Action Types

EXHIBIT 7.1 ▓ CCC System Framework Correlates with Six Standards of the Nursing Process

1. **Care Components—Assessment**

   CCC Care Components: The 21 Care Components provide the standardized framework for the CCC System and support the four CCC System Healthcare Patterns: Physiological, Functional, Psychological, and Health Behavioral. The Care Components provide the classification groups for the CCC System's two interrelated terminologies: (a) CCC of Nursing Diagnoses and Outcomes and (b) CCC of Nursing Interventions/Actions. The Care Components correlate with the first standard in the nursing process—**Assessment** of the patients' signs and symptoms.

2. **Nursing Diagnoses—Diagnosis**

   CCC Nursing Diagnoses: The CCC of Nursing Diagnoses, Version 2.5, consists of 176 (60 major categories and 116 subcategories) diagnostic concepts. The **Diagnosis** is a granular, atomic-level diagnostic condition based on the analysis and synthesis of the assessed signs and symptoms, Care Components, and problems that require therapeutic nursing care to alter the health status of the patient.

3. **Expected Outcome—Outcome Identification**

   CCC Expected Outcomes: The Expected Outcomes represent the goals of nursing care. The Expected Outcomes are identified by three nursing outcome qualifiers (see below) that maximize the **Outcome Identification** from the 176 Nursing Diagnoses to 528 Expected Outcomes. Each Nursing Diagnosis requires an Expected Outcome to achieve a measurable outcome resulting from the therapeutic nursing care that alters the health status of the patient. Three qualifiers are presented in the present tense:

   1. *Improve or Resolve* the patient's condition

   2. *Stabilize or Maintain* the patient's condition

   3. *Support the Deterioration* of the patient's condition

4. **Nursing Interventions—Planning**

   CCC Nursing Interventions: The CCC of Nursing Interventions, Version 2.5, consists of 201 (77 core categories and 124 subcategories) concepts. The Nursing Interventions are granular atomic-level services or core concepts used for **planning** and describing the proposed nursing Plan of Care (POC) for the patient. The POC is designed to treat each diagnostic condition or patient problem assessed that requires therapeutic nursing care.

5. **Action Types—Implementation**

   CCC Action Types: The four Action Types enhance the 201 Nursing Interventions to 804 Nursing Intervention/action concepts. Each nursing intervention in the POC requires an Action Type qualifier. The Action Type qualifier focuses on the specific action needed for the **implementation** of each of the Nursing Interventions in the POC. The Action Types provide the measures used to determine the status of the care process at any given point in time as well as identify nursing workload, resources, and the nursing cost of patient care. With the nursing interventions, the Action Types provide the evidence for clinical decision-making:

   1. *Assess/Monitor/Observe/Evaluate*: Action Type evaluating the patient's health status

   2. *Perform/Care/Provide/Assist*: Action Type performing therapeutic (hands-on) care

   3. *Teach/Educate/Instruct/Supervise*: Action Type educating patient and/or caregiver

   4. *Manage/Refer/Contact/Notify*: Action Type coordinating patient care (indirect care)

6. **Actual Outcomes—Evaluation**

   Actual Outcomes: The Actual Outcomes are identified by three Nursing Outcome qualifiers (see below) that maximize the 176 Nursing Diagnoses to 528 Actual Outcomes. Each Nursing Diagnosis requires an Actual Outcome as an **Evaluation** of the therapeutic care or Nursing Intervention/Actions. The same three qualifiers are used to

(continued)

EXHIBIT 7.1 (*Continued*)

determine whether the goals were met or not met. The Actual Outcomes qualifiers are presented in the past tense as follows:

1. *Improved or Resolved* the patient's condition

2. *Stabilized or Maintained* the patient's condition

3. *Supported the Deterioration* of the patient's condition or *died*

Source: American Nurses Association. (2010). Nursing: Scope and standards of practice. Silver Spring, MD: ANA.

The CCC System framework makes it possible to code, document, link, and track the patient care process for an episode of illness as well as support the data collection of nursing care through computer processing and statistical analyses. The CCC System can also be used to evaluate patient care holistically, over time, across all healthcare settings, for population groups, and for geographic locations.

Coding Process

The CCC System coding structure for each of the two interrelated terminologies: CCC of Nursing Diagnoses and Outcomes and CCC of Nursing Interventions/Actions, is an essential part of the CCC Framework for each concept. The CCC codes and framework are needed for the integration and computer processing of the POCs for EHR/HIT systems. The CCC codes also make it possible to measure and analyze patient care outcomes. Coding examples are presented below:

The CCC System Coding structure facilitates computer processing of the care component classes, provides the linkage between the two terminologies, as well as supports word mappings between and among other healthcare classifications. The CCC System coding structure facilitates the configuration of a POC, a clinical pathway, or other documentation format applications. The CCC System also supports the development of decision support, evidence-based systems, and/or expert clinical systems. Patient care that is not coded but recorded in narrative text or statements is almost impossible to automate, quantify, process, measure, analyze, or use to develop evidence-based, clinical nursing practice measures and protocols.

● "Essence of Care"

Identifying **what data should be coded** in an EHR/HIT is vital. Many of the preestablished POCs are adaptations of textbook descriptions of patient care, including all the possible conditions and actions to "remember." Designing or configuring a POC to capture all of the textbook conditions for patient care is impractical to use at the bedside—this becomes an electronic procedure manual and is impractical to use to code, process, retrieve, or analyze data. What is recommended is coding the "**essence of care**" provided to the patient. This means coding the POC based on the nurses'

TABLE 7.1 ■ Nursing Diagnosis and Outcome Coding Structure

Patient Sign/Symptom: *Unable to walk*	
Assessment:	*Activity Component (A)*
Nursing Diagnosis:	*Physical Mobility Impairment (A01.5)*
Expected Outcome:	***Improve** Physical Mobility Impairment (A01.5.**1**)*
Actual Outcome:	*Physical Mobility Impairment **Improved** (A01.5.**1**)*

TABLE 7.2 ■ Nursing Interventions/Actions Coding Structure

Therapeutic Action: *Teach Ambulation therapy*	
Component:	*Activity Component (A)*
Nursing Intervention:	*Ambulation Therapy (A03.1)*
Action Type:	***Teach** Ambulation Therapy (A03.1.**3**)*

identification of nursing diagnoses from the patient's assessed signs and symptoms, followed by the selection of the goals of care and the nursing intervention and actions needed to care for the patient. (See Tables 7.1 and 7.2.) This process requires documenting the actual outcomes of the care process. This strategy excludes **reminders** of what to look for, nice-to-know data, or other unrelated information. Such reminders could be placed in a procedure manual that can be retrieved on demand as an electronic resource. In other words, the "**essence of care**" is documenting and **coding the actual care** provided to the patient.

Essence of Care Example

Here is an illustration for documenting and coding the **essence of care** following the CCC System information model and CCC nursing process framework.

A patient has the following:

1. Sign/Symptom: *difficulty breathing (Respiratory Care Component: L)*
2. Nursing Diagnosis: *Respiration Alteration—**L26.0***
3. Expected Outcome: *Improve Respiration Alteration—L26.0.**1***
4. Nursing Intervention/Action Type: ***Teach** Breathing Exercises—**L36.1.3***

On discharge:

5. Actual Outcome: *Respiration Alteration **Improved**—L26.0.**1***

Evidence of the actual outcome is the *frequency of teaching* as well as the *frequency of Teaching Breathing Exercises* by healthcare provider, nursing unit, disease condition, and over a length of time. The coded information provides the structure for the analyses and evaluation of the care provided to the patient.

● Plan of Care Design Strategy

Nursing Focus

Many EHR systems are still developed without consideration of the nursing process and the requirements for accountable nursing documentation at the point of care. Plan-of-care applications are generally the optional applications in computerized provider order-entry systems, whose primary focus has been revenue-generating departments: pharmacy, radiology, and laboratory. As a result, nursing departments generally have not been involved in the selection of the EHR/HIT systems or in the design or prioritization of the nursing applications. Traditionally, the professional focus of nursing departments has been on delivering patient care without regard to data elements or documentation of outcomes. Nursing salaries are still embedded in the room rate, and determining the workload and resource requirements of the nursing staff including the cost of nursing care is still based on subjective assumptions. Furthermore, the nursing contribution to patient outcomes remains undocumented without EHR/HIT applications using coded, standardized nursing data, such as the CCC System in practice.

The paper POC is obsolete in the electronic healthcare environment. The "homegrown" POCs developed by nursing departments with local codes to capture regional best practices and requirements are also becoming obsolete. What is needed today is an electronic, standardized, coded, integrated POC available to the healthcare team for continuity of care. A POC developed by EHR/HIT vendors who emphasize the documentation of tasks (checklists for nursing care) or assessments owing to malpractice concerns does not support professional nursing practice as described by the professional nursing organizations.

In Stage I "Meaningful Use," required by the HITECH Act of 2009, there is an opportunity to require POC documentation for each patient to meet the requirements of integrated care. Today, professional nursing and allied health staffs involved in implementing EHR/HIT systems are insisting that various professional contributions be collected and coded. Nursing departments want to evaluate their clinical practice and demonstrate the value of nursing services to the broader healthcare community. Many healthcare facilities are starting to require the use of standardized, coded, integrated POC applications in EHR/HIT systems for Continuity of Care to meet emerging accountability organizations.

Design Strategy

To **get started** using the CCC System, the nursing members of the POC development team need to have sound nursing knowledge and an understanding of the principals of nursing practice. The team members also must have an understanding of the principles of data, data structures, and databases and how and why a standardized terminology is needed to code POC data. Team members should also understand how data are organized in a database, processed, retrieved, and aggregated. Also, members must understand the principles of the **system life cycle** and the impact these principles have on the configuration of an application for an EHR system. The system life cycle provides the outline for the sequence of activities needed to describe to the nurse executive of a hospital, healthcare facility, or EHR vendor, or an individual clinician, the steps required to meet the outlined objectives. The system life-cycle phases have been described in the literature for designing, implementing, or upgrading a nursing documentation system. The major phases of the life cycle focus on the planning, designing, implementing, and evaluating of the system (Douglas & Celli, 2006). The team should also be aware of some of the major pitfalls of developing POC applications. The major general concerns are listed as follows:

1. What degree of specificity and/or level of the care should be coded versus what information can be recorded as narrative text?

   Remember that specificity requires software programming which may increase resources and costs.

2. What data should be collected, stored, analyzed, and retrieved for decision-making?

   *Remember that "**nice to know**" data can be collected and not coded.*

3. Should reminders of diseases or medical conditions be integrated and coded in the POC software?

   *Remember that too many **reminders** can increase the overall cost of the application—an electronic policy and procedure manual can be easily accessed and achieve the same result.*

4. Do physician-to-nurse orders have to be integrated and coded in the nursing POC application?

   *Remember that the **physician-to-nurse orders** are generally in the order-entry dictionary of the EHR system.*

5. What sources of POC content should be selected?

   Content *can be selected from several sources, such as electronic evidence-based literature.*

In summary, the POC application proposed in this manual should be configured to document and code the "**essence of care**" provided by nurses and allied health professionals. The system life-cycle principles should serve as a guide for configuring the CCC System documentation and the POC application for an EHR/HIT system. The leader of the POC application team should be directed by a knowledgeable nurse informatics expert.

● **Plan of Care**

The electronic POC is configured using various formats and developmental strategies depending on the purpose, objective, and use, as well as the clinical content derived from many different sources. There are several POC types, and any one or all of the following types may be found in an EHR/HIT system. The POC types are described as **Standardized, Individualized,** and **Interactive**. These plans are described according to their format, structure, developmental strategy, source of content, and coding structure.

Standardized POC

The **Standardized** POC that provides predefined, traditional care information for a specific disease or medical condition. A standardized POC consists of time-sequenced nursing interventions with their respective nursing diagnoses represented as a clinical pathway or case study. The content for the Standardized POC generally focuses on the clinicians' standardized

EXHIBIT 7.2 ■ Standardized Plan of Care for Patient with Pneumonia

Signs/Symptoms	Care Component	Nursing Diagnoses	Expected Outcomes	Nursing Interventions/Actions	Actual Outcomes	Evidence
Pain when coughing or deep breathing	Sensory: Q	Acute pain: Q63.1	Improve Acute Pain: Q63.1.1	**Assess Acute Pain Control: Q47.1.1** Determine location and intensity of pain **Teach Acute Pain Control: Q47.1.3** Splint ribs with pillow when coughing **Perform Medication Treatment: H24.4.2** Give pain medication prn	**Acute Pain: Improved Q63.1.1**	No pain No pain when coughing Does not need pain medication
Shortness of breath when walking more than 20 feet	Respiratory: L	Breathing Pattern Impairment: L26.2	Stabilize Breathing Pattern Impairment: L26.2.2	**Perform Oxygen Therapy Care: L35.0.2** Administer oxygen therapy 10 Liters **Teach Breathing Exercises: L36.1.3** Instruct in pursed-lip breathing **Perform Medication Treatment: H24.4.2** Give nebulizer treatment	**Breathing Pattern Impairment Stabilized: L26.2.2**	Does not require oxygen Able to breath with lips pursed Able to use nebulizer
Has temperature (102 °F)	Physical Regulation: K	Hyperthermia: K25.2	Improve Hyperthermia (lower Temperature): K25.2.1	**Perform Injection Administration: H23.0.2** Give IM injection of antibiotics	**Hyperthermia Improved: K25.2.1**	Temperature normal

VKS: 2004/2006/2011

Note. This standardized POC is an example of an EHR/HIT clinical pathway format.

EHR = electronic health record; HIT = healthcare information technology; POC = plan of care.

approach to the care of the condition using the CCC System. In the example, the Nursing Interventions are documented as three discrete encounters for each of the Assessed Nursing Diagnoses. The objective is to demonstrate the time sequences for the clinical pathway. Once the Expected Outcome for each Nursing Diagnosis is **met**, its respective interventions are discontinued, and the pathway ends. (See Exhibit 7.2.)

EXHIBIT 7.3 ■ Individualized Plan of Care for Patient with Pneumonia

---

Case Study:

Mr. Jones, age 70, was admitted to a unit complaining of acute pain when coughing and/or deep breathing. He has shortness of breath when he walks more than 20 feet. Mr. Jones's physician diagnosed his patient as having Pneumonia and ordered Oxygen Therapy, Antibiotic Injection, Pain Medication, and Inhalant Mist.

Signs and Symptoms (Assessment)

- Acute pain on coughing
- Shortness of breath when walking more than 20 feet
- Temperature of 102 °F

Care Components/Nursing Diagnoses

- **Sensory Component: Q**

  Nursing Diagnosis: Acute Pain: **Q63.1**

- **Respiratory Component: L**

  Nursing Diagnosis: Breathing Pattern Impairment: **L26.2**

- **Physical Regulation Component: K**

  Nursing Diagnosis: Hyperthermia: **K25.2**

Expected Outcomes/Goals of Care

- Improve Acute Pain: Q63.1.**1**
- Stabilize Breathing Pattern Impairment: L26.2.**2**
- Improve Hyperthermia: K.25.2.**1**

Interventions/Action Types	Nursing Rationale
Assess: Acute Pain Control: Q47.1.**1**	Determine location and intensity of pain
Teach: Acute Pain Control: Q47.1.**3**	Instruct on how to splint ribs for coughing
Perform: Medication Treatment: H24.4.**2**	Give pain medication prn (as needed)
Perform: Oxygen Therapy Care: L35.0.**2**	Administer oxygen therapy
Teach: Breathing Exercises: L36.1.**3**	Instruct in breathing exercises
Perform: Medication Treatment: H24.4.**2**	Give nebulizer treatment
Perform: Injection Administration: H23.0.**2**	Give Intramuscular (IM) antibiotic injection

Actual Outcomes/Goals Met

- Nursing Diagnosis: Acute Pain Improved: Q63.1.**1**

  Evidence: no pain when coughing

- Nursing Diagnosis: Breathing Pattern Impairment Stabilized: L26.2.**2**

  Evidence: Able to walk more than 20 feet without shortness of breath

- Nursing Diagnosis: Hyperthermia Improved: K25.2.**1**

  Evidence: Temperature normal

Note. This individualized Plan of Care for a specific patient is an example of an adapted traditional Plan of Care.

Individualized POC

The **Individualized** POC is configured for an individual patient with a specific disease or medical condition. The nurse generally adapts the traditional POC format and integrates the POC with the medical therapeutic regimen for a specific patient. The nurse configures the Individualized POC in real time based on professional expertise and determines the nursing actions (nursing orders) to complement the medical orders for the specific patient. (See Exhibit 7.3.)

Interactive POC

The **Interactive POC** based on Nursing Diagnosis or patient condition with branching logic, including electronic menu-driven options for selection by the nurse to individualize the patient's POC. The POC options are selected and complied as a POC **data set**. The Interactive POC branching logic requires nursing knowledge of care content and how to build a data set. Once the Interactive POC is completed, the data set is dynamic, adaptable, and flexible in accepting frequent updates based on changes in the patient's condition. The Interactive POC is compiled for an episode of care and stored in an EHR data repository for future use. (See Exhibit 7.4.)

EXHIBIT 7.4 ■ Interactive Plan of Care for a Patient with Nursing Diagnosis of Breathing Pattern Impairment

Signs/ Symptoms	Care Component	Nursing Diagnoses	Expected Outcomes/ Goal	Nursing Interventions/ Actions	Actual Outcomes
Shortness of breath	Respiratory	Breathing Pattern Impairment:	Breathing Pattern Impairment:	Oxygen Therapy Care: Actions performed to support the administration of oxygen treatment	Breathing Pattern Impairment:
	L	L26.2	*Select ONE Below:	*Select ONE Below:	*Select ONE Below:
			Improve: L26.2.1 Stabilize: L26.2.2 Deteriorate: L26.2.3	Assess: L35.0.1.1 Perform: L35.0.2 Teach: L35.0.3 Manage: L35.0.4	Improve: L26.2.1 Stabilize: L26.2.2 Deteriorate: L26.2.3
				Breathing Exercises: Action performed to provide therapy for respiratory or lung extertion	
				*Select ONE below:	
				Assess: L36.1.1 Perform: L36.1.2 Teach: L36.1.3 Manage: L36.1.4	

Note. This interactive POC is an example of an EHR/HIT menu-driven options format. The POC selections are complied to form the POC data set.

EHR = electronic health record; HIT = healthcare information technology; POC = plan of care.

● **Discussion**

The three POCs type examples demonstrate different formats and strategies for the documentation of care. Each format demonstrates how the CCC System terminologies are unified and can be used to document and code patient care. Each example, regardless of format, depicts the "**essence of care**" by tracking and coding the documentation of the care process from admission to discharge.

● **References**

American Nurses Association. (2010). *Nursing: Scope and Standards of Practice.* Silver Spring, MD: ANA.

Douglas, M. L., & Celli, M. L. (2006). Implementing and upgrading clinical information systems. In V. K. Saba & K. A. McCormick (Eds.), *Essentials of nursing informatics* (4th ed., pp. 291–309). New York, NY: McGraw–Hill.

The Health Information Technology for Economic and Clinical Health Act. (2009). *American Recovery and Reinvestment Act of 2009.* PL-111-5. Washington, DC: Federal Register.

World Health Organization. (1992). *International classification of disease and health related problems: Tenth revision (ICD-10).* Geneva, Switzerland: WHO.

TERMINOLOGY TABLES 8

The Clinical Care Classification (CCC) System, Version 2.5, offers a unified information framework approach for documenting nursing care in electronic health record (EHR) and health information technology (HIT) systems. The CCC System consists of two inter-related terminologies, the CCC of Nursing Diagnoses and Outcomes and the CCC of Nursing Interventions/Actions, which are classified by 21 Care Components to form a single nursing terminology standard recognized in 1991 by the American Nurses Association (Zielstorff et al., 1995) and the Department of Health and Human Services (HHS, 2007). The two CCC terminologies use a five-character alphanumeric structure based in the Tenth Revision of the International Statistical Classification of Diseases and Related Health Problems (World Health Organization, 1992) to code the concepts in each of the two CCC System terminologies.

The two CCC Terminologies form the CCC System, a standardized framework that follows the six professional steps/standard of the nursing process (Figure 8.1; American Nurses Association, 2010). The nursing process is the framework of professional practice that makes it possible to code, document, link, and track patient care for an episode of illness as well as support data collection of nursing care through computer processing and statistical analyses. The CCC System can be used to evaluate patient care holistically, over time, across all health-care settings, for population groups, and for geographic locations (Saba, 1994, 1995; Saba & Sparks, 1998).

This chapter provides the appropriate and relevant CCC System, Version 2.5, Termi-nology Tables for use in documenting plans of care and/or nursing practice, education, and research. Each table focuses on a specific viewpoint for identifying the appropriate CCC of Nursing Diagnoses, CCC of Nursing Outcomes, CCC of Nursing Interventions/Actions (by Care Components with codes, with and without definitions), and/or other CCC System ter-minology views to guide the ready use of the CCC System.

● CCC Care Components

The 21 Care Components classify the two interrelated CCC Terminologies and serve as the second level of the CCC System's four-level structure. The Care Components are the frame-work for documenting patient care following the six steps/standards of the nursing process. The Care Components are used for computer processing in the electronic health record and can be used for the analyses of clinical nursing practice.

A Care Component represents a cluster of elements that depict the four Healthcare Patterns, Functional, Health Behavioral, Physiological, and Psychological, representing a holistic ap-proach to patient care (Saba, 1994, 1995; Saba & Sparks, 1998).

The 21 Care Components are grouped by the four Healthcare Patterns which represent the first level of specificity for the CCC System framework. Generally, when documenting an episode of care, research has determined that one Care Component and Nursing Diagnosis for each of the four Healthcare Patterns describes the patient condition being treated and requiring 8 to 10 nursing interventions with a specific medical condition. The 21 Care Components have been found to be the most clinically relevant classes, the best predictors of nursing care resource requirements, and the most appropriate framework for classifying patient care (Holzemer et al., 1997).

The Care Components represent the second level of the CCC System framework and also provides the framework for the patient's admission assessment, discharge summary, and/or referral of a patient to community health agencies and other organizations or settings in

FIGURE 8.1 ▨ Nursing Process Model and Clinical Care Classification System.
Source: American Nurses Association (2010). *Nursing: Scope and Standards of Practice* (p. 8). Silver Spring, MD: ANA.

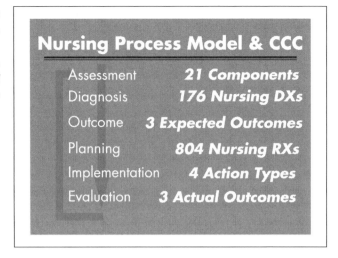

the continuum of care. By using such a framework rather than body systems, the CCC System helps focus the admission assessment on the patient's presenting condition and the reason for care. The Care Components are also used to aggregate patient care data elements to measure outcomes and determine resources and costs.

● CCC of Nursing Diagnoses

The CCC of Nursing Diagnoses, Version 2.5, consists of 176 (60 major categories and 116 subcategories) concepts that depict patient diagnoses, problems, and/or medical conditions. The CCC of Nursing Diagnoses includes unique diagnostic concepts from the original 1998 research study. The CCC System Diagnoses are compatible with the CCC Nursing Interventions and are structured as noun clauses. A diagnosis is defined by the ANA (2010) as:

> *A clinical judgement about the healthcare consumer's response to actual and potential health conditions or needs. The diagnosis provides the basis for determination of a plan to achieve expected outcomes. Registered nurses utilize nursing and medical diagnoses depending upon educational and clinical preparation and legal authority (ANA, 2010, p. 64).*

The CCC Nursing Diagnoses, which represent the third level of the CCC System framework, are used to represent the patient diagnoses, problems, and/or conditions being treated and requiring nursing care. The definition states, nursing diagnoses "**drive**" the six steps/standards of the nursing process and direct the selection of the CCC of Nursing Interventions and Action Types to accomplish the desired outcomes. The tables that are included in this chapter can be used for different purposes depending on the application being configured.

● CCC of Nursing Outcomes

The CCC of Nursing Outcomes is derived from the modification of the 176 CCC Nursing Diagnoses using the three qualifiers to depict 528 CCC Nursing Outcomes. The three qualifiers depict the **Expected Outcomes** and/or **Actual Outcomes** and represent the fourth level of the CCC System framework. The Expected Outcomes depict the **goal** of the patient care as (a) to/will **Improve**, (b) to/will **Stabilize**, or (c) to/will support **Deterioration**. These three qualifiers are written in the present and/or future tense depending on their use, whereas the **Actual Outcomes** depict whether the goals of the Nursing Diagnoses were **met** or **not met** using the same three qualifiers: (a) **Improved**, (b) **Stabilized,** or (c) **Deteriorated** and/or Died. The Actual Outcomes are used to depict Nursing Diagnoses that are resolved during the care process or on discharge. The comparison of the Expected to the Actual Outcomes provides evidence that the care was effective.

The CCC Nursing Diagnoses and Outcomes are presented in two separate tables: (a) Expected Outcomes/Goals and (b) Actual Outcomes. The outcomes are presented in these formats because the outcomes are used at different times during the care process and written in different tenses.

● CCC of Nursing Interventions/Actions

The CCC of Nursing Interventions/Actions, Version 2.5, consists of 201 (77 major categories and 124 subcategories) that depict nursing interventions, procedures, treatments, activities, and/or services provided to a patient. A Nursing Intervention is defined as follows:

A single nursing action is designed to achieve an outcome for a diagnosis (medical/nursing) for which the nurse is accountable (Saba, 2007, p.160).

Each of the CCC Nursing Interventions represents a core concept that is critical to treating the goal of a Nursing Diagnosis and also represents the third level of specificity, whereas the design of the CCC System requires that one of each of the four Action Types is required to expand the scope of the CCC of Nursing Intervention. By combining the two concepts, a new concept with a different meaning is formed that provides new data and, when added to a time factor, can be used to measure outcomes, workload, and cost. A Nursing Intervention without the Action Type is too general in scope to give the measures needed to evaluate care.

● CCC of Nursing Interventions/Actions

Each of the 804 CCC Nursing Interventions/Actions represents a core intervention with one of each of the four qualifiers, each representing a specific type of Nursing Intervention Action Type:

- **Assess or Monitor**: Collect, analyze, and monitor data on the health status
- **Perform/Care or Provide**: Perform a therapeutic action
- **Teach or Instruct**: Provide knowledge and education
- **Manage or Refer**: Coordinate care process

The four Action Types represent a fourth level of specificity and are used to modify each of the 201 core Nursing Intervention concepts. The 804 CCC Nursing Interventions/Actions depict the "essence of care." The strategy of combining the core intervention with an Action Type makes the terminology flexible, expandable, and easy to use to document, classify, retrieve, and analyze patient care.

An example of a core CCC Nursing Intervention (e.g., **Wound Care**) that has been combined with each of the four Action Types follows: (a) **Assess** Wound Care, (b) **Perform** Wound Care, (c) **Teach** Wound Care, and (d) **Manage** Wound Care. Each of the four Action Types requires different resources and different nursing skills and takes different lengths of time to perform. Another advantage of the combined concepts is that they allow for not only Action Types but also other levels of specificity to be added.

For example, if the user wants to expand "**Perform Wound Care**" to include supplies or add the different catheter sizes for "**Perform Bladder Installation**," it is possible to add and code another level of specificity. The CCC of Nursing Interventions/Actions are included and can be used for different purposes depending on the application being designed.

A comprehensive CCC System "Working Table" resource (Table 8.15) was prepared for use in selecting the appropriate CCC concepts. Table 8.15 consists of three columns: the first column lists the 21 Care Components, which can serve as an index to locate and view the Nursing Diagnoses and/or Nursing Interventions. The second and third columns present the CCC of Nursing Diagnoses side by side with the CCC of Nursing of Interventions for each of the 21 Care Components to help visualize the relationships between them.

Also presented at the top of the CCC Nursing Diagnoses column are the three Nursing Outcome qualifiers—(a) Improve(d), (b) Stabilize(d), and (c) Deteriorate(d)—to depict the Expected and/or Actual Outcomes. Additionally, at the top of the CCC of Nursing Interventions column are the four Action Types: (a) Assess, (b) Perform, (c) Teach, and (d) Manage.

● Conclusion

The CCC System, Version 2.5, Terminology Tables are presented for use either separately or in combination depending on the application being designed. The Tables offer a unified approach for documenting patient care in an electronic health record (EHR/HIT) systems and can be used to document the nursing process six steps/standards of care to each other as well as to map to other classifications and systems. The Tables serve as a resource for the configuration of any patient care documentation system/clinical application for nurses and/or allied health professionals/personnel.

● References

American Nurses Association (2010). Nursing: scope and standards of practice (p. 8). Silver Spring, MD: ANA.

Department of Health and Human Services. (2007). January 22 Letter of Secretary Michael O. Leavitt. Retrieved from http://www.hhs.gov/healthit/documents/m20070123/012207letter.html

Holzemer, W. L., Henry, S. B., Dawson, C., Sousa, K., Bain, C., & Hsieh, S. F. (1997). An evaluation of the utility of the Home Healthcare Classification for categorizing patient problems and nursing interventions from the hospital setting. In U. Gerdin, M. Tallberg, & P. Wainwright (Eds.), *NI'99: Nursing informatics: The impact of nursing knowledge on healthcare informatics* (pp. 21–26). Stockholm, Sweden: IOS Press.

Saba, V. K. (1994). Twenty nursing diagnoses home healthcare components. In R. M. Carroll–Johnson & M. Paquette (Eds.), *Classification of NURSING Diagnoses: Proceedings of the tenth conference* (p. 301). Philadelphia: J. B. Lippincott.

Saba, V. K. (1995). A new paradigm for computer-based nursing information systems: Twenty care components. In R. A. Greenes, H. E. Peterson, & D. J. Proti (Eds.), *MEDINFO'95 proceedings* (pp. 1404–1406). Edmonton, Canada: IMIA.

Saba, V. K., & Sparks, S. M. (1998). Twenty care components: An educational strategy to teach nursing science. In B. Cesnik, A. T. McCray, & J. R. Scherrer (Eds.), *Medinfo'98: Proceedings of the Ninth World Congress on Medical Informatics* (pp. 756–759). Amsterdam, Netherlands: IOS Press.

World Health Organization. (1992). *ICD-10: International statistical classification of diseases and related health problems* (10th rev., Vol. 1). Geneva, Switzerland: WHO.

Zielstorff D., Lang, N. M., Saba, V. K., McCormick, K. A., & Milholland, D. K. (1995). Toward a uniform language for nursing in the US: Work of the American Nurses Association Steering Committee on Database to Support Clinical Practice. In R. A. Greenes, H. E. Peterson, & D. J. Protti (Eds.), *MEDINFO 95 Proceedings of the 8th World Congress on Medical Informatics* (pp. 1362–1366). Amsterdam, Netherlands: North-Holland.

TABLE 8.1 ■ Clinical Care Classification System 21 Care Components, Version 2.5: Coded by Four Healthcare Patterns[1,2]

Health Behavior Components

1. Medication (H)

2. Safety (N)

3. Health Behavior (G)

Functional Components

4. Activity (A)

5. Fluid Volume (F)

6. Nutritional (J)

7. Self-Care (O)

8. Sensory (Q)

Physiological Components

9. Bowel/Gastric (B)

10. Cardiac (C)

11. Respiratory (L)

12. Metabolic (I)

13. Physical Regulation (K)

14. Skin Integrity (R)

15. Tissue Perfusion (S)

16. Urinary (T)

17. Life Cycle (U)

Psychological Components

10. Cognitive/Neuro Component (D)

11. Coping (E)

12. Role Relationship (M)

13. Self-Concept (P)

[1] Clinical Care Classification (CCC) System, Version 2.5 (previously known as: (a) Clinical Care Classification (CCC) System, Version 2.0, Copyright © 2004; and (b) Home Healthcare Classification (HHCC) System, Version 1.0, Copyright © 1994] pending Copyright © 2012 by Virginia K. Saba. EdD, RN, FAAN, FACMI, LL, may be used ONLY with written Permission by Dr. Virginia K. Saba. (Permission Form available from website <http://www.sabacare.com>)

[2] Revised 1992, 1994, 2004, 2006, and 2011.

TABLE 8.2 ▦ Clinical Care Classification System 21 Care Components, Version 2.5: Coded by Alphabetic Classes[1,2]

A	Activity Component
B	Bowel/Gastric Component
C	Cardiac Component
D	Cognitive/Neuro Component
E	Coping Component
F	Fluid Volume Component
G	Health Behavior Component
H	Medication Component
I	Metabolic Component
J	Nutritional Component
K	Physical Regulation Component
L	Respiratory Component
M	Role Relationship Component
N	Safety Component
O	Self-Care Component
P	Self-Concept Component
Q	Sensory Component
R	Skin Integrity Component
S	Tissue Perfusion Component
T	Urinary Component
U	Life Cycle Component

[1] Clinical Care Classification (CCC) System, Version 2.5 (previously known as: (a) Clinical Care Classification (CCC) System, Version 2.0, Copyright © 2004; and (b) Home Healthcare Classification (HHCC) System, Version 1.0, Copyright © 1994] pending Copyright © 2012 by Virginia K. Saba. EdD, RN, FAAN, FACMI, LL, may be used ONLY with written Permission by Dr. Virginia K. Saba. (Permission Form available from website <http://www.sabacare.com>)

[2] Revised 1992, 1994, 2004, 2006, and 2011.

TABLE 8.3 ▧ Clinical Care Classification System 21 Care Components, Version 2.5: Coded by Alphabetic Classes with Definitions[1,2]

A   Activity Component
   Cluster of elements that involve the use of energy in carrying out musculoskeletal and bodily actions

B   Bowel/Gastric Component
   Cluster of elements that involve the gastrointestinal system

C   Cardiac Component
   Cluster of elements that involve the heart and blood vessels.

D   Cognitive/Neuro Component
   Cluster of elements that involve the cognitive, mental, cerebral, and neurological processes

E   Coping Component
   Cluster of elements that involve the ability to deal with responsibilities, problems, or difficulties

F   Fluid Volume Component
   Cluster of elements that involve liquid consumption

G   Health Behavior Component
   Cluster of elements that involve actions to sustain, maintain, or regain health

H   Medication Component
   Cluster of elements that involve medicinal substances

I   Metabolic Component
   Cluster of elements that involve the endocrine and immunological processes

J   Nutritional Component
   Cluster of elements that involve the intake of food and nutrients

K   Physical Regulation Component
   Cluster of elements that involve bodily processes

L   Respiratory Component
   Cluster of elements that involve breathing and the pulmonary system

M   Role Relationship Component
   Cluster of elements involving interpersonal, work, social, family, and sexual interactions

N   Safety Component
   Cluster of elements that involve prevention of injury, danger, loss, or abuse

O   Self-Care Component
   Cluster of elements that involve the ability to carry out activities to maintain oneself

P   Self-Concept Component
   Cluster of elements that involve an individual's mental image of oneself.

Q   Sensory Component
   Cluster of elements that involve the senses, including pain

R   Skin Integrity Component
   Cluster of elements that involve the mucous membrane, corneal, integumentary, or subcutaneous structures of the body

S   Tissue Perfusion Component
   Cluster of elements that involve the oxygenation of tissues, including the circulatory and vascular systems

T   Urinary Component
   Cluster of elements that involve the genitourinary system

U   Life Cycle Component
   Cluster of elements that involve the life span of individuals

[1] Clinical Care Classification (CCC) System, Version 2.5 (previously known as: (a) Clinical Care Classification (CCC) System, Version 2.0, Copyright © 2004; and (b) Home Healthcare Classification (HHCC) System, Version 1.0, Copyright © 1994] pending Copyright © 2012 by Virginia K. Saba. EdD, RN, FAAN, FACMI, LL, may be used ONLY with written Permission by Dr. Virginia K. Saba. (Permission Form available from website <http://www.sabacare.com>)

[2] Revised 1992, 1994, 2004, 2006, and 2011.

TABLE 8.4 ◼ Clinical Care Classification of 176 Nursing Diagnoses, Version 2.5: Coded and Classified by 21 Care Components[1,2]

A. Activity Component

01.0   Activity Alteration
      01.1   Activity Intolerance
      01.2   Activity Intolerance Risk
      01.3   Diversional Activity Deficit
      01.4   Fatigue
      01.5   Physical Mobility Impairment
      01.6   Sleep Pattern Disturbance
      01.7   Sleep Deprivation
02.0   Musculoskeletal Alteration

B. Bowel/Gastric Component

03.0   Bowel Elimination Alteration
      03.1   Bowel Incontinence
      03.3   Diarrhea
      03.4   Fecal Impaction
      03.5   Perceived Constipation
      03.6   Constipation
04.0   Gastrointestinal Alteration
      04.1   Nausea
      04.2   Vomiting

C. Cardiac Component

05.0   Cardiac Output Alteration
06.0   Cardiovascular Alteration
      06.1   Blood Pressure Alteration
      06.2   Bleeding Risk

D. Cognitive/Neuro Component

07.0   Cerebral Alteration
      07.1   Confusion
08.0   Knowledge Deficit
      08.1   Knowledge Deficit of Diagnostic Test
      08.2   Knowledge Deficit of Dietary Regimen
      08.3   Knowledge Deficit of Disease Process
      08.4   Knowledge Deficit of Fluid Volume
      08.5   Knowledge Deficit of Medication Regimen
      08.6   Knowledge Deficit of Safety Precautions
      08.7   Knowledge Deficit of Therapeutic Regimen
09.0   Thought Process Alteration
      09.1   Memory Impairment

E. Coping Component

10.0   Dying Process
52.0   Community Coping Impairment
11.0   Family Coping Impairment
      11.2   Disabled Family Coping
12.0   Individual Coping Impairment
      12.1   Adjustment Impairment
      12.2   Decisional Conflict
      12.3   Defensive Coping
      12.4   Denial
13.0   Posttrauma Response
      13.1   Rape Trauma Syndrome

TABLE 8.4 ▦ (*Continued*)

14.0 Spiritual State Alteration
    14.1 Spiritual Distress
53.0 Grieving
    53.1 Anticipatory Grieving
    53.2 Dysfunctional Grieving

F. Fluid Volume Component

15.0 Fluid Volume Alteration
    15.1 Fluid Volume Deficit
    15.2 Fluid Volume Deficit Risk
    15.3 Fluid Volume Excess
    15.4 Fluid Volume Excess Risk
62.0 Electrolyte Imbalance

G. Health Behavior Component

17.0 Health Maintenance Alteration
    17.1 Failure to Thrive
18.0 Health-Seeking Behavior Alteration
19.0 Home Maintenance Alteration
20.0 Noncompliance
    20.1 Noncompliance of Diagnostic Test
    20.2 Noncompliance of Dietary Regimen
    20.3 Noncompliance of Fluid Volume
    20.4 Noncompliance of Medication Regimen
    20.5 Noncompliance of Safety Precautions
    20.6 Noncompliance of Therapeutic Regimen

H. Medication Component

21.0 Medication Risk
    21.1 Polypharmacy

I. Metabolic Component

22.0 Endocrine Alteration
23.0 Immunologic Alteration

J. Nutritional Component

24.0 Nutrition Alteration
    24.1 Body Nutrition Deficit
    24.2 Body Nutrition Deficit Risk
    24.3 Body Nutrition Excess
    24.4 Body Nutrition Excess Risk
    24.5 Swallowing Impairment
54.0 Infant Feeding Pattern Impairment
55.0 Breastfeeding Impairment

K. Physical Regulation Component

25.0 Physical Regulation Alteration
    25.1 Autonomic Dysreflexia
    25.2 Hyperthermia
    25.3 Hypothermia
    25.4 Thermoregulation Impairment
    25.5 Infection Risk
    25.6 Infection
    25.7 Intracranial Adaptive Capacity Impairment

(*Continued*)

TABLE 8.4 ■ Clinical Care Classification of 176 Nursing Diagnoses, Version 2.5: Coded and Classified by 21 Care Components[1,2] (*Continued*)

L. Respiratory Component

26.0   Respiration Alteration
    26.1   Airway Clearance Impairment
    26.2   Breathing Pattern Impairment
    26.3   Gas Exchange Impairment
56.0   Ventilatory Weaning Impairment

M. Role Relationship Component

27.0   Role Performance Alteration
    27.1   Parental Role Conflict
    27.2   Parenting Alteration
    27.3   Sexual Dysfunction
    27.4   Caregiver Role Strain
28.0   Communication Impairment
    28.1   Verbal Impairment
29.0   Family Process Alteration
31.0   Sexuality Pattern Alteration
32.0   Socialization Alteration
    32.1   Social Interaction Alteration
    32.2   Social Isolation
    32.3   Relocation Stress Syndrome

N. Safety Component

33.0   Injury Risk
    33.1   Aspiration Risk
    33.2   Disuse Syndrome
    33.3   Poisoning Risk
    33.4   Suffocation Risk
    33.5   Trauma Risk
    33.6   Fall Risk
34.0   Violence Risk
    34.1   Suicide Risk
    34.2   Self-Mutilation Risk
57.0   Perioperative Injury Risk
    57.1   Perioperative Positioning Injury
    57.2   Surgical Recovery Delay
58.0   Substance Abuse
    58.1   Tobacco Abuse
    58.2   Alcohol Abuse
    58.3   Drug Abuse

O. Self-Care Component

35.0   Bathing/Hygiene Deficit
36.0   Dressing/Grooming Deficit
37.0   Feeding Deficit
38.0   Self-Care Deficit
    38.1   Activities of Daily Living Alteration
    38.2   Instrumental Activities of Daily Living Alteration
39.0   Toileting Deficit

P. Self-Concept Component

40.0   Anxiety
41.0   Fear
42.0   Meaningfulness Alteration
    42.1   Hopelessness
    42.2   Powerlessness

TABLE 8.4 ▨ (*Continued*)

43.0	Self-Concept Alteration	
	43.1	Body Image Disturbance
	43.2	Personal Identity Disturbance
	43.3	Chronic Low Self-Esteem Disturbance
	43.4	Situational Self-Esteem Disturbance

Q. Sensory Component

44.0	Sensory Perceptual Alteration	
	44.1	Auditory Alteration
	44.2	Gustatory Alteration
	44.3	Kinesthetic Alteration
	44.4	Olfactory Alteration
	44.5	Tactile Alteration
	44.6	Unilateral Neglect
	44.7	Visual Alteration
45.0	Comfort Alteration	
63.0	Pain	
	63.1	Acute Pain
	63.2	Chronic Pain

R. Skin Integrity Component

46.0	Skin Integrity Alteration	
	46.1	Oral Mucous Membrane Impairment
	46.2	Skin Integrity Impairment
	46.3	Skin Integrity Impairment Risk
	46.4	Skin Incision
	46.5	Latex Allergy Response
47.0	Peripheral Alteration	

S. Tissue Perfusion Component

48.0	Tissue Perfusion Alteration	

T. Urinary Elimination Component

49.0	Urinary Elimination Alteration	
	49.1	Functional Urinary Incontinence
	49.2	Reflex Urinary Incontinence
	49.3	Stress Urinary Incontinence
	49.5	Urge Urinary Incontinence
	49.6	Urinary Retention
50.0	Renal Alteration	

U. Life Cycle Component

59.0	Reproductive Risk	
	59.1	Fertility Risk
	59.2	Infertility Risk
	59.3	Contraception Risk
60.0	Perinatal Risk	
	60.1	Pregnancy Risk
	60.2	Labor Risk
	60.3	Delivery Risk
	60.4	Postpartum Risk
61.0	Growth and Development Alteration	

[1] Clinical Care Classification (CCC) System, Version 2.5 (previously known as: (a) Clinical Care Classification (CCC) System, Version 2.0, Copyright © 2004; and (b) Home Healthcare Classification (HHCC) System, Version 1.0, Copyright © 1994] pending Copyright © 2012 by Virginia K. Saba. EdD, RN, FAAN, FACMI, LL, may be used ONLY with written Permission by Dr. Virginia K. Saba. (Permission Form available from website <http://www.sabacare.com>)

[2] Revised 1992, 1994, 2004, 2006, and 2011.

TABLE 8.5 ■ Clinical Care Classification of 176 Nursing Diagnoses, Version 2.5: Coded with Definitions and Classified by 21 Care Components[1,2]

A. Activity Component

Cluster of elements that involve the use of energy in carrying out musculoskeletal and bodily actions
Activity Alteration—A01.0
Change in or modification of energy used by the body
    Activity Intolerance—A01.1
    Incapacity to carry out physiological or psychological daily activities
    Activity Intolerance Risk—A01.2
    Increased chance of an incapacity to carry out physiological or psychological daily activities
    Diversional Activity Deficit—A01.3
    Lack of interest or engagement in leisure activities
    Fatigue—A01.4
    Exhaustion that interferes with physical and mental activities
    Physical Mobility Impairment—A01.5
    Diminished ability to perform independent movement
    Sleep Pattern Disturbance—A01.6
    Imbalance in the normal sleep/wake cycle
    Sleep Deprivation—A01.7
    Lack of a normal sleep/wake cycle
Musculoskeletal Alteration—A02.0
Change in or modification of the muscles, bones, or support structures

B. Bowel/Gastric Component

Cluster of elements that involve the gastrointestinal system
Bowel Elimination Alteration—B03.0
Change in or modification of the gastrointestinal system
    Bowel Incontinence—B03.1
    Involuntary defecation
    Diarrhea—B03.3
    Abnormal frequency and fluidity of feces
    Fecal Impaction—B03.4
    Feces wedged in intestines
    Perceived Constipation—B03.5
    Impression of infrequent or difficult passage of hard, dry feces without cause
    Constipation—B03.6
    Difficult passage of hard, dry feces
Gastrointestinal Alteration—B04.0
Change in or modification of the stomach or intestines
    Nausea—B04.1
    Distaste for food/fluids and an urge to vomit
    Vomiting—B04.2
    Expulsion of stomach contents through the mouth

C. Cardiac Component

Cluster of elements that involve the heart and blood vessels
Cardiac Output Alteration—C05.0
Change in or modification of the pumping action of the heart
Cardiovascular Alteration—C06.0
Change in or modification of the heart or blood vessels
    Blood Pressure Alteration—C06.1
    Change in or modification of the systolic or diastolic pressure
    Bleeding Risk—C06.2
    Increased chance of loss of blood volume

TABLE 8.5 ▓ (*Continued*)

D. Cognitive/Neuro Component

Cluster of elements that involve the cognitive, mental, cerebral, and neurological processes
Cerebral Alteration—D07.0
Change in or modification of mental processes
    Confusion—D07.1
    State of being disoriented (mixed up)
Knowledge Deficit—D08.0
Lack of information, understanding, or comprehension
    Knowledge Deficit of Diagnostic Test—D08.1
    Lack of information on test(s) to identify disease or assess health condition
    Knowledge Deficit Dietary Regimen—D08.2
    Lack of information on the prescribed diet/ food intake
    Knowledge Deficit of Disease Process—D08.3
    Lack of information on the morbidity, course, or treatment of the health condition
    Knowledge Deficit of Fluid Volume—D08.4
    Lack of information on fluid volume intake requirements
    Knowledge Deficit of Medication Regimen—D08.5
    Lack of information on prescribed regulated course of medicinal substances
    Knowledge Deficit of Safety Precautions—D08.6
    Lack of information on measures to prevent injury, danger, or loss
    Knowledge Deficit of Therapeutic Regimen—D08.7
    Lack of information on regulated course of treating disease
Thought Process Alteration—D09.0
Change in or modification of thought and cognitive processes
    Memory Impairment—D09.1
    Diminished ability or inability to recall past events

E. Coping Component

Cluster of elements that involve the ability to deal with responsibilities, problems, or difficulties
Dying Process—E10.0
Physical and behavioral responses associated with death
Community Coping Impairment—E52.0
Inadequate community response to problems or difficulties
Family Coping Impairment—E11.0
Inadequate family response to problems or difficulties
    Disabled Family Coping—E11.2
    Inability of family to function optimally
Individual Coping Impairment—E12.0
Inadequate personal response to problems or difficulties
    Adjustment Impairment—E12.1
    Inadequate adjustment to condition or change in health status
    Decisional Conflict—E12.2
    Struggle related to determining a course of action
    Defensive Coping—E12.3
    Self-protective strategies to guard against threats to self
    Denial—E12.4
    Attempt to reduce anxiety by refusal to accept thoughts, feelings, or facts
Posttrauma Response—E13.0
Sustained behavior related to a traumatic event
    Rape Trauma Syndrome—E13.1
    Group of symptoms related to a forced sexual act
Spiritual State Alteration—E14.0
Change in or modification of the spirit or soul
    Spiritual Distress—E14.1
    Anguish related to the spirit or soul

(Continued)

TABLE 8.5 ■ Clinical Care Classification of 176 Nursing Diagnoses, Version 2.5: Coded with Definitions and Classified by 21 Care Components[1,2] (*Continued*)

Grieving—E53.0
Feeling of great sorrow
    Anticipatory Grieving—E53.1
    Feeling great sorrow before the event or loss
    Dysfunctional Grieving—E53.2
    Prolonged feeling of great sorrow

F. Fluid Volume Component

Cluster of elements that involve liquid consumption
Fluid Volume Alteration—F15.0
Change in or modification of bodily fluid
    Fluid Volume Deficit—F15.1
    Dehydration or fluid loss
    Fluid Volume Deficit Risk—F15.2
    Increased chance of dehydration or fluid loss
    Fluid Volume Excess—F15.3
    Fluid retention, overload, or edema
    Fluid Volume Excess Risk—F15.4
    Increased chance of fluid retention, overload, or edema
Electrolyte Imbalance—F62.0
Higher or lower body electrolyte levels

G. Health Behavior Component

Cluster of elements that involve actions to sustain, maintain, or regain health
Health Maintenance Alteration—G17.0
Change in or modification of ability to manage health-related needs
    Failure to Thrive—G17.1
    Inability to grow and develop normally
Health-Seeking Behavior Alteration—G18.0
Change in or modification of actions needed to improve health state
Home Maintenance Alteration—G19.0
Inability to sustain a safe, healthy environment
Noncompliance—G20.0
Failure to follow therapeutic recommendations
    Noncompliance of Diagnostic Test—G20.1
    Failure to follow therapeutic recommendations on tests to identify disease or assess health condition
    Noncompliance of Dietary Regimen—G20.2
    Failure to follow the prescribed diet/food intake
    Noncompliance of Fluid Volume—G20.3
    Failure to follow fluid volume intake requirements
    Noncompliance of Medication Regimen—G20.4
    Failure to follow prescribed regulated course of medicinal substances
    Noncompliance of Safety Precautions—G20.5
    Failure to follow measures to prevent injury, danger, or loss
    Noncompliance of Therapeutic Regimen—G20.6
    Failure to follow regulated course of treating disease or health condition

H. Medication Component

Cluster of elements that involve medicinal substances
Medication Risk—H21.0
Increased chance of negative response to medicinal substances
    Polypharmacy—H21.1
    Use of two or more drugs together

TABLE 8.5 ■ (*Continued*)

I.   Metabolic Component

Cluster of elements that involve the endocrine and immunologic processes
Endocrine Alteration—I22.0
Change in or modification of internal secretions or hormones
Immunologic Alteration—I23.0
Change in or modification of the immune systems

J.   Nutritional Component

Cluster of elements that involve the intake of food and nutrients
Nutrition Alteration—J24.0
Change in or modification of food and nutrients
   Body Nutrition Deficit—J24.1
   Less than adequate intake or absorption of food or nutrients
   Body Nutrition Deficit Risk—J24.2
   Increased chance of less than adequate intake or absorption of food or nutrients
   Body Nutrition Excess—J24.3
   More than adequate intake or absorption of food or nutrients
   Body Nutrition Excess Risk—J24.4
   Increased chance of more than adequate intake or absorption of food or nutrients
   Swallowing Impairment—J24.5
   Inability to move food from mouth to stomach
Infant Feeding Pattern Impairment—J54.0
Imbalance in the normal feeding habits of an infant
Breastfeeding Impairment—J55.0
Diminished ability to nourish infant at the breast

K.   Physical Regulation Component

Cluster of elements that involve bodily processes
Physical Regulation Alteration—K25.0
Change in or modification of somatic control
   Autonomic Dysreflexia—K25.1
   Life-threatening inhibited sympathetic response to noxious stimuli in a person with a spinal cord injury at or above T7
   Hyperthermia—K25.2
   Abnormally high body temperature
   Hypothermia—K25.3
   Abnormally low body temperature
   Thermoregulation Impairment—K25.4
   Fluctuation of temperature between hypothermia and hyperthermia
   Infection Risk—K25.5
   Increased chance of contamination with disease-producing germs
   Infection—K25.6
   Contamination with disease-producing germs
   Intracranial Adaptive Capacity Impairment—K25.7
   Intracranial fluid volumes are compromised

L.   Respiratory Component

Cluster of elements that involve breathing and the pulmonary system
Respiration Alteration—L26.0
Change in or modification of the breathing function
   Airway Clearance Impairment—L26.1
   Inability to clear secretions/obstructions in airway
   Breathing Pattern Impairment—L26.2
   Inadequate inhalation or exhalation

(Continued)

TABLE 8.5 ■ Clinical Care Classification of 176 Nursing Diagnoses, Version 2.5: Coded with Definitions and Classified by 21 Care Components[1,2] (*Continued*)

Gas Exchange Impairment—L26.3
Imbalance of oxygen and carbon dioxide transfer between lung and vascular system
Ventilatory Weaning Impairment—L56.0
Inability to tolerate decreased levels of ventilator support

M. Role Relationship Component

Cluster of elements involving interpersonal work, social, family, and sexual interactions
Role Performance Alteration—M27.0
Change in or modification of carrying out responsibilities
    Parental Role Conflict—M27.1
    Struggle with parental position and responsibilities
    Parenting Alteration—M27.2
    Change in or modification of nurturing figure's ability to promote growth
    Sexual Dysfunction—M27.3
    Deleterious change in sexual response
    Caregiver Role Strain—M27.4
    Excessive tension of one who gives physical or emotional care and support to another person or patient
Communication Impairment—M28.0
Diminished ability to exchange thoughts, opinions, or information
    Verbal Impairment—M28.1
    Diminished ability to exchange thoughts, opinions, or information through speech
Family Process Alteration—M29.0
Change in or modification of usual functioning of a related group
Sexuality Pattern Alteration—M31.0
Change in or modification of a person's sexual response
Socialization Alteration—M32.0
Change in or modification of personal identity
    Social Interaction Alteration—M32.1
    Change in or modification of inadequate quantity or quality of personal relations
    Social Isolation—M32.2
    State of aloneness; lack of interaction with others
    Relocation Stress Syndrome—M32.3
    Excessive tension from moving to a new location

N. Safety Component

Cluster of elements that involve prevention of injury, danger, loss, or abuse
Injury Risk—N33.0
Increased chance of danger or loss
    Aspiration Risk—N33.1
    Increased chance of material into trachea–bronchial passages
    Disuse Syndrome—N33.2
    Group of symptoms related to effects of immobility
    Poisoning Risk—N33.3
    Exposure to or ingestion of dangerous products
    Suffocation Risk—N33.4
    Increased chance of inadequate air for breathing
    Trauma Risk—N33.5
    Increased chance of accidental tissue processes
    Fall Risk—N33.6
    Increased chance of conditions that result in falls
Violence Risk—N34.0
Increased chance of harming self or others
    Suicide Risk—N34.1
    Increased chance of taking one's life intentionally

TABLE 8.5 ■ (*Continued*)

Self-Mutilation Risk—N34.2
Increased chance of destroying a limb or essential part of the body
Perioperative Injury Risk—N57.0
Increased chance of injury during the operative processes
    Perioperative Positioning Injury—N57.1
    Damages from operative process positioning
    Surgical Recovery Delay—N57.2
    Slow or delayed recovery from a surgical procedure
Substance Abuse—N58.0
Excessive use of harmful bodily materials
    Tobacco Abuse—N58.1
    Excessive use of tobacco products
    Alcohol Abuse—N58.2
    Excessive use of distilled liquors
    Drug Abuse—N58.3
    Excessive use of habit-forming medications

O. Self-Care Component

Cluster of elements that involve the ability to carry out activities to maintain oneself
Bathing/Hygiene Deficit—O35.0
Impaired ability to cleanse oneself
Dressing/Grooming Deficit—O36.0
Inability to clothe and groom oneself
Feeding Deficit—O37.0
Impaired ability to feed oneself
Self-Care Deficit—O38.0
Impaired ability to maintain oneself
    Activities of Daily Living Alteration—O38.1
    Change in or modification of ability to maintain oneself
    Instrumental Activities of Daily Living Alteration—O38.2
    Change in or modification of more complex activities than those needed to maintain oneself
Toileting Deficit—O39.0
Impaired ability to urinate or defecate for oneself

P. Self-Concept Component

Cluster of elements that involve an individual mental image of oneself
Anxiety—P40.0
Feeling of distress or apprehension whose source is unknown
Fear—P41.0
Feeling of dread or distress whose cause can be identified
Meaningfulness Alteration—P42.0
Change in or modification of the ability to see the significance, purpose, or value in something
    Hopelessness—P42.1
    Feeling of despair or futility and passive involvement
    Powerlessness—P42.2
    Feeling of helplessness or inability to act
Self-Concept Alteration—P43.0
Change in or modification of ability to maintain one's image of self
    Body Image Disturbance—P43.1
    Imbalance in the perception of the way one's body looks
    Personal Identity Disturbance—P43.2
    Imbalance in the ability to distinguish between the self and the nonself
    Chronic Low Self-Esteem Disturbance—P43.3
    Persistent negative evaluation of oneself
    Situational Self-Esteem Disturbance—P43.4
    Negative evaluation of oneself in response to a loss or change

(*Continued*)

TABLE 8.5 ■ Clinical Care Classification of 176 Nursing Diagnoses, Version 2.5: Coded with Definitions and Classified by 21 Care Components[1,2] (*Continued*)

Q.   Sensory Component

Cluster of elements that involve the senses, including pain
Sensory Perceptual Alteration—Q44.0
Change in or modification of the response to stimuli
    Auditory Alteration—Q44.1
    Change in or modification of diminished ability to hear
    Gustatory Alteration—Q44.2
    Change in or modification of diminished ability to taste
    Kinesthetic Alteration—Q44.3
    Change in or modification of diminished balance
    Olfactory Alteration—Q44.4
    Change in or modification of diminished ability to smell
    Tactile Alteration—Q44.5
    Change in or modification of diminished ability to feel
    Unilateral Neglect—Q44.6
    Lack of awareness of one side of the body
    Visual Alteration—Q44.7
    Change in or modification of diminished ability to see
Comfort Alteration—Q45.0
Change in or modification of sensation that is distressing
Pain—Q63.0
Physical suffering or distress; to hurt
    Acute Pain—Q63.1
    Severe pain of limited duration
    Chronic Pain—Q63.2
    Pain that persists over time

R.   Skin Integrity Component

Cluster of elements that involve the mucous membrane, corneal, integumentary, or subcutaneous structures of the body
Skin Integrity Alteration—R46.0
Change in or modification of skin conditions
    Oral Mucous Membrane Impairment—R46.1
    Diminished ability to maintain the tissues of the oral cavity
    Skin Integrity Impairment—R46.2
    Decreased ability to maintain the integument
    Skin Integrity Impairment Risk—R46.3
    Increased chance of skin breakdown
    Skin Incision—R46.4
    Cutting of the integument/skin
    Latex Allergy Response—R46.5
    Pathological reaction to latex products
Peripheral Alteration—R47.0
Change in or modification of neurovascularization of the extremities

S.   Tissue Perfusion Component

Cluster of elements that involve the oxygenation of tissues, including the circulatory and vascular systems
Tissue Perfusion Alteration—S48.0
Change in or modification of the oxygenation of tissues

TABLE 8.5 ▦ (*Continued*)

T.   Urinary Elimination Component

Cluster of elements that involve the genitourinary systems
Urinary Elimination Alteration—T49.0
Change in or modification of excretion of the waste matter of the kidneys
 Functional Urinary Incontinence—T49.1
 Involuntary, unpredictable passage of urine
 Reflex Urinary Incontinence—T49.2
 Involuntary passage of urine occurring at predictable intervals
 Stress Urinary Incontinence—T49.3
 Loss of urine occurring with increased abdominal pressure
 Urge Urinary Incontinence—T49.5
 Involuntary passage of urine following a sense of urgency to void
 Urinary Retention—T49.6
 Incomplete emptying of the bladder
Renal Alteration—T50.0
Change in or modification of kidney function

U.   Life Cycle Component

Cluster of elements that involve the life span of individuals
Reproductive Risk—U59.0
Increased chance of harm in the process of replicating or giving rise to an offspring/child
 Fertility Risk—U59.1
 Increased chance of conception to develop an offspring/child
 Infertility Risk—U59.2
 Decreased chance of conception to develop an offspring/child
 Contraception Risk—U59.3
 Increased chance of harm preventing the conception of an offspring/child
Perinatal Risk—U60.0
Increased chance of harm before, during, and immediately after the creation of an offspring/child
 Pregnancy Risk—U60.1
 Increased chance of harm during the gestational period of the formation of an offspring/child
 Labor Risk—U60.2
 Increased chance of harm during the period supporting the bringing forth of an offspring/child
 Delivery Risk—U60.3
 Increased chance of harm during the period supporting the expulsion of an offspring/child
 Postpartum Risk—U60.4
 Increased chance of harm during the period immediately following the delivery of an offspring/child
Growth and Development Alteration—U61.0
Change in or modification of age-specific normal growth standards and/or developmental skills

---

[1] Clinical Care Classification (CCC) System, Version 2.5 (previously known as: (a) Clinical Care Classification (CCC) System, Version 2.0, Copyright © 2004; and (b) Home Healthcare Classification (HHCC) System, Version 1.0, Copyright © 1994] pending Copyright © 2012 by Virginia K. Saba. EdD, RN, FAAN, FACMI, LL, may be used ONLY with written Permission by Dr. Virginia K. Saba. (Permission Form available from website <http://www.sabacare.com>)

[2] Revised 1992, 1994, 2004, 2006, and 2011.

TABLE 8.6 ■ Clinical Care Classification of 176 Nursing Diagnoses, Version 2.5: Coded Alphabetically with Definitions[1,2]

A01.0	**Activity Alteration**
	Change in or modification of energy used by the body
A01.1	**Activity Intolerance**
	Incapacity to carry out physiological or psychological daily activities
A01.2	**Activity Intolerance Risk**
	Increased chance of an incapacity to carry out physiological or psychological daily activities
O38.1	**Activities of Daily Living Alteration**
	Change in modification of ability to maintain oneself
Q63.1	**Acute Pain**
	Severe pain of limited duration
E12.1	**Adjustment Impairment**
	Inadequate adaptation to condition or change in health status
L26.1	**Airway Clearance Impairment**
	Inability to clear secretions/obstructions in airway
N58.2	**Alcohol Abuse**
	Excessive use of distilled liquors
E53.1	**Anticipatory Grieving**
	Feeling great sorrow before the event or loss
P40.0	**Anxiety**
	Feeling of distress or apprehension whose source is unknown
N33.1	**Aspiration Risk**
	Increased chance of material into trachea–bronchial passages
Q44.1	**Auditory Alteration**
	Change in or modification of diminished ability to hear
K25.1	**Autonomic Dysreflexia**
	Life-threatening inhibited sympathetic response to noxious stimuli in a person with a spinal cord injury at or above T7
O35.0	**Bathing/Hygiene Deficit**
	Impaired ability to cleanse oneself
C06.2	**Bleeding Risk**
	Increased chance of loss of blood volume
C06.1	**Blood Pressure Alteration**
	Change in or modification of the systolic or diastolic pressure
P43.1	**Body Image Disturbance**
	Imbalance in the perception of the way one's body looks
J24.1	**Body Nutrition Deficit**
	Less than adequate intake or absorption of food or nutrients
J24.2	**Body Nutrition Deficit Risk**
	Increased chance of less than adequate intake or absorption of food or nutrients
J24.3	**Body Nutrition Excess**
	More than adequate intake or absorption of food or nutrients
J24.4	**Body Nutrition Excess Risk**
	Increased chance of more than adequate intake or absorption of food or nutrients
B03.0	**Bowel Elimination Alteration**
	Change in or modification of the gastrointestinal system

TABLE 8.6 ▮ (*Continued*)

B03.1   **Bowel Incontinence**
Involuntary defecation

J55.0   **Breastfeeding Impairment**
Diminished ability to nourish infant at the breast

L26.2   **Breathing Pattern Impairment**
Inadequate inhalation or exhalation

C05.0   **Cardiac Output Alteration**
Change in or modification of the pumping action of the heart

C06.0   **Cardiovascular Alteration**
Change in or modification of the heart or blood vessels

M27.4   **Caregiver Role Strain**
Excessive tension of one who gives physical or emotional care and support to another person or patient

D07.0   **Cerebral Alteration**
Change in or modification of mental processes

P43.3   **Chronic Low Self-Esteem Disturbance**
Persistent negative evaluation of oneself

Q63.2   **Chronic Pain**
Pain that persists over time

Q45.0   **Comfort Alteration**
Change in or modification of sensation that is distressing

M28.0   **Communication Impairment**
Diminished ability to exchange thoughts, opinions, or information

E52.0   **Community Coping Impairment**
Inadequate community response to problems or difficulties

D07.1   **Confusion**
State of being disoriented (mixed up)

B03.6   **Constipation**
Difficult passage of hard, dry feces

U59.3   **Contraception Risk**
Increased chance of harm by preventing the conception of an offspring/child

E12.2   **Decisional Conflict**
Struggle related to determining a course of action

E12.3   **Defensive Coping**
Self-protective strategies to guard against threats to self

U60.3   **Delivery Risk**
Increased chance of harm during the period supporting the expulsion of an offspring/child at birth.

E12.4   **Denial**
Attempt to reduce anxiety by refusal to accept thoughts, feelings, or facts

B03.3   **Diarrhea**
Abnormal frequency and fluidity of feces

E11.2   **Disabled Family Coping**
Inability of family to function optimally

N33.2   **Disuse Syndrome**
Group of symptoms related to effects of immobility

(Continued)

TABLE 8.6 ■ Clinical Care Classification of 176 Nursing Diagnoses, Version 2.5: Coded Alphabetically with Definitions[1,2] (*Continued*)

A01.3	**Diversional Activity Deficit**	Lack of interest or engagement in leisure activities
O36.0	**Dressing/Grooming Deficit**	Impaired ability to clothe and groom oneself
N58.3	**Drug Abuse**	Excessive use of habit-forming medications
E10.0	**Dying Process**	Physical and behavioral responses associated with death
E53.2	**Dysfunctional Grieving**	Prolonged feeling of great sorrow
F62.0	**Electrolyte Imbalance**	Higher or lower body electrolyte levels
I22.0	**Endocrine Alteration**	Change in or modification of internal secretions or hormones
G17.1	**Failure to Thrive**	Inability to grow and develop normally
N33.6	**Fall Risk**	Increased chance of conditions that result in falls
E11.0	**Family Coping Impairment**	Inadequate family response to problems or difficulties
M29.0	**Family Processes Alteration**	Change in or modification of usual functioning of a related group
A01.4	**Fatigue**	Exhaustion that interferes with physical and mental activities
P41.0	**Fear**	Feeling of dread or distress whose cause can be identified
B03.4	**Fecal Impaction**	Feces wedged in intestine
O37.0	**Feeding Deficit**	Impaired ability to feed oneself
U59.1	**Fertility Risk**	Increased chance of conception to develop an offspring/child
F15.0	**Fluid Volume Alteration**	Change in or modification of bodily fluid
F15.1	**Fluid Volume Deficit**	Dehydration or fluid loss
F15.2	**Fluid Volume Deficit Risk**	Increased chance of dehydration or fluid loss
F15.3	**Fluid Volume Excess**	Fluid retention, overload, or edema
F15.4	**Fluid Volume Excess Risk**	Increased chance of fluid retention, overload, or edema
T49.1	**Functional Urinary Incontinence**	Involuntary, unpredictable passage of urine
L26.3	**Gas Exchange Impairment**	Imbalance of oxygen and carbon dioxide transfer between lung and vascular system

TABLE 8.6 ▨ (*Continued*)

B04.0	**Gastrointestinal Alteration**
	Change in or modification of the stomach or intestines
E53.0	**Grieving**
	Feeling of great sorrow
U61.0	**Growth and Development Alteration**
	Change in or modification of age-specific normal growth standards and/or developmental skills
Q44.2	**Gustatory Alteration**
	Change in or modification of diminished ability to taste
G17.0	**Health Maintenance Alteration**
	Change in or modification of ability to manage health-related needs.
G18.0	**Health-Seeking Behavior Alteration**
	Change in or modification of actions needed to improve health state
G19.0	**Home Maintenance Alteration**
	Inability to sustain a safe, healthy environment
P42.1	**Hopelessness**
	Feeling of despair or futility and passive abandonment
K25.2	**Hyperthermia**
	Abnormally high body temperature
K25.3	**Hypothermia**
	Abnormally low body temperature
I23.0	**Immunologic Alteration**
	Change in or modification of the immune system
E12.0	**Individual Coping Impairment**
	Inadequate personal response to problems or difficulties
J54.0	**Infant Feeding Pattern Impairment**
	Imbalance in the normal feeding habits of an infant
K25.5	**Infection Risk**
	Increased change of contamination with disease-producing germs
K25.6	**Infection**
	Contamination with disease-producing germs
U59.2	**Infertility Risk**
	Decreased chance of conception to develop an offspring/child
N33.0	**Injury Risk**
	Increased chance of danger or loss
O38.2	**Instrumental Activities of Daily Living Alteration**
	Change in or modification of more complex activities than those needed to maintain oneself
K25.7	**Intracranial Adaptive Capacity Impairment**
	Intracranial fluid volumes are compromised
Q44.3	**Kinesthetic Alteration**
	Change in or modification of diminished balance
D08.0	**Knowledge Deficit**
	Lack of information, understanding, or comprehension
D08.1	**Knowledge Deficit of Diagnostic Test**
	Lack of information on tests to identify disease or assess health condition

(*Continued*)

TABLE 8.6 ■ Clinical Care Classification of 176 Nursing Diagnoses, Version 2.5: Coded Alphabetically with Definitions[1,2] (*Continued*)

D08.2	**Knowledge Deficit of Dietary Regimen**
	Lack of information on the prescribed diet/food intake
D08.3	**Knowledge Deficit of Disease Process**
	Lack of information on the morbidity, course, or treatment of the health condition
D08.4	**Knowledge Deficit of Fluid Volume**
	Lack of information on fluid volume intake requirements
D08.5	**Knowledge Deficit of Medication Regimen**
	Lack of information on prescribed regulated course of medicinal substances
D08.6	**Knowledge Deficit of Safety Precautions**
	Lack of information on measures to prevent injury, danger, or loss
D08.7	**Knowledge Deficit of Therapeutic Regimen**
	Lack of information on regulated course of treating disease
U60.2	**Labor Risk**
	Increased chance of harm during the period supporting the bringing forth of an offspring/child
R46.5	**Latex Allergy Response**
	Pathological reaction to latex products
P42.0	**Meaningfulness Alteration**
	Change in or modification of the ability to see the significance, purpose, or value in something
H21.0	**Medication Risk**
	Increased chance of negative response to medicinal substance
D09.1	**Memory Impairment**
	Diminished or inability to recall past events
A02.0	**Musculoskeletal Alteration**
	Change in or modification of the muscles, bones, or support structures
B04.1	**Nausea**
	Distaste for food/fluids and an urge to vomit
G20.0	**Noncompliance**
	Failure to follow therapeutic recommendations
G20.1	**Noncompliance of Diagnostic Test**
	Failure to follow therapeutic recommendations on tests to identify disease or assess health condition
G20.2	**Noncompliance of Dietary Regimen**
	Failure to follow the prescribed diet/food intake
G20.3	**Noncompliance of Fluid Volume**
	Failure to follow fluid volume intake requirements
G20.4	**Noncompliance of Medication Regimen**
	Failure to follow prescribed regulated course of medicinal substances
G20.5	**Noncompliance of Safety Precautions**
	Failure to follow measures to prevent injury, danger, or loss
G20.6	**Noncompliance of Therapeutic Regimen**
	Failure to follow regulated course of treating disease
J24.0	**Nutrition Alteration**
	Change in or modification of food or nutrients

TABLE 8.6 ▨ (*Continued*)

Q44.4　**Olfactory Alteration**
Change in or modification of diminished ability to smell

R46.1　**Oral Mucous Membrane Impairment**
Diminished ability to maintain the tissues of the oral cavity

Q63.0　**Pain**
Physical suffering or distress; to hurt

M27.1　**Parental Role Conflict**
Struggle with parental position and responsibilities

M27.2　**Parenting Alteration**
Change in or modification of nurturing figure's ability to promote growth and
development of infant/child

B03.5　**Perceived Constipation**
Impression of infrequent or difficult passage of hard, dry feces without cause

U60.0　**Perinatal Risk**
Increased chance of harm before, during, and immediately after the creation of an
offspring/child

N57.0　**Perioperative Injury Risk**
Increased chance of injury during the operative processes

N57.1　**Perioperative Positioning Injury**
Damages from operative process positioning

R47.0　**Peripheral Alteration**
Change in or modification of neurovascularization of the extremities

P43.2　**Personal Identity Disturbance**
Imbalance in the ability to distinguish between the self and the nonself

A01.5　**Physical Mobility Impairment**
Diminished ability to perform independent movement

K25.0　**Physical Regulation Alteration**
Change in or modification of somatic control

N33.3　**Poisoning Risk**
Exposure to or ingestion of dangerous products

H21.1　**Polypharmacy**
Use of two or more drugs together

U60.4　**Postpartum Risk**
Increased chance of harm during the period immediately following the delivery of an
offspring/child

E13.0　**Posttrauma Response**
Sustained behavior related to a traumatic event

P42.2　**Powerlessness**
Feeling of helplessness or inability to act

U60.1　**Pregnancy Risk**
Increased chance of harm during the gestational period of the formation of an
offspring/child

E13.1　**Rape Trauma Syndrome**
Group of symptoms related to a forced sexual act

T49.2　**Reflex Urinary Incontinence**
Involuntary passage of urine occurring at predictable intervals

M32.3　**Relocation Stress Syndrome**
Excessive tension from moving to a new location

(*Continued*)

TABLE 8.6 ■ Clinical Care Classification of 176 Nursing Diagnoses, Version 2.5: Coded Alphabetically with Definitions[1,2] (*Continued*)

T50.0	**Renal Alteration**	
	Change in or modification of kidney function	
U59.0	**Reproductive Risk**	
	Increased chance of harm in the process of replicating or giving rise to an offspring/child	
L26.0	**Respiration Alteration**	
	Change in or modification of the breathing function	
M27.0	**Role Performance Alteration**	
	Change in or modification of carrying out responsibilities	
O38.0	**Self-Care Deficit**	
	Impaired ability to maintain oneself	
P43.0	**Self-Concept Alteration**	
	Change in or modification of ability to maintain one's image of self	
N34.2	**Self-Mutilation Risk**	
	Increased chance of destroying a limb or essential part of the body	
Q44.0	**Sensory Perceptual Alteration**	
	Change in or modification of the response to stimuli	
M27.3	**Sexual Dysfunction**	
	Deleterious change in sexual response	
M31.0	**Sexuality Patterns Alteration**	
	Change in or modification of person's sexual response	
P43.4	**Situational Self-Esteem Disturbance**	
	Negative evaluation of oneself in response to a loss or change	
R46.0	**Skin Integrity Alteration**	
	Change in or modification of skin conditions	
R46.2	**Skin Integrity Impairment**	
	Diminished ability to maintain the integument	
R46.3	**Skin Integrity Impairment Risk**	
	Increased chance of skin breakdown	
R46.4	**Skin Incision**	
	Cutting of the integument/skin	
A01.7	**Sleep Deprivation**	
	Lack of a normal sleep/wake cycle	
A01.6	**Sleep Pattern Disturbance**	
	Imbalance in the normal sleep/wake cycle	
M32.1	**Social Interaction Alteration**	
	Inadequate quantity or quality of personal relations	
M32.2	**Social Isolation**	
	State of aloneness; lack of interaction with others	
M32.0	**Socialization Alteration**	
	Change in or modification of personal identity	
E14.1	**Spiritual Distress**	
	Anguish related to the spirit or soul	
E14.0	**Spiritual State Alteration**	
	Change in or modification of the spirit or soul	
T49.3	**Stress Urinary Incontinence**	
	Loss of urine occurring with increased abdominal pressure	
N58.0	**Substance Abuse**	
	Excessive use of harmful bodily materials	

TABLE 8.6 ▨ (*Continued*)

N33.4	**Suffocation Risk**
	Increased chance of inadequate air for breathing
N34.1	**Suicide Risk**
	Increased chance of taking one's life intentionally
N57.2	**Surgical Recovery Delay**
	Slow or delayed recovery from a surgical procedure
J24.5	**Swallowing Impairment**
	Inability to move food from mouth to stomach
Q44.5	**Tactile Alteration**
	Change in or modification of diminished ability to feel
K25.4	**Thermoregulation Impairment**
	Fluctuation of temperature between hypothermia and hyperthermia
S48.0	**Tissue Perfusion Alteration**
	Change in or modification of the oxygenation of tissues
N58.1	**Tobacco Abuse**
	Excessive use of tobacco products
O39.0	**Toileting Deficit**
	Impaired ability to urinate or defecate for oneself
D09.0	**Thought Processes Alteration**
	Change in or modification of thought and cognitive processes
N33.5	**Trauma Risk**
	Increased chance of accidental tissue injury
Q44.6	**Unilateral Neglect**
	Lack of awareness of one side of the body
T49.0	**Urinary Elimination Alteration**
	Change in or modification of excretion of the waste matter of the kidneys
T49.6	**Urinary Retention**
	Incomplete emptying of the bladder
T49.5	**Urge Urinary Incontinence**
	Involuntary passage of urine following a sense of urgency to void
L56.0	**Ventilatory Weaning Impairment**
	Inability to tolerate decreased levels of ventilator support
M28.1	**Verbal Impairment**
	Diminished ability to exchange thoughts, opinions, or information through speech
N34.0	**Violence Risk**
	Increased chance of harming self or others
Q44.7	**Visual Alteration**
	Change in or modification of diminished ability to see
B04.2	**Vomiting**
	Expulsion of stomach contents through the mouth

[1] Clinical Care Classification (CCC) System, Version 2.5 (previously known as: (a) Clinical Care Classification (CCC) System, Version 2.0, Copyright © 2004; and (b) Home Healthcare Classification (HHCC) System, Version 1.0, Copyright © 1994] pending Copyright © 2012 by Virginia K. Saba. EdD, RN, FAAN, FACMI, LL, may be used ONLY with written Permission by Dr. Virginia K. Saba. (Permission Form available from website <http://www.sabacare.com>).

[2] Revised 1992, 1994, 2004, 2006, and 2011.

TABLE 8.7 ■ Clinical Care Classification of 176 Nursing Diagnoses, Version 2.5: Listed Alphabetically by Code Numbers[1,2]

Activities of Daily Living Alteration	O38.1
Activity Alteration	A01.0
Activity Intolerance	A01.1
Activity Intolerance Risk	A01.2
Acute Pain	Q63.1
Adjustment Impairment	E12.1
Airway Clearance Impairment	L26.1
Alcohol Abuse	N58.2
Anticipatory Grieving	E53.1
Anxiety	P40.0
Aspiration Risk	N33.1
Auditory Alteration	Q44.1
Autonomic Dysreflexia	K25.1
Bathing/Hygiene Deficit	O35.0
Bleeding Risk	C06.2
Blood Pressure Alteration	C06.1
Body Image Distribution	P43.1
Body Nutrition Deficit	J24.1
Body Nutrition Deficit Risk	J24.2
Body Nutrition Excess	J24.3
Body Nutrition Excess Risk	J24.4
Bowel Elimination Alteration	B03.0
Bowel Incontinence	B03.1
Breastfeeding Impairment	J55.0
Breathing Pattern Impairment	L26.2
Cardiac Alteration	C05.0
Cardiovascular Alteration	C06.0
Caregiver Role Strain	M27.4
Cerebral Alteration	D07.0
Chronic Low Self-Esteem Disturbance	P43.3
Chronic Pain	Q63.2
Comfort Alteration	Q45.0
Communication Impairment	M28.0
Community Coping Impairment	E52.0
Confusion	D07.1
Constipation	B03.6
Contraceptive Risk	U59.3
Decisional Conflict	E12.2
Defensive Coping	E12.3
Delivery Risk	U60.3
Denial	E12.4
Diarrhea	B03.3
Disabled Family Coping	E11.2
Disuse Syndrome	N33.2
Diversional Activity Deficit	A01.3
Dressing/Grooming Deficit	O36.0
Drug Abuse	N58.3
Dying Process	E10.0
Dysfunctional Grieving	E53.2

TABLE 8.7 ■ (*Continued*)

Electrolyte Imbalance	F62.0
Endocrine Alteration	I22.0
Failure to Thrive	G17.1
Fall Risk	N33.6
Family Coping Impairment	E11.0
Family Process Alteration	M29.0
Fatigue	A01.4
Fear	P41.0
Fecal Impaction	B03.4
Feeding Deficit	O37.0
Fertility Risk	U59.1
Fluid Volume Alteration	F15.0
Fluid Volume Deficit	F15.1
Fluid Volume Deficit Risk	F15.2
Fluid Volume Excess	F15.3
Fluid Volume Excess Risk	F15.4
Functional Urinary Incontinence	T49.1
Gas Exchange Impairment	L26.3
Gastrointestinal Alteration	B04.0
Grieving	E53.0
Growth and Development Alteration	U61.0
Gustatory Alteration	Q44.2
Health Maintenance Alteration	G17.0
Health-Seeking Behavior Alteration	G18.0
Home Maintenance Alteration	G19.0
Hopelessness	P42.1
Hyperthermia	K25.2
Hypothermia	K25.3
Immunologic Alteration	I23.0
Individual Coping Impairment	E12.0
Infant Feeding Pattern Impairment	J54.0
Infection	K25.6
Infection Risk	K25.5
Infertility Risk	U59.2
Injury Risk	N33.0
Instrumental Activities of Daily Living Alteration	O38.2
Intracranial Adaptive Capacity Impairment	K25.7
Kinesthetic Alteration	Q44.3
Knowledge Deficit	D08.0
Knowledge Deficit of Diagnostic Test	D08.1
Knowledge Deficit of Dietary Regimen	D08.2
Knowledge Deficit of Disease Process	D08.3
Knowledge Deficit of Fluid Volume	D08.4
Knowledge Deficit of Medication Regimen	D08.5
Knowledge Deficit of Safety Precautions	D08.6
Knowledge Deficit of Therapeutic Regimen	D08.7

(*Continued*)

TABLE 8.7 ■ Clinical Care Classification of 176 Nursing Diagnoses, Version 2.5: Listed Alphabetically by Code Numbers[1,2] (*Continued*)

Labor Risk U60.2
Latex Allergy Response R46.5

Meaningfulness Alteration P42.0
Medication Risk H21.0
Memory Impairment D09.1
Musculoskeletal Alteration A02.0

Nausea B04.1
Noncompliance G20.0
Noncompliance of Diagnostic Test G20.1
Noncompliance of Dietary Regimen G20.2
Noncompliance of Fluid Volume G20.3
Noncompliance of Medication Regimen G20.4
Noncompliance of Safety Precautions G20.5
Noncompliance of Therapeutic Regimen G20.6
Nutrition Alteration J24.0

Olfactory Alteration Q44.4
Oral Mucous Membrane Impairment R46.1

Pain Q63.0
Parental Role Conflict M27.1
Parenting Alteration M27.2
Perceived Constipation B03.5
Perinatal Risk U60.0
Perioperative Injury Risk N57.0
Perioperative Positioning Injury N57.1
Peripheral Alteration R47.0
Personal Identity Disturbance P43.2
Physical Mobility Impairment A01.5
Physical Regulation Alteration K25.0
Poisoning Risk N33.3
Polypharmacy H21.1
Postpartum Risk U60.4
Posttrauma Response E13.0
Powerlessness P42.2
Pregnancy Risk U60.1

Rape Trauma Syndrome E13.1
Reflex Urinary Incontinence T49.2
Relocation Stress Syndrome M32.3
Renal Alteration T50.0
Reproductive Risk U59.0
Respiration Alteration L26.0
Role Performance Alteration M27.0

Self-Care Deficit O38.0
Self-Concept Alteration P43.0
Self-Mutilation Risk N34.2
Sensory Perceptual Alteration Q44.0
Sexual Dysfunction M27.3

TABLE 8.7 ▪ (*Continued*)

Sexuality Patterns Alteration	M31.0
Situational Self-Esteem Disturbance	P43.4
Skin Incision	R46.4
Skin Integrity Alteration	R46.0
Skin Integrity Impairment	R46.2
Skin Integrity Impairment Risk	R46.3
Sleep Deprivation	A01.7
Sleep Pattern Disturbance	A01.6
Social Interaction Alteration	M32.1
Social Isolation	M32.2
Socialization Alteration	M32.0
Spiritual Distress	E14.1
Spiritual State Alteration	E14.0
Stress Urinary Incontinence	T49.3
Substance Abuse	N58.0
Suffocation Risk	N33.4
Suicide Risk	N34.1
Surgical Recovery Delay	N57.2
Swallowing Impairment	J24.5
Tactile Alteration	Q44.5
Thermoregulation Impairment	K25.4
Thought Processes Alteration	D09.0
Tissue Perfusion Alteration	S48.0
Tilting Deficit	O39.0
Tobacco Abuse	N58.1
Trauma Risk	N33.5
Unilateral Neglect	Q44.6
Urge Urinary Incontinence	T49.5
Urinary Elimination Alteration	T49.0
Urinary Retention	T49.6
Ventilatory Weaning Impairment	L56.0
Verbal Impairment	M28.1
Violence Risk	N34.0
Visual Alteration	Q44.7
Vomiting	B04.2

[1] Clinical Care Classification (CCC) System, Version 2.5 (previously known as: (a) Clinical Care Classification (CCC) System, Version 2.0, Copyright © 2004; and (b) Home Healthcare Classification (HHCC) System, Version 1.0, Copyright © 1994] pending Copyright © 2012 by Virginia K. Saba. EdD, RN, FAAN, FACMI, LL, may be used ONLY with written Permission by Dr. Virginia K. Saba. (Permission Form available from website <http://www.sabacare.com>)

[2] Revised 1992, 1994, 2004, 2006, and 2011.

TABLE 8.8 ■ Clinical Care Classification of 176 Nursing Diagnoses, Version 2.5: Coded with Definitions and Three Expected Outcomes and Classified by 21 Care Components[1,2]

A.   Activity Component

Cluster of elements that involve the use of energy in carrying out musculoskeletal and bodily actions

Activity Alteration—A01.0
Change in or modification of energy used by the body
A01.0.1   Improve
A01.0.2   Stabilize
A01.0.3   Deteriorate

Activity Intolerance—A01.1
Incapacity to carry out physiological or psychological daily activities
A01.1.1   Improve
A01.1.2   Stabilize
A01.1.3   Deteriorate

Activity Intolerance Risk—A01.2
Increased chance of an incapacity to carry out physiological or psychological daily activities
A01.2.1   Improve
A01.2.2   Stabilize
A01.2.3   Deteriorate

Diversional Activity Deficit—A01.3
Lack of interest or engagement in leisure activities
A01.3.1   Improve
A01.3.2   Stabilize
A01.3.3   Deteriorate

Fatigue—A01.4
Exhaustion that interferes with physical and mental activities
A01.4.1   Improve
A01.4.2   Stabilize
A01.4.3   Deteriorate

Physical Mobility Impairment—A01.5
Diminished ability to perform independent movement
A01.5.1   Improve
A01.5.2   Stabilize
A01.5.3   Deteriorate

Sleep Pattern Disturbance—A01.6
Imbalance in the normal sleep/wake cycle
A01.6.1   Improve
A01.6.2   Stabilize
A01.6.3   Deteriorate

Sleep Deprivation—A01.7
Lack of a normal sleep/wake cycle
A01.7.1   Improve
A01.7.2   Stabilize
A01.7.3   Deteriorate

Musculoskeletal Alteration—A02.0
Change in or modification of the muscles, bones, or support structures
A02.0.1   Improve
A02.0.2   Stabilize
A02.0.3   Deteriorate

B.   Bowel/Gastric Component

Cluster of elements that involve the gastrointestinal system

Bowel Elimination Alteration—B03.0
Change in or modification of the gastrointestinal system
B03.0.1   Improve
B03.0.2   Stabilize
B03.0.3   Deteriorate

TABLE 8.8 ▦ (*Continued*)

Bowel Incontinence—B03.1
Involuntary defecation
B03.1.1   Improve
B03.1.2   Stabilize
B03.1.3   Deteriorate
Diarrhea—B03.3
Abnormal frequency and fluidity of feces
B03.2.1   Improve
B03.2.2   Stabilize
B03.2.3   Deteriorate
Fecal Impaction—B03.4
Feces wedged in intestines
B03.4.1   Improve
B03.4.2   Stabilize
B03.4.3   Deteriorate
Perceived Constipation—B03.5
Impression of infrequent or difficult passage of hard, dry, feces without cause
B03.5.1   Improve
B03.5.2   Stabilize
B03.5.3   Deteriorate
Constipation—B03.6
Difficult passage of hard, dry feces
B03.6.1   Improve
B03.6.2   Stabilize
B03.6.3   Deteriorate
Gastrointestinal Alteration—B04.0
Change in or modification of the stomach or intestines
B04.0.1   Improve
B04.0.2   Stabilize
B04.0.3   Deteriorate
Nausea—B04.1
Distaste for food/fluids and an urge to vomit
B04.1.1   Improve
B04.1.2   Stabilize
B04.1.3   Deteriorate
Vomiting—B04.2
Expulsion of stomach contents through the mouth
B04.2.1   Improve
B04.2.2   Stabilize
B04.2.3   Deteriorate

C.   Cardiac Component

Cluster of elements that involve the heart and blood vessels
Cardiac Output Alteration—C05.0
Change in or modification of the pumping action of the heart
C05.0.1   Improve
C05.0.2   Stabilize
C05.0.3   Deteriorate
Cardiovascular Alteration—C06.0
Change in or modification of the heart or blood vessels
C06.0.1   Improve
C06.0.2   Stabilize
C06.0.3   Deteriorate

(*Continued*)

TABLE 8.8 ▥ Clinical Care Classification of 176 Nursing Diagnoses, Version 2.5: Coded with Definitions and Three Expected Outcomes and Classified by 21 Care Components[1,2] (*Continued*)

Blood Pressure Alteration—C06.1
Change in or modification of the systolic or diastolic pressure
C06.1.1 Improve
C06.1.2 Stabilize
C06.1.3 Deteriorate
Bleeding Risk—C06.2
Increased chance of loss of blood volume
C06.2.1 Improve
C06.2.2 Stabilize
C06.2.3 Deteriorate

D. Cognitive/Neuro Component

Cluster of elements that involve cognitive, mental, cerebral, and neurological processes
Cerebral Alteration—D07.0
Change in or modification of mental processes
D07.0.1 Improve
D07.0.2 Stabilize
D07.0.3 Deteriorate
Confusion—D07.1
State of being disoriented (mixed up)
D07.1.1 Improve
D07.1.2 Stabilize
D07.1.3 Deteriorate
Knowledge Deficit—D08.0
Lack of information, understanding, or comprehension
D08.0.1 Improve
D08.0.2 Stabilize
D08.0.3 Deteriorate
Knowledge Deficit of Diagnostic Test—D08.1
Lack of information on test(s) to identify disease or assess health condition
D08.1.1 Improve
D08.1.2 Stabilize
D08.1.3 Deteriorate
Knowledge Deficit of Dietary Regimen—D08.2
Lack of information on the prescribed diet/food intake
D08.2.1 Improve
D08.2.2 Stabilize
D08.2.3 Deteriorate
Knowledge Deficit of Disease Process—D08.3
Lack of information on the morbidity, course, or treatment of the health condition
D08.3.1 Improve
D08.3.2 Stabilize
D08.3.3 Deteriorate
Knowledge Deficit of Fluid Volume—D08.4
Lack of information on fluid volume intake requirements
D08.4.1 Improve
D08.4.2 Stabilize
D08.4.3 Deteriorate
Knowledge Deficit of Medication Regimen—D08.5
Lack of information on prescribed regulated course of medicinal substances
D08.5.1 Improve
D08.5.2 Stabilize
D08.5.3 Deteriorate

TABLE 8.8 ▦ (*Continued*)

Knowledge Deficit of Safety Precautions—D08.6
Lack of information on measures to prevent injury, danger, or loss
D08.6.1 Improve
D08.6.2 Stabilize
D08.6.3 Deteriorate
Knowledge Deficit of Therapeutic Regimen—D08.7
Lack of information on regulated course of treating disease
D08.7.1 Improve
D08.7.2 Stabilize
D08.7.3 Deteriorate
Thought Process Alteration—D09.0
Change in or modification of thought and cognitive processes
D09.0.1 Improve
D09.0.2 Stabilize
D09.0.3 Deteriorate
Memory Impairment—D09.1
Diminished ability or inability to recall past events
D09.1.1 Improve
D09.1.2 Stabilize
D09.1.3 Deteriorate

E. Coping Component

Cluster of elements that involve the ability to deal with responsibilities, problems, or difficulties
Dying Process—E10.0
Physical and behavioral responses associated with death
E10.0.1 Improve
E10.0.2 Stabilize
E10.0.3 Deteriorate
Community Coping Impairment—E52.0
Inadequate community response to problems or difficulties
E52.0.1 Improve
E52.0.2 Stabilize
E52.0.3 Deteriorate
Family Coping Impairment—E11.0
Inadequate family response to problems or difficulties
E11.0.1 Improve
E11.0.2 Stabilize
E11.0.3 Deteriorate
Disabled Family Coping—E11.2
Inability of family to function optimally
E11.2.1 Improve
E11.2.2 Stabilize
E11.2.3 Deteriorate
Individual Coping Impairment—E12.0
Inadequate personal response to problems or difficulties
E12.0.1 Improve
E12.0.2 Stabilize
E12.0.3 Deteriorate
Adjustment Impairment—E12.1
Inadequate adjustment to condition or change in health status
E12.1.1 Improve
E12.1.2 Stabilize
E12.1.3 Deteriorate

(*Continued*)

TABLE 8.8 ■ Clinical Care Classification of 176 Nursing Diagnoses, Version 2.5: Coded with Definitions and Three Expected Outcomes and Classified by 21 Care Components[1,2] (*Continued*)

Decisional Conflict—E12.2
Struggle related to determining a course of action
E12.2.1 Improve
E12.2.2 Stabilize
E12.2.3 Deteriorate

Defensive Coping—E12.3
Self-protective strategies to guard against threats to self
E12.3.1 Improve
E12.3.2 Stabilize
E12.3.3 Deteriorate

Denial—E12.4
Attempt to reduce anxiety by refusal to accept thoughts, feelings, or facts
E12.4.1 Improve
E12.4.2 Stabilize
E12.4.3 Deteriorate

Posttrauma Response—E13.0
Sustained behavior related to a traumatic event
E13.0.1 Improve
E13.0.2 Stabilize
E13.0.3 Deteriorate

Rape Trauma Syndrome—E13.1
Group of symptoms related to a forced sexual act
E13.1.1 Improve
E13.1.2 Stabilize
E13.1.3 Deteriorate

Spiritual State Alteration—E14.0
Change in or modification of the spirit or soul
E14.0.1 Improve
E14.0.2 Stabilize
E14.0.3 Deteriorate

Spiritual Distress—E14.1
Anguish related to the spirit or soul
E14.1.1 Improve
E14.1.2 Stabilize
E14.1.3 Deteriorate

Grieving—E53.0
Feeling of great sorrow
E53.0.1 Improve
E53.0.2 Stabilize
E43.0.3 Deteriorate

Anticipatory Grieving—E53.1
Feeling great sorrow before the event or loss
E53.1.1 Improve
E53.1.2 Stabilize
E53.1.3 Deteriorate

Dysfunctional Grieving—E53.2
Prolonged feeling of great sorrow
E53.2.1 Improve
E53.2.2 Stabilize
E53.2.3 Deteriorate

TABLE 8.8 ▓ (*Continued*)

F.   Fluid Volume Component

Cluster of elements that involve liquid consumption

Fluid Volume Alteration—F15.0

Change in or modification of bodily fluid

F15.0.1   Improve
F15.0.2   Stabilize
F15.0.3   Deteriorate

   Fluid Volume Deficit—F15.1

   Dehydration or fluid loss

   F15.1.1   Improve
   F15.1.2   Stabilize
   F15.1.3   Deteriorate

Fluid Volume Deficit Risk—F15.2

Increased chance of dehydration or fluid loss

F15.2.1   Improve
F15.2.2   Stabilize
F15.2.3   Deteriorate

Fluid Volume Excess—F15.3

Fluid retention, overload, or edema

F15.3.1   Improve
F15.3.2   Stabilize
F15.3.3   Deteriorate

Fluid Volume Excess Risk—F15.4

Increased chance of fluid retention, overload, or edema

F15.4.1   Improve
F15.4.2   Stabilize
F15.4.3   Deteriorate

Electrolyte Imbalance—F62.0

Higher or lower body electrolyte levels

F62.0.1   Improve
F62.0.2   Stabilize
F62.0.3   Deteriorate

G.   Health Behavior Component

Cluster of elements that involve actions to sustain, maintain, or regain health

Health Maintenance Alteration—G17.0

Change in or modification of ability to manage health-related needs

G17.0.1   Improve
G17.0.2   Stabilize
G17.0.3   Deteriorate

   Failure to Thrive—G17.1

   Inability to grow and develop normally

   G17.1.1   Improve
   G17.1.2   Stabilize
   G17.1.3   Deteriorate

Health-Seeking Behavior Alteration—G18.0

Change in or modification of actions needed to improve health state

G18.0.1   Improve
G18.0.2   Stabilize
G18.0.3   Deteriorate

(Continued)

TABLE 8.8 ■ Clinical Care Classification of 176 Nursing Diagnoses, Version 2.5: Coded with Definitions and Three Expected Outcomes and Classified by 21 Care Components[1,2] (*Continued*)

Home Maintenance Alteration—G19.0
Inability to sustain a safe, healthy environment
G19.0.1   Improve
G19.0.2   Stabilize
G19.0.3   Deteriorate

Noncompliance—G20.0
Failure to follow therapeutic recommendations
G20.0.1   Improve
G20.0.2   Stabilize
G20.0.3   Deteriorate

   Noncompliance of Diagnostic Test—G20.1
   Failure to follow therapeutic recommendations on tests to identify disease or assess health condition
   G20.1.1   Improve
   G20.1.2   Stabilize
   G20.1.3   Deteriorate

   Noncompliance of Dietary Regimen—G20.2
   Failure to follow the prescribed diet/food intake
   G20.2.1   Improve
   G20.2.2   Stabilize
   G20.2.3   Deteriorate

   Noncompliance of Fluid Volume—G20.3
   Failure to follow fluid volume intake requirements
   G20.3.1   Improve
   G20.3.2   Stabilize
   G20.3.3   Deteriorate

   Noncompliance of Medication Regimen—G20.4
   Failure to follow prescribed regulated course of medicinal substances
   G20.4.1   Improve
   G20.4.2   Stabilize
   G20.4.3   Deteriorate

   Noncompliance of Safety Precautions—G20.5
   Failure to follow measures to prevent injury, danger, or loss
   G20.5.1   Improve
   G20.5.2   Stabilize
   G20.5.3   Deteriorate

   Noncompliance of Therapeutic Regimen—G20.6
   Failure to follow regulated course of treating disease or health condition
   G20.6.1   Improve
   G20.6.2   Stabilize
   G20.6.3   Deteriorate

H.   Medication Component

Cluster of elements that involve medicinal substances
Medication Risk—H21.0
Increased chance of negative response to medicinal substances
H21.0.1   Improve
H21.0.2   Stabilize
H21.0.3   Deteriorate

   Polypharmacy—H21.1
   Use of two or more drugs together
   H21.1.1   Improve
   H21.1.2   Stabilize
   H21.1.3   Deteriorate

TABLE 8.8 ▓ (*Continued*)

I. Metabolic Component

Cluster of elements that involve the endocrine and immunologic processes
Endocrine Alteration—I22.0
Change in or modification of internal secretions or hormones
I22.0.1 Improve
I22.0.2 Stabilize
I22.0.3 Deteriorate
Immunologic Alteration—I23.0
Change in or modification of the immune systems
I23.0.1 Improve
I23.0.2 Stabilize
I23.0.3 Deteriorate

J. Nutritional Component

Cluster of elements that involve the intake of food and nutrients
Nutrition Alteration—J24.0
Change in or modification of food and nutrients.
J24.0.1 Improve
J24.0.2 Stabilize
J24.0.3 Deteriorate
  Body Nutrition Deficit—J24.1
  Less than adequate intake or absorption of food or nutrients
  J24.1.1 Improve
  J24.1.2 Stabilize
  J24.1.3 Deteriorate
  Body Nutrition Deficit Risk—J24.2
  Increased chance of less than adequate intake or absorption of food or nutrients
  J24.2.1 Improve
  J24.2.2 Stabilize
  J24.2.3 Deteriorate
  Body Nutrition Excess—J24.3
  More than adequate intake or absorption of food or nutrients
  J24.3.1 Improve
  J24.3.2 Stabilize
  J24.3.3 Deteriorate
  Body Nutrition Excess Risk—J24.4
  Increased chance of more than adequate intake or absorption of food or nutrients
  J24.4.1 Improve
  J24.4.2 Stabilize
  J24.4.3 Deteriorate
  Swallowing Impairment—J24.5
  Inability to move food from mouth to stomach
  J24.5.1 Improve
  J24.5.2 Stabilize
  J24.5.3 Deteriorate
Infant Feeding Pattern Impairment—J54.0
Imbalance in the normal feeding habits of an infant
J54.0.1 Improve
J54.0.2 Stabilize
J54.0.3 Deteriorate
Breastfeeding Impairment—J55.0
Diminished ability to nourish infant at the breast
J55.0.1 Improve
J55.0.2 Stabilize
J55.0.3 Deteriorate

(*Continued*)

TABLE 8.8 ▆ Clinical Care Classification of 176 Nursing Diagnoses, Version 2.5: Coded with Definitions and Three Expected Outcomes and Classified by 21 Care Components[1,2] (*Continued*)

K. Physical Regulation Component

Cluster of elements that involve bodily processes
Physical Regulation Alteration—K25.0
Change in or modification of somatic control
K25.0.1   Improve
K25.0.2   Stabilize
K25.0.3   Deteriorate

Autonomic Dysreflexia—K25.1
Life-threatening inhibited sympathetic response to noxious stimuli in a person with a spinal cord injury at or above T7
K25.1.1   Improve
K25.1.2   Stabilize
K25.1.3   Deteriorate

Hyperthermia—K25.2
Abnormally high body temperature
K25.2.1   Improve
K25.2.2   Stabilize
K25.2.3   Deteriorate

Hypothermia—K25.3
Abnormally low body temperature
K25.3.1   Improve
K25.3.2   Stabilize
K25.3.3   Deteriorate

Thermoregulation Impairment—K25.4
Fluctuation of temperature between hypothermia and hyperthermia
K25.4.1   Improve
K25.4.2   Stabilize
K25.4.3   Deteriorate

Infection Risk—K25.5
Increased chance of contamination with disease-producing germs
K25.5.1   Improve
K25.5.2   Stabilize
K25.5.3   Deteriorate

Infection—K25.6
Contamination with disease-producing germs
K25.6.1   Improve
K25.6.2   Stabilize
K25.6.3   Deteriorate

Intracranial Adaptive Capacity Impairment—K25.7
Intracranial fluid volumes are compromised
K25.7.1   Improve
K25.7.2   Stabilize
K25.7.3   Deteriorate

L. Respiratory Component

Cluster of elements that involve breathing and the pulmonary system
Respiration Alteration—L26.0
Change in or modification of the breathing function
L26.0.1   Improve
L26.0.2   Stabilize
L26.0.3   Deteriorate

TABLE 8.8 ▨ (*Continued*)

Airway Clearance Impairment—L26.1
Inability to clear secretions/obstructions in airway
L26.1.1   Improve
L26.1.2   Stabilize
L26.1.3   Deteriorate
Breathing Pattern Impairment—L26.2
Inadequate inhalation or exhalation
L26.2.1   Improve
L26.2.2   Stabilize
L26.2.3   Deteriorate
Gas Exchange Impairment—L26.3
Imbalance of oxygen and carbon dioxide transfer between lung and vascular system
L26.3.1   Improve
L26.3.2   Stabilize
L26.3.3   Deteriorate
Ventilatory Weaning Impairment—L56.0
Inability to tolerate decreased levels of ventilator support
L56.0.1   Improve
L56.0.2   Stabilize
L56.0.3   Deteriorate

M.   Role Relationship Component

Cluster of elements involving interpersonal work, social, family, and sexual interactions
Role Performance Alteration—M27.0
Change in or modification of carrying out responsibilities
M27.0.1   Improve
M27.0.2   Stabilize
M27.0.3   Deteriorate
Parental Role Conflict—M27.1
Struggle with parental position and responsibilities
M27.1.1   Improve
M27.1.2   Stabilize
M27.1.3   Deteriorate
Parenting Alteration—M27.2
Change in or modification of nurturing figure's ability to promote growth
M27.2.1   Improve
M27.2.2   Stabilize
M27.2.3   Deteriorate
Sexual Dysfunction—M27.3
Deleterious change in sexual response
M27.3.1   Improve
M27.3.2   Stabilize
M27.3.3   Deteriorate
Caregiver Role Strain—M27.4
Excessive tension of one who gives physical or emotional care and support to another person or patient
M27.4.1   Improve
M27.4.2   Stabilize
M27.4.3   Deteriorate
Communication Impairment—M28.0
Diminished ability to exchange thoughts, opinions, or information
M28.0.1   Improve
M28.0.2   Stabilize
M28.0.3   Deteriorate

(*Continued*)

TABLE 8.8 ■ Clinical Care Classification of 176 Nursing Diagnoses, Version 2.5: Coded with Definitions and Three Expected Outcomes and Classified by 21 Care Components[1,2] (*Continued*)

Communication Impairment—M28.0
Diminished ability to exchange thoughts, opinions, or information
    Verbal Impairment—M28.1
    Diminished ability to exchange thoughts, opinions, or information through speech
    M28.1.1   Improve
    M28.1.2   Stabilize
    M28.1.3   Deteriorate
Family Process Alteration—M29.0
Change in or modification of usual functioning of a related group
M29.0.1   Improve
M29.0.2   Stabilize
M29.0.3   Deteriorate
Sexuality Pattern Alteration—M31.0
Change in or modification of person's sexual response
M31.0.1   Improve
M31.0.2   Stabilize
M31.0.3   Deteriorate
Socialization Alteration—M32.0
Change in or modification of personal identity
M32.0.1   Improve
M32.0.2   Stabilize
M32.0.3   Deteriorate
    Social Interaction Alteration—M32.1
    Change in or modification of inadequate quantity or quality of personal relations
    M32.1.1   Improve
    M32.1.2   Stabilize
    M32.1.3   Deteriorate
    Social Isolation—M32.2
    State of aloneness; lack of interaction with others
    M32.2.1   Improve
    M32.2.2   Stabilize
    M32.2.3   Deteriorate
    Relocation Stress Syndrome—M32.3
    Excessive tension from moving to a new location
    M32.3.1   Improve
    M32.3.2   Stabilize
    M32.3.3   Deteriorate

N. Safety Component

Cluster of elements that involve prevention of injury, danger, loss, or abuse
Injury Risk—N33.0
Increased chance of danger or loss
N33.0.1   Improve
N33.0.2   Stabilize
N33.0.3   Deteriorate
    Aspiration Risk—N33.1
    Increased chance of material into trachea–bronchial passages
    N33.1.1   Improve
    N33.1.2   Stabilize
    N33.1.3   Deteriorate
    Disuse Syndrome—N33.2
    Group of symptoms related to effects of immobility
    N33.2.1   Improve
    N33.2.2   Stabilize
    N33.2.3   Deteriorate

TABLE 8.8 ■ (*Continued*)

Poisoning Risk—N33.3
Exposure to or ingestion of dangerous products
N33.3.1   Improve
N33.3.2   Stabilize
N33.3.3   Deteriorate
Suffocation Risk—N33.4
Increased chance of inadequate air for breathing
N33.4.1   Improve
N33.4.2   Stabilize
N33.4.3   Deteriorate
Trauma Risk—N33.5
Increased chance of accidental tissue processes
N33.5.1   Improve
N33.5.2   Stabilize
N33.5.3   Deteriorate
Fall Risk—N33.6
Increased the chance of conditions that result in falls
N33.6.1   Improve
N33.6.2   Stabilize
N33.6.3   Deteriorate
Violence Risk—N34.0
Increased chance of harming self or others
N34.0.1   Improve
N34.0.2   Stabilize
N34.0.3   Deteriorate
Suicide Risk—N34.1
Increased chance of taking one's life intentionally
N34.1.1   Improve
N34.1.2   Stabilize
N34.1.3   Deteriorate
Self-Mutilation Risk—N34.2
Increased chance of destroying a limb or essential part of the body
N34.2.1   Improve
N34.2.2   Stabilize
N34.2.3   Deteriorate
Perioperative Injury Risk—N57.0
Increased chance of injury during the operative processes
N57.0.1   Improve
N57.0.2   Stabilize
N57.0.3   Deteriorate
Perioperative Positioning Injury—N57.1
Damages from operative process positioning
N57.1.1   Improve
N57.1.2   Stabilize
N57.1.3   Deteriorate
Surgical Recovery Delay—N57.2
Slow or delayed recovery from a surgical procedure
N57.2.1   Improve
N57.2.2   Stabilize
N57.2.3   Deteriorate
Substance Abuse—N58.0
Excessive use of harmful bodily materials
N58.0.1 Improve
N58.0.2 Stabilize
N58.0.3 Deteriorate

(Continued)

TABLE 8.8 ■ Clinical Care Classification of 176 Nursing Diagnoses, Version 2.5: Coded with Definitions and Three Expected Outcomes and Classified by 21 Care Components[1,2] (*Continued*)

Tobacco Abuse—N58.1
Excessive use of tobacco products
N58.1.1   Improve
N58.1.2   Stabilize
N58.1.3   Deteriorate

Alcohol Abuse—N58.2
Excessive use of distilled liquors
N58.2.1   Improve
N58.2.2   Stabilize
N58.2.3   Deteriorate

Drug Abuse—N58.3
Excessive use of habit-forming medications
N58.3.1   Improve
N58.3.2   Stabilize
N58.3.3   Deteriorate

O.   Self-Care Component

Cluster of elements that involve the ability to carry out activities to maintain oneself

Bathing/Hygiene Deficit—O35.0
Impaired ability to cleanse oneself
O35.0.1   Improve
O35.0.2   Stabilize
O35.0.3   Deteriorate

Dressing/Grooming Deficit—O36.0
Inability to clothe and groom oneself
O36.0.1   Improve
O36.0.2   Stabilize
O36.0.3   Deteriorate

Feeding Deficit—O37.0
Impaired ability to feed oneself
O37.0.1   Improve
O37.0.2   Stabilize
O37.0.3   Deteriorate

Self-Care Deficit—O38.0
Impaired ability to maintain oneself
O38.0.1   Improve
O38.0.2   Stabilize
O38.0.3   Deteriorate

    Activities of Daily Living Alteration—O38.1
    Change in or modification of ability to maintain oneself
    O38.1.1   Improve
    O38.1.2   Stabilize
    O38.1.3   Deteriorate

    Instrumental Activities of Daily Living Alteration—O38.2
    Change in or modification of more complex activities than those needed to maintain oneself
    O38.2.1   Improve
    O38.2.2   Stabilize
    O38.2.3   Deteriorate

Toileting Deficit—O39.0
Impaired ability to urinate or defecate for oneself
O39.0.1   Improve
O39.0.2   Stabilize
O39.0.3   Deteriorate

TABLE 8.8 ■ (*Continued*)

P.   Self-Concept Component

Cluster of elements that involve an individual's mental image of oneself
Anxiety—P40.0
Feeling of distress or apprehension whose source is unknown
P40.0.1   Improve
P40.0.2   Stabilize
P40.0.3   Deteriorate
Fear—P41.0
Feeling of dread or distress whose cause can be identified
P41.0.1   Improve
P41.0.2   Stabilize
P41.0.3   Deteriorate
Meaningfulness Alteration—P42.0
Change in or modification of the ability to see the significance, purpose, or value in something
P42.0.1   Improve
P42.0.2   Stabilize
P42.0.3   Deteriorate
   Hopelessness—P42.1
   Feeling of despair or futility and passive involvement
   P42.1.1   Improve
   P42.1.2   Stabilize
   P42.1.3   Deteriorate
   Powerlessness—P42.2
   Feeling of helplessness or inability to act
   P42.2.1   Improve
   P42.2.2   Stabilize
   P42.2.3   Deteriorate
Self-Concept Alteration—P43.0
Change in or modification of ability to maintain one's image of self
P43.0.1   Improve
P43.0.2   Stabilize
P43.0.3   Deteriorate
   Body Image Disturbance—P43.1
   Imbalance in the perception of the way one's body looks
   P43.1.1   Improve
   P43.1.2   Stabilize
   P43.1.3   Deteriorate
   Personal Identity Disturbance—P43.2
   Imbalance in the ability to distinguish between the self and the nonself
   P43.2.1   Improve
   P43.2.2   Stabilize
   P43.2.3   Deteriorate
   Chronic Low Self-Esteem Disturbance—P43.3
   Persistent negative evaluation of oneself
   P43.3.1   Improve
   P43.3.2   Stabilize
   P43.3.3   Deteriorate
   Situational Self-Esteem Disturbance—P43.4
   Negative evaluation of oneself in response to a loss or change
   P43.4.1   Improve
   P43.4.2   Stabilize
   P43.4.3   Deteriorate

(Continued)

TABLE 8.8 ■ Clinical Care Classification of 176 Nursing Diagnoses, Version 2.5: Coded with Definitions and Three Expected Outcomes and Classified by 21 Care Components[1,2] (*Continued*)

Q. Sensory Component

Cluster of elements that involve the senses, including pain

Sensory Perceptual Alteration—Q44.0

Change in or modification of the response to stimuli

Q44.0.1 Improve
Q44.0.2 Stabilize
Q44.0.3 Deteriorate

Auditory Alteration—Q44.1

Change in or modification of diminished ability to hear

Q44.1.1 Improve
Q44.1.2 Stabilize
Q44.1.3 Deteriorate

Gustatory Alteration—Q44.2

Change in or modification of diminished balance

Q44.2.1 Improve
Q44.2.2 Stabilize
Q44.2.3 Deteriorate

Kinesthetic Alteration—Q44.3

Change in or modification of diminished ability to move

Q44.3.1 Improve
Q44.3.2 Stabilize
Q44.3.3 Deteriorate

Olfactory Alteration—Q44.4

Change in or modification of diminished ability to smell

Q44.4.1 Improve
Q44.4.2 Stabilize
Q44.4.3 Deteriorate

Tactile Alteration—Q44.5

Change in or modification of diminished ability to feel

Q44.5.1 Improve
Q44.5.2 Stabilize
Q44.5.3 Deteriorate

Unilateral Neglect—Q44.6

Lack of awareness of one side of the body

Q44.6.1 Improve
Q44.6.2 Stabilize
Q44.6.3 Deteriorate

Visual Alteration—Q44.7

Change in or modification of diminished ability to see

Q44.7.1 Improve
Q44.7.2 Stabilize
Q44.7.3 Deteriorate

Comfort Alteration—Q45.0

Change in or modification of sensation that is distressing

Q45.0.1 Improve
Q45.0.2 Stabilize
Q45.0.3 Deteriorate

Pain—Q63.0

Physical suffering or distress; to hurt

Q63.0.1 Improve
Q63.0.2 Stabilize
Q63.0.3 Deteriorate

TABLE 8.8 ■ (*Continued*)

R.   Skin Integrity Component

Acute Pain—Q63.1
Severe pain of limited duration
Q63.1.1   Improve
Q63.1.2   Stabilize
Q63.1.3   Deteriorate
Chronic Pain—Q63.2
Pain that persists over time
Q63.2.1   Improve
Q63.2.2   Stabilize
Q63.2.3   Deteriorate
Cluster of elements that involve the mucous membrane, corneal, integumentary, or subcutaneous structures of the body
Skin Integrity Alteration—R46.0
Change in or modification of skin conditions
R46.0.1   Improve
R46.0.2   Stabilize
R46.0.3   Deteriorate
  Oral Mucous Membrane Impairment—R46.1
  Diminished ability to maintain the tissues of the oral cavity
  R46.1.1   Improve
  R46.1.2   Stabilize
  R46.1.3   Deteriorate
  Skin Integrity Impairment—R46.2
  Decreased ability to maintain the integument
  R46.2.1   Improve
  R46.2.2   Stabilize
  R46.2.3   Deteriorate
  Skin Integrity Impairment Risk—R46.3
  Increased chance of skin breakdown
  R46.3.1   Improve
  R46.3.2   Stabilize
  R46.3.3   Deteriorate
  Skin Incision—R46.4
  Cutting of the integument
  R46.4.1   Improve
  R46.4.2   Stabilize
  R46.4.3   Deteriorate
  Latex Allergy Response—R46.5
  Pathological reaction to latex products
  R46.5.1   Improve
  R46.5.2   Stabilize
  R46.5.3   Deteriorate
Peripheral Alteration—R47.0
Change in or modification of neurovascularization of the extremities
R47.0.1   Improve
R47.0.2   Stabilize
R47.0.3   Deteriorate

(*Continued*)

TABLE 8.8 ■ Clinical Care Classification of 176 Nursing Diagnoses, Version 2.5: Coded with Definitions and Three Expected Outcomes and Classified by 21 Care Components[1,2] (*Continued*)

S. Tissue Perfusion Component

Cluster of elements that involve the oxygenation of tissues, including the circulatory and vascular systems

Tissue Perfusion Alteration—S48.0
Change in or modification of the oxygenation of tissues
S48.0.1   Improve
S48.0.2   Stabilize
S48.0.3   Deteriorate

T. Urinary Elimination Component

Cluster of elements that involve the genitourinary systems

Urinary Elimination Alteration—T49.0
Change in or modification of excretion of the waste matter of the kidneys
T49.0.1   Improve
T49.0.2   Stabilize
T49.0.3   Deteriorate

    Functional Urinary Incontinence—T49.1
    Involuntary, unpredictable passage of urine
    T49.1.1   Improve
    T49.1.2   Stabilize
    T49.1.3   Deteriorate

    Reflex Urinary Incontinence—T49.2
    Involuntary passage of urine occurring at predictable intervals
    T49.2.1   Improve
    T49.2.2   Stabilize
    T49.2.3   Deteriorate

    Stress Urinary Incontinence—T49.3
    Loss of urine occurring with increased abdominal pressure
    T49.3.1   Improve
    T49.3.2   Stabilize
    T49.3.3   Deteriorate

    Urge Urinary Incontinence—T49.5
    Involuntary passage of urine following a sense of urgency to void
    T49.5.1   Improve
    T49.5.2   Stabilize
    T49.5.3   Deteriorate

    Urinary Retention—T49.6
    Incomplete emptying of the bladder
    T49.6.1   Improve
    T49.6.2   Stabilize
    T49.6.3   Deteriorate

Renal Alteration—T50.0
Change in or modification of kidney function
T50.0.1   Improve
T50.0.2   Stabilize
T50.0.3   Deteriorate

U. Life Cycle Component

Cluster of elements that involve the life span of individuals

Reproductive Risk—U59.0
Increased chance of harm in the process of replicating or giving rise to an offspring/child
U59.0.1   Improve
U59.0.2   Stabilize
U59.0.3   Deteriorate

TABLE 8.8 ▨ (*Continued*)

Fertility Risk—U59.1
Increased chance of conception to develop an offspring/child
U59.1.1   Improve
U59.1.2   Stabilize
U59.1.3   Deteriorate

Infertility Risk—U59.2
Decreased chance of conception to develop an offspring/child
U59.2.1   Improve
U59.2.2   Stabilize
U59.2.3   Deteriorate

Contraception Risk—U59.3
Increased chance of harm preventing the conception of an offspring/child
U59.3.1   Improve
U59.3.2   Stabilize
U59.3.3   Deteriorate

Perinatal Risk—U60.0
Increased chance of harm before, during, and immediately after the creation of an offspring/child
U60.1.1   Improve
U60.1.2   Stabilize
U60.1.3   Deteriorate

Pregnancy Risk—U60.1
Increased chance of harm during the gestational period of the formation of an offspring/child
U60.1.1   Improve
U60.1.2   Stabilize
U60.1.3   Deteriorate

Labor Risk—U60.2
Increased chance of harm during the period supporting the bringing forth of an offspring/child
U60.2.1   Improve
U60.2.2   Stabilize
U60.2.3   Deteriorate

Delivery Risk—U60.3
Increased chance of harm during the period supporting the expulsion of an offspring/child
U60.3.1   Improve
U60.3.2   Stabilize
U60.3.3   Deteriorate

Postpartum Risk—U60.4
Increased chance of harm during the period immediately following the delivery of an offspring/child
U60.4.1   Improve
U60.4.2   Stabilize
U60.4.3   Deteriorate

Growth and Development Alteration—U61.0
Change in or modification of age-specific normal growth standards and/or developmental skills.
U61.0.1   Improve
U61.0.2   Stabilize
U61.0.3   Deteriorate

---

[1] Clinical Care Classification (CCC) System, Version 2.5 (previously known as: (a) Clinical Care Classification (CCC) System, Version 2.0, Copyright © 2004; and (b) Home Healthcare Classification (HHCC) System, Version 1.0, Copyright © 1994] pending Copyright © 2012 by Virginia K. Saba. EdD, RN, FAAN, FACMI, LL, may be used ONLY with written Permission by Dr. Virginia K. Saba. (Permission Form available from website <http://www.sabacare.com>)

[2] Revised 1992, 1994, 2004, 2006, and 2011.

TABLE 8.9 ■ Clinical Care Classification of 176 Nursing Diagnoses, Version 2.5: Coded with Definitions and Three Actual Outcomes and Classified by 21 Care Components[1,2]

A. Activity Component

Cluster of elements that involve the use of energy in carrying out musculoskeletal and bodily actions
Activity Alteration—A01.0
Change in or modification of energy used by the body
A01.0.1 Improved
A01.0.2 Stabilized
A01.0.3 Deteriorated
  Activity Intolerance—A01.1
  Incapacity to carry out physiological or psychological daily activities
  A01.1.1 Improved
  A01.1.2 Stabilized
  A01.1.3 Deteriorated
  Activity Intolerance Risk—A01.2
  Increased chance of an incapacity to carry out physiological or psychological daily activities
  A01.2.1 Improved
  A01.2.2 Stabilized
  A01.2.3 Deteriorated
  Diversional Activity Deficit—A01.3
  Lack of interest or engagement in leisure activities
  A01.3.1 Improved
  A01.3.2 Stabilized
  A01.3.3 Deteriorated
  Fatigue—A01.4
  Exhaustion that interferes with physical and mental activities
  A01.4.1 Improved
  A01.4.2 Stabilized
  A01.4.3 Deteriorated
  Physical Mobility Impairment—A01.5
  Diminished ability to perform independent movement
  A01.5.1 Improved
  A01.5.2 Stabilized
  A01.5.3 Deteriorated
  Sleep Pattern Disturbance—A01.6
  Imbalance in the normal sleep/wake cycle
  A01.6.1 Improved
  A01.6.2 Stabilized
  A01.6.3 Deteriorated
  Sleep Deprivation—A01.7
  Lack of a normal sleep/wake cycle
  A01.7.1 Improved
  A01.7.2 Stabilized
  A01.7.3 Deteriorated
Musculoskeletal Alteration—A02.0
Change in or modification of the muscles, bones, or support structures
A02.0.1 Improved
A02.0.2 Stabilized
A02.0.3 Deteriorated

B. Bowel/Gastric Component

Cluster of elements that involve the gastrointestinal system
Bowel Elimination Alteration—B03.0
Change in or modification of the gastrointestinal system
B03.0.1 Improved
B03.0.2 Stabilized
B03.0.3 Deteriorated

TABLE 8.9 ■ *(Continued)*

Bowel Incontinence—B03.1
Involuntary defecation
B03.1.1   Improved
B03.1.2   Stabilized
B03.1.3   Deteriorated
Diarrhea—B03.3
Abnormal frequency and fluidity of feces
B03.2.1   Improved
B03.2.2   Stabilized
B03.2.3   Deteriorated
Fecal Impaction—B03.4
Feces wedged in intestines
B03.4.1   Improved
B03.4.2   Stabilized
B03.4.3   Deteriorated
Perceived Constipation—B03.5
Impression of infrequent or difficult passage of hard, dry, feces without cause
B03.5.1   Improved
B03.5.2   Stabilized
B03.5.3   Deteriorated
Constipation—B03.6
Difficult passage of hard, dry feces
B03.6.1   Improved
B03.6.2   Stabilized
B03.6.3   Deteriorated
Gastrointestinal Alteration—B04.0
Change in or modification of the stomach or intestines
B04.0.1   Improved
B04.0.2   Stabilized
B04.0.3   Deteriorated
Nausea—B04.1
Distaste for food/fluids and an urge to vomit
B04.1.1   Improved
B04.1.2   Stabilized
B04.1.3   Deteriorated
Vomiting—B04.2
Expulsion of stomach contents through the mouth
B04.2.1   Improved
B04.2.2   Stabilized
B04.2.3   Deteriorated

C.   Cardiac Component

Cluster of elements that involve the heart and blood vessels
Cardiac Output Alteration—C05.0
Change in or modification of the pumping action of the heart
C05.0.1   Improved
C05.0.2   Stabilized
C05.0.3   Deteriorated
Cardiovascular Alteration—C06.0
Change in or modification of the heart or blood vessels
C06.0.1   Improved
C06.0.2   Stabilized
C06.0.3   Deteriorated

(Continued)

TABLE 8.9 ■ Clinical Care Classification of 176 Nursing Diagnoses, Version 2.5: Coded with Definitions and Three Actual Outcomes and Classified by 21 Care Components[1,2] (*Continued*)

Blood Pressure Alteration—C06.1
Change in or modification of the systolic or diastolic pressure
C06.1.1 Improved
C06.1.2 Stabilized
C06.1.3 Deteriorated
Bleeding Risk—C06.2
Increased chance of loss of blood volume
C06.2.1 Improved
C06.2.2 Stabilized
C06.2.3 Deteriorated

D. Cognitive/Neuro Component

Cluster of elements that involve cognitive, mental, cerebral, and neurological processes
Cerebral Alteration—D07.0
Change in or modification of mental processes
D07.0.1 Improved
D07.0.2 Stabilized
D07.0.3 Deteriorated
Confusion—D07.1
State of being disoriented (mixed up)
D07.1.1 Improved
D07.1.2 Stabilized
D07.1.3 Deteriorated
Knowledge Deficit—D08.0
Lack of information, understanding, or comprehension
D08.0.1 Improved
D08.0.2 Stabilized
D08.0.3 Deteriorated
Knowledge Deficit of Diagnostic Test—D08.1
Lack of information on test(s) to identify disease or assess health condition
D08.1.1 Improved
D08.1.2 Stabilized
D08.1.3 Deteriorated
Knowledge Deficit of Dietary Regimen—D08.2
Lack of information on the prescribed diet/food intake
D08.2.1 Improved
D08.2.2 Stabilized
D08.2.3 Deteriorated
Knowledge Deficit of Disease Process—D08.3
Lack of information on the morbidity, course, or treatment of the health condition
D08.3.1 Improved
D08.3.2 Stabilized
D08.3.3 Deteriorated
Knowledge Deficit of Fluid Volume—D08.4
Lack of information on fluid volume intake requirements
D08.4.1 Improved
D08.4.2 Stabilized
D08.4.3 Deteriorated
Knowledge Deficit of Medication Regimen—D08.5
Lack of information on prescribed regulated course of medicinal substances
D08.5.1 Improved
D08.5.2 Stabilized
D08.5.3 Deteriorated

TABLE 8.9 ▪ (*Continued*)

Knowledge Deficit of Safety Precautions—D08.6
Lack of information on measures to prevent injury, danger, or loss
D08.6.1   Improved
D08.6.2   Stabilized
D08.6.3   Deteriorated
Knowledge Deficit of Therapeutic Regimen—D08.7
Lack of information on regulated course of treating disease
D08.7.1   Improved
D08.7.2   Stabilized
D08.7.3   Deteriorated
Thought Process Alteration—D09.0
Change in or modification of thought and cognitive processes
D09.0.1   Improved
D09.0.2   Stabilized
D09.0.3   Deteriorated
  Memory Impairment—D09.1
  Diminished ability or inability to recall past events
  D09.1.1   Improved
  D09.1.2   Stabilized
  D09.1.3   Deteriorated

E.   Coping Component

Cluster of elements that involve the ability to deal with responsibilities, problems, or difficulties
Dying Process—E10.0
Physical and behavioral responses associated with death
E10.0.1   Improved
E10.0.2   Stabilized
E10.0.3   Deteriorated
Community Coping Impairment—E52.0
Inadequate community response to problems or difficulties
E52.0.1   Improved
E52.0.2   Stabilized
E52.0.3   Deteriorated
Family Coping Impairment—E11.0
Inadequate family response to problems or difficulties
E11.0.1   Improved
E11.0.2   Stabilized
E11.0.3   Deteriorated
  Disabled Family Coping—E11.2
  Inability of family to function optimally
  E11.2.1   Improved
  E11.2.2   Stabilized
  E11.2.3   Deteriorated
Individual Coping Impairment—E12.0
Inadequate personal response to problems or difficulties
E12.0.1   Improved
E12.0.2   Stabilized
E12.0.3   Deteriorated
  Adjustment Impairment—E12.1
  Inadequate adjustment to condition or change in health status
  E12.1.1   Improved
  E12.1.2   Stabilized
  E12.1.3   Deteriorated

(*Continued*)

TABLE 8.9 ▪ Clinical Care Classification of 176 Nursing Diagnoses, Version 2.5: Coded with Definitions and Three Actual Outcomes and Classified by 21 Care Components[1,2] (*Continued*)

Decisional Conflict—E12.2
Struggle related to determining a course of action
E12.2.1 Improved
E12.2.2 Stabilized
E12.2.3 Deteriorated

Defensive Coping—E12.3
Self-protective strategies to guard against threats to self
E12.3.1 Improved
E12.3.2 Stabilized
E12.3.3 Deteriorated

Denial—E12.4
Attempt to reduce anxiety by refusal to accept thoughts, feelings, or facts
E12.4.1 Improved
E12.4.2 Stabilized
E12.4.3 Deteriorated

Posttrauma Response—E13.0
Sustained behavior related to a traumatic event
E13.0.1 Improved
E13.0.2 Stabilized
E13.0.3 Deteriorated

Rape Trauma Syndrome—E13.1
Group of symptoms related to a forced sexual act
E13.1.1 Improved
E13.1.2 Stabilized
E13.1.3 Deteriorated

Spiritual State Alteration—E14.0
Change in or modification of the spirit or soul
E14.0.1 Improved
E14.0.2 Stabilized
E14.0.3 Deteriorated

Spiritual Distress—E14.1
Anguish related to the spirit or soul
E14.1.1 Improved
E14.1.2 Stabilized
E14.1.3 Deteriorated

Grieving—E53.0
Feeling of great sorrow
E53.0.1 Improved
E53.0.2 Stabilized
E43.0.3 Deteriorated

Anticipatory Grieving E53.1
Feeling great sorrow before the event or loss
E53.1.1 Improved
E53.1.2 Stabilized
E53.1.3 Deteriorated

Dysfunctional Grieving—E53.2
Prolonged feeling of great sorrow
E53.2.1 Improved
E53.2.2 Stabilized
E53.2.3 Deteriorated

TABLE 8.9 ■ (*Continued*)

F. Fluid Volume Component

Cluster of elements that involve liquid consumption
Fluid Volume Alteration—F15.0
Change in or modification of bodily fluid
F15.0.1 Improved
F15.0.2 Stabilized
F15.0.3 Deteriorated
   Fluid Volume Deficit—F15.1
   Dehydration or fluid loss
   F15.1.1 Improved
   F15.1.2 Stabilized
   F15.1.3 Deteriorated
   Fluid Volume Deficit Risk—F15.2
   Increased chance of dehydration or fluid loss
   F15.2.1 Improved
   F15.2.2 Stabilized
   F15.2.3 Deteriorated
   Fluid Volume Excess—F15.3
   Fluid retention, overload, or edema
   F15.3.1 Improved
   F15.3.2 Stabilized
   F15.3.3 Deteriorated
   Fluid Volume Excess Risk—F15.4
   Increased chance of fluid retention, overload, or edema
   F15.4.1 Improved
   F15.4.2 Stabilized
   F15.4.3 Deteriorated
Electrolyte Imbalance—F62.0
Higher or lower body electrolyte levels
F62.0.1 Improved
F62.0.2 Stabilized
F62.0.3 Deteriorated

G. Health Behavior Component

Cluster of elements that involve actions to sustain, maintain, or regain health
Health Maintenance Alteration—G17.0
Change in or modification of ability to manage health-related needs
G17.0.1 Improved
G17.0.2 Stabilized
G17.0.3 Deteriorated
   Failure to Thrive—G17.1
   Inability to grow and develop normally
   G17.1.1 Improved
   G17.1.2 Stabilized
   G17.1.3 Deteriorated
Health-Seeking Behavior Alteration—G18.0
Change in or modification of actions needed to improve health state
G18.0.1 Improved
G18.0.2 Stabilized
G18.0.3 Deteriorated
Home Maintenance Alteration—G19.0
Inability to sustain a safe, healthy environment
G19.0.1 Improved
G19.0.2 Stabilized
G19.0.3 Deteriorated

(*Continued*)

TABLE 8.9 ■ Clinical Care Classification of 176 Nursing Diagnoses, Version 2.5: Coded with Definitions and Three Actual Outcomes and Classified by 21 Care Components[1,2] (*Continued*)

Noncompliance—G20.0
Failure to follow therapeutic recommendations
G20.0.1   Improved
G20.0.2   Stabilized
G20.0.3   Deteriorated

> **Noncompliance of Diagnostic Test—G20.1**
> *Failure to follow therapeutic recommendations on tests to identify disease or assess health condition*
> G20.1.1   Improved
> G20.1.2   Stabilized
> G20.1.3   Deteriorated

> **Noncompliance of Dietary Regimen—G20.2**
> *Failure to follow the prescribed diet/food intake*
> G20.2.1   Improved
> G20.2.2   Stabilized
> G20.2.3   Deteriorated

> **Noncompliance of Fluid Volume—G20.3**
> *Failure to follow fluid volume intake requirements*
> G20.3.1   Improved
> G20.3.2   Stabilized
> G20.3.3   Deteriorated

> **Noncompliance of Medication Regimen—G20.4**
> *Failure to follow prescribed regulated course of medicinal substances*
> G20.4.1   Improved
> G20.4.2   Stabilized
> G20.4.3   Deteriorated

> **Noncompliance of Safety Precautions—G20.5**
> *Failure to follow measures to prevent injury, danger, or loss*
> G20.5.1   Improved
> G20.5.2   Stabilized
> G20.5.3   Deteriorated

> **Noncompliance of Therapeutic Regimen—G20.6**
> *Failure to follow regulated course of treating disease or health condition*
> G20.6.1   Improved
> G20.6.2   Stabilized
> G20.6.3   Deteriorated

H.   Medication Component

Cluster of elements that involve medicinal substances
Medication Risk—H21.0
Increased chance of negative response to medicinal substances
H21.0.1   Improved
H21.0.2   Stabilized
H21.0.3   Deteriorated

> **Polypharmacy—H21.1**
> *Use of two or more drugs together*
> H21.1.1   Improved
> H21.1.2   Stabilized
> H21.1.3   Deteriorated

I.   Metabolic Component

Cluster of elements that involve the endocrine and immunologic processes
Endocrine Alteration—I22.0
Change in or modification of internal secretions or hormones
I22.0.1   Improved
I22.0.2   Stabilized
I22.0.3   Deteriorated

TABLE 8.9 ■ (*Continued*)

Immunologic Alteration—I23.0
Change in or modification of the immune systems
I23.0.1 Improved
I23.0.2 Stabilized
I23.0.3 Deteriorated

J. Nutritional Component

Cluster of elements that involve the intake of food and nutrients
Nutrition Alteration—J24.0
Change in or modification of food and nutrients
J24.0.1 Improved
J24.0.2 Stabilized
J24.0.3 Deteriorated

  Body Nutrition Deficit—J24.1
Less than adequate intake or absorption of food or nutrients
J24.1.1 Improved
J24.1.2 Stabilized
J24.1.3 Deteriorated

  Body Nutrition Deficit Risk—J24.2
Increased chance of less than adequate intake or absorption of food or nutrients
J24.2.1 Improved
J24.2.2 Stabilized
J24.2.3 Deteriorated

  Body Nutrition Excess—J24.3
More than adequate intake or absorption of food or nutrients
J24.3.1 Improved
J24.3.2 Stabilized
J24.3.3 Deteriorated

  Body Nutrition Excess Risk—J24.4
Increased chance of more than adequate intake or absorption of food or nutrients
J24.4.1 Improved
J24.4.2 Stabilized
J24.4.3 Deteriorated

  Swallowing Impairment—J24.5
Inability to move food from mouth to stomach
J24.5.1 Improved
J24.5.2 Stabilized
J24.5.3 Deteriorated

Infant Feeding Pattern Impairment—J54.0
Imbalance in the normal feeding habits of an infant
J54.0.1 Improved
J54.0.2 Stabilized
J54.0.3 Deteriorated

Breastfeeding Impairment—J55.0
Diminished ability to nourish infant at the breast
J55.0.1 Improved
J55.0.2 Stabilized
J55.0.3 Deteriorated

K. Physical Regulation Component

Cluster of elements that involve bodily processes
Physical Regulation Alteration—K25.0
Change in or modification of somatic control
K25.0.1 Improved
K25.0.2 Stabilized
K25.0.3 Deteriorated

(Continued)

TABLE 8.9 ■ Clinical Care Classification of 176 Nursing Diagnoses, Version 2.5: Coded with Definitions and Three Actual Outcomes and Classified by 21 Care Components[1,2] (*Continued*)

Autonomic Dysreflexia—K25.1
Life-threatening inhibited sympathetic response to noxious stimuli in a person with a spinal cord injury at or above T7
K25.1.1   Improved
K25.1.2   Stabilized
K25.1.3   Deteriorated
Hyperthermia—K25.2
Abnormally high body temperature
K25.2.1   Improved
K25.2.2   Stabilized
K25.2.3   Deteriorated
Hypothermia—K25.3
Abnormally low body temperature
K25.3.1   Improved
K25.3.2   Stabilized
K25.3.3   Deteriorated
Thermoregulation Impairment—K25.4
Fluctuation of temperature between hypothermia and hyperthermia
K25.4.1   Improved
K25.4.2   Stabilized
K25.4.3   Deteriorated
Infection Risk—K25.5
Increased chance of contamination with disease-producing germs
K25.5.1   Improved
K25.5.2   Stabilized
K25.5.3   Deteriorated
Infection—K25.6
Contamination with disease-producing germs
K25.6.1   Improved
K25.6.2   Stabilized
K25.6.3   Deteriorated
Intracranial Adaptive Capacity Impairment—K25.7
Intracranial fluid volumes are compromised
K25.7.1   Improved
K25.7.2   Stabilized
K25.7.3   Deteriorated

L.   Respiratory Component

Cluster of elements that involve breathing and the pulmonary system
Respiration Alteration—L26.0
Change in or modification of the breathing function
L26.0.1   Improved
L26.0.2   Stabilized
L26.0.3   Deteriorated
Airway Clearance Impairment—L26.1
Inability to clear secretions/obstructions in airway
L26.1.1   Improved
L26.1.2   Stabilized
L26.1.3   Deteriorated
Breathing Pattern Impairment—L26.2
Inadequate inhalation or exhalation
L26.2.1   Improved
L26.2.2   Stabilized
L26.2.3   Deteriorated

TABLE 8.9 ▩ (*Continued*)

Gas Exchange Impairment—L26.3
Imbalance of oxygen and carbon dioxide transfer between lung and vascular system
L26.3.1   Improved
L26.3.2   Stabilized
L26.3.3   Deteriorated
Ventilatory Weaning Impairment—L56.0
Inability to tolerate decreased levels of ventilator support
L56.0.1   Improved
L56.0.2   Stabilized
L56.0.3   Deteriorated

M.   Role Relationship Component

Cluster of elements involving interpersonal work, social, family, and sexual interactions
Role Performance Alteration—M27.0
Change in or modification of carrying out responsibilities
M27.0.1   Improved
M27.0.2   Stabilized
M27.0.3   Deteriorated
  Parental Role Conflict—M27.1
  Struggle with parental position and responsibilities
  M27.1.1   Improved
  M27.1.2   Stabilized
  M27.1.3   Deteriorated
  Parenting Alteration—M27.2
  Change in or modification of nurturing figure's ability to promote growth
  M27.2.1   Improved
  M27.2.2   Stabilized
  M27.2.3   Deteriorated
  Sexual Dysfunction—M27.3
  Deleterious change in sexual response
  M27.3.1   Improved
  M27.3.2   Stabilized
  M27.3.3   Deteriorated
  Caregiver Role Strain—M27.4
  Excessive tension of one who gives physical or emotional care and support to another person or patient
  M27.4.1   Improved
  M27.4.2   Stabilized
  M27.4.3   Deteriorated
Communication Impairment—M28.0
Diminished ability to exchange thoughts, opinions, or information
M28.0.1   Improved
M28.0.2   Stabilized
M28.0.3   Deteriorated
  Verbal Impairment—M28.1
  Diminished ability to exchange thoughts, opinions, or information through speech
  M28.1.1   Improved
  M28.1.2   Stabilized
  M28.1.3   Deteriorated
Family Process Alteration—M29.0
Change in or modification of usual functioning of a related group
M29.0.1   Improved
M29.0.2   Stabilized
M29.0.3   Deteriorated

(*Continued*)

TABLE 8.9 ■ Clinical Care Classification of 176 Nursing Diagnoses, Version 2.5: Coded with Definitions and Three Actual Outcomes and Classified by 21 Care Components[1,2] (*Continued*)

Sexuality Pattern Alteration—M31.0
Change in or modification of person's sexual response
M31.0.1   Improved
M31.0.2   Stabilized
M31.0.3   Deteriorated

Socialization Alteration—M32.0
Change in or modification of personal identity
M32.0.1   Improved
M32.0.2   Stabilized
M32.0.3   Deteriorated

> **Social Interaction Alteration—M32.1**
> *Change in or modification of inadequate quantity or quality of personal relations*
> M32.1.1   Improved
> M32.1.2   Stabilized
> M32.1.3   Deteriorated
>
> **Social Isolation—M32.2**
> *State of aloneness; lack of interaction with others*
> M32.2.1   Improved
> M32.2.2   Stabilized
> M32.2.3   Deteriorated
>
> **Relocation Stress Syndrome—M32.3**
> *Excessive tension from moving to a new location*
> M32.3.1   Improved
> M32.3.2   Stabilized
> M32.3.3   Deteriorated

N.   Safety Component

Cluster of elements that involve prevention of injury, danger, loss, or abuse
Injury Risk—N33.0
Increased chance of danger or loss
N33.0.1   Improved
N33.0.2   Stabilized
N33.0.3   Deteriorated

> **Aspiration Risk—N33.1**
> *Increased chance of material into trachea–bronchial passages*
> N33.1.1   Improved
> N33.1.2   Stabilized
> N33.1.3   Deteriorated
>
> **Disuse Syndrome—N33.2**
> *Group of symptoms related to effects of immobility*
> N33.2.1   Improved
> N33.2.2   Stabilized
> N33.2.3   Deteriorated
>
> **Poisoning Risk—N33.3**
> *Exposure to or ingestion of dangerous products*
> N33.3.1   Improved
> N33.3.2   Stabilized
> N33.3.3   Deteriorated
>
> **Suffocation Risk—N33.4**
> *Increased chance of inadequate air for breathing*
> N33.4.1   Improved
> N33.4.2   Stabilized
> N33.4.3   Deteriorated

TABLE 8.9 ■ (*Continued*)

Trauma Risk—N33.5
Increased chance of accidental tissue processes
N33.5.1   Improved
N33.5.2   Stabilized
N33.5.3   Deteriorated

Fall Risk—N33.6
Increased the chance of conditions that result in falls
N33.6.1   Improved
N33.6.2   Stabilized
N33.6.3   Deteriorated

Violence Risk—N34.0
Increased chance of harming self or others
N34.0.1   Improved
N34.0.2   Stabilized
N34.0.3   Deteriorated

Suicide Risk—N34.1
Increased chance of taking one's life intentionally
N34.1.1   Improved
N34.1.2   Stabilized
N34.1.3   Deteriorated

Self-Mutilation Risk—N34.2
Increased chance of destroying a limb or essential part of the body
N34.2.1   Improved
N34.2.2   Stabilized
N34.2.3   Deteriorated

Perioperative Injury Risk—N57.0
Increased chance of injury during the operative processes
N57.0.1   Improved
N57.0.2   Stabilized
N57.0.3   Deteriorated

Perioperative Positioning Injury—N57.1
Damages from operative process positioning
N57.1.1   Improved
N57.1.2   Stabilized
N57.1.3   Deteriorated

Surgical Recovery Delay—N57.2
Slow or delayed recovery from a surgical procedure
N57.2.1   Improved
N57.2.2   Stabilized
N57.2.3   Deteriorated

Substance Abuse—N58.0
Excessive use of harmful bodily materials
N58.0.1   Improved
N58.0.2   Stabilized
N58.0.3   Deteriorated

Tobacco Abuse—N58.1
Excessive use of tobacco products
N58.1.1   Improved
N58.1.2   Stabilized
N58.1.3   Deteriorated

Alcohol Abuse—N58.2
Excessive use of distilled liquors
N58.2.1   Improved
N58.2.2   Stabilized
N58.2.3   Deteriorated

(*Continued*)

TABLE 8.9 ■ Clinical Care Classification of 176 Nursing Diagnoses, Version 2.5: Coded with Definitions and Three Actual Outcomes and Classified by 21 Care Components[1,2] (*Continued*)

Drug Abuse—N58.3
Excessive use of habit-forming medications
N58.3.1   Improved
N58.3.2   Stabilized
N58.3.3   Deteriorated

O.   Self-Care Component

Cluster of elements that involve the ability to carry out activities to maintain oneself
Bathing/Hygiene Deficit—O35.0
Impaired ability to cleanse oneself
O35.0.1   Improved
O35.0.2   Stabilized
O35.0.3   Deteriorated
Dressing/Grooming Deficit—O36.0
Inability to clothe and groom oneself
O36.0.1   Improved
O36.0.2   Stabilized
O36.0.3   Deteriorated
Feeding Deficit—O37.0
Impaired ability to feed oneself
O37.0.1   Improved
O37.0.2   Stabilized
O37.0.3   Deteriorated
Self-Care Deficit—O38.0
Impaired ability to maintain oneself
O38.0.1   Improved
O38.0.2   Stabilized
O38.0.3   Deteriorated

> **Activities of Daily Living Alteration—O38.1**
> *Change in or modification of ability to maintain oneself*
> O38.1.1   Improved
> O38.1.2   Stabilized
> O38.1.3   Deteriorated
> **Instrumental Activities of Daily Living Alteration—O38.2**
> *Change in or modification of more complex activities than those needed to maintain oneself*
> O38.2.1   Improved
> O38.2.2   Stabilized
> O38.2.3   Deteriorated

Toileting Deficit—O39.0
Impaired ability to urinate or defecate for oneself
O39.0.1   Improved
O39.0.2   Stabilized
O39.0.3   Deteriorated

P.   Self-Concept Component

Cluster of elements that involve an individual's mental image of oneself
Anxiety—P40.0
Feeling of distress or apprehension whose source is unknown
P40.0.1   Improved
P40.0.2   Stabilized
P40.0.3   Deteriorated
Fear—P41.0
Feeling of dread or distress whose cause can be identified
P41.0.1   Improved
P41.0.2   Stabilized
P41.0.3   Deteriorated

TABLE 8.9 ▥ (*Continued*)

Meaningfulness Alteration—P42.0
Change in or modification of the ability to see the significance, purpose, or value in something
P42.0.1   Improved
P42.0.2   Stabilized
P42.0.3   Deteriorated
  Hopelessness—P42.1
  Feeling of despair or futility and passive involvement
  P42.1.1   Improved
  P42.1.2   Stabilized
  P42.1.3   Deteriorated
  Powerlessness—P42.2
  Feeling of helplessness or inability to act
  P42.2.1   Improved
  P42.2.2   Stabilized
  P42.2.3   Deteriorated
Self-Concept Alteration—P43.0
Change in or modification of ability to maintain one's image of self
P43.0.1   Improved
P43.0.2   Stabilized
P43.0.3   Deteriorated
  Body Image Disturbance—P43.1
  Imbalance in the perception of the way one's body looks
  P43.1.1   Improved
  P43.1.2   Stabilized
  P43.1.3   Deteriorated
  Personal Identity Disturbance—P43.2
  Imbalance in the ability to distinguish between the self and the nonself
  P43.2.1   Improved
  P43.2.2   Stabilized
  P43.2.3   Deteriorated
  Chronic Low Self-Esteem Disturbance—P43.3
  Persistent negative evaluation of oneself
  P43.3.1   Improved
  P43.3.2   Stabilized
  P43.3.3   Deteriorated
  Situational Self-Esteem Disturbance—P43.4
  Negative evaluation of oneself in response to a loss or change
  P43.4.1   Improved
  P43.4.2   Stabilized
  P43.4.3   Deteriorated

Q.   Sensory Component

Cluster of elements that involve the senses, including pain
Sensory Perceptual Alteration—Q44.0
Change in or modification of the response to stimuli
Q44.0.1   Improved
Q44.0.2   Stabilized
Q44.0.3   Deteriorated
  Auditory Alteration—Q44.1
  Change in or modification of diminished ability to hear
  Q44.1.1   Improved
  Q44.1.2   Stabilized
  Q44.1.3   Deteriorated

(*Continued*)

TABLE 8.9 ■ Clinical Care Classification of 176 Nursing Diagnoses, Version 2.5: Coded with Definitions and Three Actual Outcomes and Classified by 21 Care Components[1,2] (*Continued*)

Gustatory Alteration—Q44.2
Change in or modification of diminished ability to taste
Q44.2.1 Improved
Q44.2.2 Stabilized
Q44.2.3 Deteriorated

Kinesthetic Alteration—Q44.3
Change in or modification of diminished balance
Q44.3.1 Improved
Q44.3.2 Stabilized
Q44.3.3 Deteriorated

Olfactory Alteration—Q44.4
Change in or modification of diminished ability to smell
Q44.4.1 Improved
Q44.4.2 Stabilized
Q44.4.3 Deteriorated

Tactile Alteration—Q44.5
Change in or modification of diminished ability to feel
Q44.5.1 Improved
Q44.5.2 Stabilized
Q44.5.3 Deteriorated

Unilateral Neglect—Q44.6
Lack of awareness of one side of the body
Q44.6.1 Improved
Q44.6.2 Stabilized
Q44.6.3 Deteriorated

Visual Alteration—Q44.7
Change in or modification of diminished ability to see
Q44.7.1 Improved
Q44.7.2 Stabilized
Q44.7.3 Deteriorated

Comfort Alteration—Q45.0
Change in or modification of sensation that is distressing
Q45.0.1 Improved
Q45.0.2 Stabilized
Q45.0.3 Deteriorated

Pain—Q63.0
Physical suffering or distress; to hurt
Q63.0.1 Improved
Q63.0.2 Stabilized
Q63.0.3 Deteriorated

Acute Pain—Q63.1
Severe pain of limited duration
Q63.1.1 Improved
Q63.1.2 Stabilized
Q63.1.3 Deteriorated

Chronic Pain—Q63.2
Pain that persists over time
Q63.2.1 Improved
Q63.2.2 Stabilized
Q63.2.3 Deteriorated

TABLE 8.9 ▦ (*Continued*)

R.   Skin Integrity Component

Cluster of elements that involve the mucous membrane, corneal, integumentary, or subcutaneous structures of the body
Skin Integrity Alteration—R46.0
Change in or modification of skin conditions
R46.0.1   Improved
R46.0.2   Stabilized
R46.0.3   Deteriorated
  Oral Mucous Membrane Impairment—R46.1
  Diminished ability to maintain the tissues of the oral cavity
  R46.1.1   Improved
  R46.1.2   Stabilized
  R46.1.3   Deteriorated
  Skin Integrity Impairment—R46.2
  Decreased ability to maintain the integument
  R46.2.1   Improved
  R46.2.2   Stabilized
  R46.2.3   Deteriorated
  Skin Integrity Impairment Risk—R46.3
  Increased chance of skin breakdown
  R46.3.1   Improved
  R46.3.2   Stabilized
  R46.3.3   Deteriorated
  Skin Incision—R46.4
  Cutting of the integument
  R46.4.1   Improved
  R46.4.2   Stabilized
  R46.4.3   Deteriorated
  Latex Allergy Response—R46.5
  Pathological reaction to latex products
  R46.5.1   Improved
  R46.5.2   Stabilized
  R46.5.3   Deteriorated
Peripheral Alteration—R47.0
Change in or modification of neurovascularization of the extremities
R47.0.1   Improved
R47.0.2   Stabilized
R47.0.3   Deteriorated

S.   Tissue Perfusion Component

Cluster of elements that involve the oxygenation of tissues, including the circulatory and vascular systems
Tissue Perfusion Alteration—S48.0
Change in or modification of the oxygenation of tissues
S48.0.1   Improved
S48.0.2   Stabilized
S48.0.3   Deteriorated

T.   Urinary Elimination Component

Cluster of elements that involve the genitourinary systems
Urinary Elimination Alteration—T49.0
Change in or modification of excretion of the waste matter of the kidneys
T49.0.1   Improved
T49.0.2   Stabilized
T49.0.3   Deteriorated

(*Continued*)

TABLE 8.9 ■ Clinical Care Classification of 176 Nursing Diagnoses, Version 2.5: Coded with Definitions and Three Actual Outcomes and Classified by 21 Care Components[1,2] (*Continued*)

Functional Urinary Incontinence—T49.1
Involuntary, unpredictable passage of urine
T49.1.1   Improved
T49.1.2   Stabilized
T49.1.3   Deteriorated
Reflex Urinary Incontinence—T49.2
Involuntary passage of urine occurring at predictable intervals
T49.2.1   Improved
T49.2.2   Stabilized
T49.2.3   Deteriorated
Stress Urinary Incontinence—T49.3
Loss of urine occurring with increased abdominal pressure
T49.3.1   Improved
T49.3.2   Stabilized
T49.3.3   Deteriorated
Urge Urinary Incontinence—T49.5
Involuntary passage of urine following a sense of urgency to void
T49.5.1   Improved
T49.5.2   Stabilized
T49.5.3   Deteriorated
Urinary Retention—T49.6
Incomplete emptying of the bladder
T49.6.1   Improved
T49.6.2   Stabilized
T49.6.3   Deteriorated
Renal Alteration—T50.0
Change in or modification of kidney function
T50.0.1   Improved
T50.0.2   Stabilized
T50.0.3   Deteriorated

U.   Life Cycle Component

Cluster of elements that involve the life span of individuals
Reproductive Risk—U59.0
Increased chance of harm in the process of replicating or giving rise to an offspring/child
U59.0.1   Improved
U59.0.2   Stabilized
U59.0.3   Deteriorated
Fertility Risk—U59.1
Increased chance of conception to develop an offspring/child
U59.1.1   Improved
U59.1.2   Stabilized
U59.1.3   Deteriorated
Infertility Risk—U59.2
Decreased chance of conception to develop an offspring/child
U59.2.1   Improved
U59.2.2   Stabilized
U59.2.3   Deteriorated
Contraception Risk—U59.3
Increased chance of harm preventing the conception of an offspring/child
U59.3.1   Improved
U59.3.2   Stabilized
U59.3.3   Deteriorated

TABLE 8.9 ■ (*Continued*)

Perinatal Risk—U60.0
Increased chance of harm before, during, and immediately after the creation of an offspring/child
U60.1.1   Improved
U60.1.2   Stabilized
U60.1.3   Deteriorated
   Pregnancy Risk—U60.1
   Increased chance of harm during the gestational period of the formation of an offspring/child
   U60.1.1   Improved
   U60.1.2   Stabilized
   U60.1.3   Deteriorated
   Labor Risk—U60.2
   Increased chance of harm during the period supporting the bringing forth of an offspring/child
   U60.2.1   Improved
   U60.2.2   Stabilized
   U60.2.3   Deteriorated
   Delivery Risk—U60.3
   Increased chance of harm during the period supporting the expulsion of an offspring/child
   U60.3.1   Improved
   U60.3.2   Stabilized
   U60.3.3   Deteriorated
   Postpartum Risk—U60.4
   Increased chance of harm during the period immediately following the delivery of an offspring/child
   U60.4.1   Improved
   U60.4.2   Stabilized
   U60.4.3   Deteriorated
Growth and Development Alteration—U61.0
Change in or modification of age-specific normal growth standards and/or developmental skills
U61.0.1   Improved
U61.0.2   Stabilized
U61.0.3   Deteriorated

[1] Clinical Care Classification (CCC) System, Version 2.5 (previously known as: (a) Clinical Care Classification (CCC) System, Version 2.0, Copyright © 2004; and (b) Home Healthcare Classification (HHCC) System, Version 1.0, Copyright © 1994] pending Copyright © 2012 by Virginia K. Saba. EdD, RN, FAAN, FACMI, LL, may be used ONLY with written Permission by Dr. Virginia K. Saba. (Permission Form available from website <http://www.sabacare.com>)

[2] Revised 1992, 1994, 2004, 2006, and 2011.

TABLE 8.10 ▪ Clinical Care Classification of 201 Nursing Interventions, Version 2.5: Coded and Classified by 21 Care Components[1,2]

A. Activity Component

01.0   Activity Care
     01.2   Energy Conservation
02.0   Fracture Care
     02.1   Cast Care
     02.2   Immobilizer Care
03.0   Mobility Therapy
     03.1   Ambulation Therapy
     03.2   Assistive Device Therapy
     03.3   Transfer Care
04.0   Sleep Pattern Control
05.0   Musculoskeletal Care
     05.1   Range of Motion
     05.2   Rehabilitation Exercise
61.0   Bedbound Care
     61.1   Positioning Therapy
77.0   Diversional Care

B. Bowel/Gastric Component

06.0   Bowel Care
     06.1   Bowel Training
     06.2   Disimpaction
     06.3   Enema
     06.4   Diarrhea Care
07.0   Bowel Ostomy Care
     07.1   Bowel Ostomy Irrigation
62.0   Gastric Care
     62.1   Nausea Care

C. Cardiac Component

08.0   Cardiac Care
     08.1   Cardiac Rehabilitation
09.0   Pacemaker Care

D. Cognitive/Neuro Component

10.0   Behavior Care
11.0   Reality Orientation
63.0   Wandering Control
64.0   Memory Loss Care
78.0   Neurological System Care

E. Coping Component

12.0   Counseling Service
     12.1   Coping Support
     12.2   Stress Control
     12.3   Crisis Therapy
13.0   Emotional Support
     13.1   Spiritual Comfort
14.0   Terminal Care
     14.1   Bereavement Support
     14.2   Dying/Death Measures
     14.3   Funeral Arrangements

TABLE 8.10 ▦ (*Continued*)

F. Fluid Volume Component

15.0 Fluid Therapy
    15.1 Hydration Control
    15.3 Intake
    15.4 Output
79.0 Hemodynamic Care
    79.1 Intravenous Care
    79.2 Venous Catheter Care
    79.3 Arterial Catheter Care

G. Health Behavior Component

17.0 Community Special Services
    17.1 Adult Day Center
    17.2 Hospice
    17.3 Meals on Wheels
18.0 Compliance Care
    18.1 Compliance with Diet
    18.2 Compliance with Fluid Volume
    18.3 Compliance with Medical Regimen
    18.4 Compliance with Medication Regimen
    18.5 Compliance with Safety Precautions
    18.6 Compliance with Therapeutic Regimen
19.0 Nursing Contact
    19.1 Bill of Rights
    19.2 Nursing Care Coordination
    19.3 Nursing Status Report
20.0 Physician Contact
    20.1 Medical Regimen Orders
    20.2 Physician Status Report
21.0 Professional/Ancillary Services
    21.1 Health Aide Service
    21.2 Social Worker Service
    21.3 Nurse Specialist Service
    21.4 Occupational Therapist Service
    21.5 Physical Therapist Service
    21.6 Speech Therapist Service
    21.7 Respiratory Therapist Service

H. Medication Component

22.0 Chemotherapy Care
23.0 Injection Administration
24.0 Medication Care
    24.1 Medication Actions
    24.2 Medication Prefill Preparation
    24.3 Medication Side Effects
    24.4 Medication Treatment
25.0 Radiation Therapy Care

I. Metabolic Component

26.0 Allergic Reaction Control
27.0 Diabetic Care
65.0 Immunologic Care

(*Continued*)

TABLE 8.10 ■ Clinical Care Classification of 201 Nursing Interventions, Version 2.5: Coded and Classified by 21 Care Components[1,2] (*Continued*)

J. Nutritional Component

28.0 Enteral Tube Care
    28.1 Enteral Tube Insertion
    28.2 Enteral Tube Irrigation
29.0 Nutrition Care
    29.2 Feeding Technique
    29.3 Regular Diet
    29.4 Special Diet
    29.5 Enteral Feeding
    29.6 Parenteral Feeding
66.0 Breastfeeding Support
67.0 Weight Control

K. Physical Regulation Component

30.0 Infection Control
    30.1 Universal Precautions
31.0 Physical Healthcare
    31.1 Health History
    31.2 Health Promotion
    31.3 Physical Examination
    31.4 Clinical Measurements
32.0 Specimen Care
    32.1 Blood Specimen Care
    32.2 Stool Specimen Care
    32.3 Urine Specimen Care
    32.5 Sputum Specimen Care
33.0 Vital Signs
    33.1 Blood Pressure
    33.2 Temperature
    33.3 Pulse
    33.4 Respiration

L. Respiratory Component

35.0 Oxygen Therapy Care
36.0 Pulmonary Care
    36.1 Breathing Exercises
    36.2 Chest Physiotherapy
    36.3 Inhalation Therapy
    36.4 Ventilator Care
37.0 Tracheostomy Care

M. Role Relationship Component

38.0 Communication Care
39.0 Psychosocial Care
    39.1 Home Situation Analysis
    39.2 Interpersonal Dynamics Analysis
    39.3 Family Process Analysis
    39.4 Sexual Behavior Analysis
    39.5 Social Network Analysis

N. Safety Component

40.0 Substance Abuse Control
    40.1 Tobacco Abuse Control
    40.2 Alcohol Abuse Control
    40.3 Drug Abuse Control

TABLE 8.10 ▦ (*Continued*)

41.0 Emergency Care
42.0 Safety Precautions
    42.1 Environmental Safety
    42.2 Equipment Safety
    42.3 Individual Safety
68.0 Violence Control
80.0 Perioperative Injury Care

O.   Self-Care Component

43.0 Personal Care
    43.1 Activities of Daily Living
    43.2 Instrumental Activities of Daily Living

P.   Self-Concept Component

45.0 Mental Healthcare
    45.1 Mental Health History
    45.2 Mental Health Promotion
    45.3 Mental Health Screening
    45.4 Mental Health Treatment

Q.   Sensory Component

47.0 Pain Control
    47.1 Acute Pain Control
    47.2 Chronic Pain Control
48.0 Comfort Care
49.0 Ear Care
    49.1 Hearing Aid Care
    49.2 Wax Removal
50.0 Eye Care
    50.1 Cataract Care
    50.2 Vision Care

R.   Skin Integrity Component

51.0 Pressure Ulcer Care
    51.1 Pressure Ulcer Stage 1 Care
    51.2 Pressure Ulcer Stage 2 Care
    51.3 Pressure Ulcer Stage 3 Care
    51.4 Pressure Ulcer Stage 4 Care
53.0 Mouth Care
    53.1 Denture Care
54.0 Skin Care
    54.1 Skin Breakdown Control
55.0 Wound Care
    55.1 Drainage Tube Care
    55.2 Dressing Change
    55.3 Incision Care
81.0 Burn Care

S.   Tissue Perfusion Component

56.0 Foot Care
57.0 Perineal Care
69.0 Edema Control
70.0 Circulatory Care
82.0 Vascular System Care

(*Continued*)

TABLE 8.10 ▧ Clinical Care Classification of 201 Nursing Interventions, Version 2.5: Coded and Classified by 21 Care Components[1,2] (*Continued*)

T. Urinary Elimination Component

- 58.0 Bladder Care
  - 58.1 Bladder Instillation
  - 58.2 Bladder Training
- 59.0 Dialysis Care
  - 59.1 Hemodialysis Care
  - 59.2 Peritoneal Dialysis Care
- 60.0 Urinary Catheter Care
  - 60.1 Urinary Catheter Insertion
  - 60.2 Urinary Catheter Irrigation
- 72.0 Urinary Incontinence Care
- 73.0 Renal Care
- 83.0 Bladder Ostomy Care
  - 83.1 Bladder Ostomy Irrigation

U. Life Cycle Component

- 74.0 Reproductive Care
  - 74.1 Fertility Care
  - 74.2 Infertility Care
  - 74.3 Contraception Care
- 75.0 Perinatal Care
  - 75.1 Pregnancy Care
  - 75.2 Labor Care
  - 75.3 Delivery Care
  - 75.4 Postpartum Care
- 76.0 Growth and Development Care

[1] Clinical Care Classification (CCC) System, Version 2.5 (previously known as: (a) Clinical Care Classification (CCC) System, Version 2.0, Copyright © 2004; and (b) Home Healthcare Classification (HHCC) System, Version 1.0, Copyright © 1994] pending Copyright © 2012 by Virginia K. Saba. EdD, RN, FAAN, FACMI, LL, may be used ONLY with written Permission by Dr. Virginia K. Saba. (Permission Form available from website <http://www.sabacare.com>)

[2] Revised 1992, 1994, 2004, 2006, and 2011.

TABLE 8.11 ▦ Clinical Care Classification of 201 Nursing Interventions, Version 2.5: Coded with Definitions and Classified by 21 Care Components[1,2]

A. Activity Component

Cluster of elements that involve the use of energy in carrying out musculoskeletal and bodily actions
Activity Care—A01.0
Activities performed to carry out physiological or psychological daily activities
    Energy Conservation—A01.2
    Actions performed taken to preserve energy
Fracture Care—A02.0
Actions performed to control broken bones
    Cast Care—A02.1
    Actions performed to control a rigid dressing
    Immobilizer Care—A02.2
    Actions performed to control a splint, cast, or prescribed bed rest
Mobility Therapy—A03.0
Actions performed to advise and instruct on mobility deficits
    Ambulation Therapy—A03.1
    Actions performed to promote walking
    Assistive Device Therapy—A03.2
    Actions performed to support the use of products to aid in caring for oneself
    Transfer Care—A03.3
    Actions performed to assist in moving from one place to another
Sleep Pattern Control—A04.0
Actions performed to support the sleep/wake cycle
Musculoskeletal Care—A05.0
Actions performed to restore physical functioning
    Range of Motion—A05.1
    Actions performed to provide active and passive exercises to maintain joint function
    Rehabilitation Exercise—A05.2
    Actions performed to promote physical functioning
Bedbound Care—A61.0
Actions performed to support an individual confined to bed
    Positioning Therapy—A61.1
    Process to support changes in body positioning
Diversional Care—A77.0
Actions performed to support interest in leisure activities or play

B. Bowel/Gastric Component

Cluster of elements that involve the gastrointestinal system
Bowel Care—B06.0
Actions performed to control and restore the functioning of the bowel
    Bowel Training—B06.1
    Actions performed to provide instruction on bowel elimination conditions
    Disimpaction—B06.2
    Actions performed to manually remove feces
    Enema—B06.3
    Actions performed to give fluid rectally
    Diarrhea Care—B06.4
    Actions performed to control the abnormal frequency and fluidity of feces
Bowel Ostomy Care—B07.0
Actions performed to maintain the artificial opening that removes bowel waste products
    Bowel Ostomy Irrigation—B07.1
    Actions performed to flush or wash out the artificial opening that removes bowel waste products
Gastric Care—B62.0
Actions performed to control changes in the stomach and intestines
    Nausea Care—B62.1
    Actions performed to control the distaste for food and desire to vomit

(Continued)

TABLE 8.11 ▦ Clinical Care Classification of 201 Nursing Interventions, Version 2.5: Coded with Definitions and Classified by 21 Care Components[1,2] (*Continued*)

C. Cardiac Component

Cluster of elements that involve the heart and blood vessels
Cardiac Care—C08.0
Actions performed to control changes in the heart or blood vessels
    Cardiac Rehabilitation—C08.1
    Actions performed to restore cardiac health
Pacemaker Care—C09.0
Actions performed to control the use of an electronic device that provides a normal heartbeat

D. Cognitive/Neuro Component

Cluster of elements involving the cognitive, mental, cerebral, and neurological processes
Behavior Care—D10.0
Actions performed to support observable responses to internal and external stimuli
Reality Orientation—D11.0
Actions performed to promote the ability to locate oneself in an environment.
Wandering Control—D63.0
Actions performed to control abnormal movability
Memory Loss Care—D64.0
Actions performed to control a person's inability to recall ideas and/or events
Neurological System Care—D78.0
Actions performed to control problems of the neurological system

E. Coping Component

Cluster of elements that involve the ability to deal with responsibilities, problems, or difficulties
Counseling Service—E12.0
Actions performed to provide advice or instruction to help another
    Coping Support—E12.1
    Actions performed to sustain a person dealing with responsibilities, problems, or difficulties
    Stress Control—E12.2
    Actions performed to support the physiological response of the body to a stimulus
    Crisis Therapy—E12.3
    Actions performed to sustain a person dealing with a condition, event, or radical change in status
Emotional Support—E13.0
Actions performed to maintain a positive affective state
    Spiritual Comfort—E13.1
    Actions performed to console, restore, or promote spiritual health
Terminal Care—E14.0
Actions performed in the period surrounding death
    Bereavement Support—E14.1
    Actions performed to provide comfort to the family/friends of the person who died
    Dying/Death Measures—E14.2
    Actions performed to support the dying process
    Funeral Arrangements—E14.3
    Actions performed to direct the preparation of measures for burial

F. Fluid Volume Component

Cluster of elements that involve liquid consumption
Fluid Therapy—F15.0
Actions performed to provide liquid volume intake
    Hydration Control—F15.1
    Actions performed to control the state of fluid balance

TABLE 8.11 ■ (*Continued*)

Intake—F15.3
Actions performed to measure the amount of fluid volume taken into the body
Output—F15.4
Actions performed to measure the amount of fluid volume removed from the body
Hemodynamic Care—F79.0
Actions performed to support the movement of solutions through the blood
Intravenous Care—F79.1
Actions performed to support the use of infusion equipment
Venous Catheter Care—F79.2
Actions performed to support the use of a venous infusion site
Arterial Catheter Care—F79.3
Actions performed to support the use of an arterial infusion site

G.   Health Behavior Component

Cluster of elements that involve actions to sustain, maintain, or regain health
Community Special Services—G17.0
Actions performed to provide advice or information about special community services
  Adult Day Center—G17.1
  Actions performed to direct the provision of a day program for adults in a specific location
  Hospice—G17.2
  Actions performed to support the provision of offering and/or providing care for terminally ill persons
  Meals on Wheels—G17.3
  Actions performed to direct the provision of a community program of delivering meals to the home
Compliance Care—G18.0
Actions performed to encourage adherence to care regimen
  Compliance with Diet—G18.1
  Actions performed to encourage adherence to diet/food intake
  Compliance with Fluid Volume—G18.2
  Actions performed to encourage adherence to therapeutic intake of liquids
  Compliance with Medical Regimen—G18.3
  Actions performed to encourage adherence to physician's/provider's treatment plan
  Compliance with Medication Regimen—G18.4
  Actions performed to encourage adherence to prescribed course of medicinal substances
  Compliance with Safety Precaution—G18.5
  Actions performed to encourage adherence with measures to protect self or others from injury, danger, or loss
  Compliance with Therapeutic Regimen—G18.6
  Actions performed to encourage adherence with plan of care
Nursing Contact—G19.0
Actions performed to communicate with another nurse
  Bill of Rights—G19.1
  Statements related to entitlements during an episode of illness
  Nursing Care Coordination—G19.2
  Actions performed to synthesize all plans of care by a nurse
  Nursing Status Report—G19.3
  Actions performed to document patient condition by a nurse
Physician Contact—G20.0
Actions performed to communicate with a physician/provider
  Medical Regimen Orders—G20.1
  Actions performed to support the physician's/provider's plan of treatment
  Physician Status Report—G20.2
  Actions performed to document patient condition by a physician/provider
Professional/Ancillary Service—G21.0
Actions performed to support the duties performed by health team members

(Continued)

TABLE 8.11 ▦ Clinical Care Classification of 201 Nursing Interventions, Version 2.5: Coded with Definitions and Classified by 21 Care Components[1,2] (*Continued*)

Health Aide Service—G21.1
Actions performed to support care services by a health aide
Social Worker Service—G21.2
Actions performed to provide advice or instruction by a social worker
Nurse Specialist Service—G21.3
Actions performed to provide advice or instruction by an advanced practice nurse or nurse practitioner
Occupational Therapist Service—G21.4
Actions performed to provide advice or instruction by an occupational therapist
Physical Therapist Service—G21.5
Actions performed to provide advice or instruction by a physical therapist
Speech Therapist Service—G21.6
Actions performed to provide advice or instruction by a speech therapist
Respiratory Therapist Service—G21.7
Actions performed to provide advice or instruction by a respiratory therapist

H.   Medication Component

Cluster of elements that involve medicinal substances
Chemotherapy Care—H22.0
Actions performed to control and monitor antineoplastic agents
Injection Administration—H23.0
Actions performed to dispense a medication by a hypodermic
Medication Care—H24.0
  Actions performed to support use of prescribed drugs or remedies regardless of route
  Medication Actions—H24.1
  Actions performed to support and monitor the intended responses to prescribed drugs
  Medication Prefill Preparation—H24.2
  Actions performed to ensure the continued supply of prescribed drugs
  Medication Side Effects—H24.3
  Actions performed to control adverse untoward reactions or conditions to prescribed drugs
  Medication Treatment—H23.4
  Actions performed to administer/give drugs or remedies regardless of route
Radiation Therapy Care—H25.0
Actions performed to control and monitor radiation therapy

I.   Metabolic Component

Cluster of elements that involve the endocrine and immunologic processes
Allergic Reaction Care—I26.0
Actions performed to reduce symptoms or precautions to reduce allergies
Diabetic Care—I27.0
Actions performed to support the control of diabetic conditions
Immunologic Care—I65.0
Actions performed to protect against a particular disease

J.   Nutritional Component

Cluster of elements that involve the intake of food and nutrients
Enteral Tube Care—J28.0
Actions performed to control the use of an enteral drainage tube
  Enteral Tube Insertion—J28.1
  Actions performed to support the placement of an enteral drainage tube
  Enteral Tube Irrigation—J28.2
  Actions performed to flush or wash out an enteral tube
Nutrition Care—J29.0
Actions performed to support the intake of food and nutrients

TABLE 8.11 ■ *(Continued)*

Feeding Technique—J29.2
Actions performed to provide special measures to provide nourishment
Regular Diet—J29.3
Actions performed to support the ingestion of food and nutrients from established nutrition standards
Special Diet—J29.4
Actions performed to support the ingestion of food and nutrients prescribed for a specific purpose
Enteral Feeding—J29.5
Actions performed to provide nourishment through a gastrointestinal route
Parenteral Feeding—J29.6
Actions performed to provide nourishment through intravenous or subcutaneous routes
Breastfeeding Support—J66.0
Actions performed to provide nourishment of an infant at the breast
Weight Control—J67.0
Actions performed to control obesity or debilitation

K. Physical Regulation Component

Cluster of elements that involve bodily processes
Infection Control—K30.0
Actions performed to contain a communicable disease
   Universal Precautions—K30.1
   Practices to prevent the spread of infections and infectious diseases
Physical Healthcare—K31.0
Actions performed to support somatic problems
   Health History—K31.1
   Actions performed to obtain information about past illness and health status
   Health Promotion—K31.2
   Actions performed to encourage behaviors to enhance health state
   Physical Examination—K31.3
   Actions performed to observe somatic events
   Clinical Measurements—K31.4
   Actions performed to conduct procedures to evaluate somatic events
Specimen Care—K32.0
Actions performed to direct the collection and/or the examination of a bodily specimen
   Blood Specimen Care—K32.1
   Actions performed to collect and/or examine a sample of blood
   Stool Specimen Care—K32.2
   Actions performed to collect and/or examine a sample of feces
   Urine Specimen Care—K32.3
   Actions performed to collect and/or examine a sample of urine
   Sputum Specimen Care—K32.5
   Actions performed to collect and/or examine a sample of sputum
Vital Signs—K33.0
Actions performed to measure temperature, pulse, respiration, and blood pressure
   Blood Pressure—K33.1
   Actions performed to measure the diastolic and systolic pressure of the blood
   Temperature—K33.2
   Actions performed to measure body temperature
   Pulse—K33.3
   Actions performed to measure rhythmic beats of the heart
   Respiration—K33.4
   Actions performed to measure the function of breathing

(Continued)

TABLE 8.11 ■ Clinical Care Classification of 201 Nursing Interventions, Version 2.5: Coded with Definitions and Classified by 21 Care Components[1,2] (*Continued*)

L.   Respiratory Component

Cluster of elements that involve breathing and the pulmonary system
Oxygen Therapy Care—L35.0
Actions performed to support the administration of oxygen treatment
Pulmonary Care—L36.0
Actions performed to support pulmonary hygiene
    Breathing Exercises—L36.1
    Actions performed to provide therapy on respiratory or lung exertion
    Chest Physiotherapy—L36.2
    Actions performed to provide exercises to provide postural drainage of lungs
    Inhalation Therapy—L36.3
    Actions performed to support breathing treatments
    Ventilator Care—L36.4
    Actions performed to control and monitor the use of a ventilator
Tracheostomy Care—L37.0
Actions performed to support a tracheostomy

M.   Role Relationship Component

Cluster of elements involving interpersonal, work, social, family, and sexual interactions
Communication Care—M38.0
Actions performed to exchange verbal/nonverbal and/or translation of information
Psychosocial Care—M39.0
Actions performed to support the study of psychological and social factors
    Home Situation Analysis—M39.1
    Actions performed to analyze the living environment
    Interpersonal Dynamics Analysis—M39.2
    Actions performed to support the analysis of the driving forces in a relationship between people
    Family Process Analysis—M39.3
    Actions performed to support the change and/or modification of a related group
    Sexual Behavior Analysis—M39.4
    Actions performed to support the change and/or modification of a person's sexual response
    Social Network Analysis—M39.5
    Actions performed to improve the quantity or quality of personal relationships

N.   Safety Component

Cluster of elements that involve prevention of injury, danger, loss, or abuse
Substance Abuse Control—N40.0
Actions performed to control substances to avoid, detect, or minimize harm
    Tobacco Abuse Control—N40.1
    Actions performed to avoid, minimize, or control the use of tobacco
    Alcohol Abuse Control—N40.2
    Actions performed to avoid, minimize, or control the use of distilled liquors
    Drug Abuse Control—N40.3
    Actions performed to avoid, minimize, or control the use of any habit-forming medication
Emergency Care—N41.0
Actions performed to support a sudden or unexpected occurrence
Safety Precautions—N42.0
Actions performed to advance measures to avoid, danger, or harm
    Environmental Safety—N42.1
    Precautions recommended to prevent or reduce environmental injury
    Equipment Safety—N42.2
    Precautions recommended to prevent or reduce equipment injury
    Individual Safety—N42.3
    Precautions to reduce individual injury

TABLE 8.11 ▦ (*Continued*)

Violence Control—N68.0
Actions performed to control behaviors that may cause harm to oneself or others
Perioperative Injury Care—N80.0
Actions performed to support perioperative care requirements

O. Self-Care Component

Cluster of elements that involve the ability to carry out activities to maintain oneself
Personal Care—O43.0
Actions performed to care for oneself
   Activities of Daily Living—O43.1
   Actions performed to support personal activities to maintain oneself
   Instrumental Activities of Daily Living—043.2
   Complex activities performed to support basic life skills

P. Self-Concept Component

Cluster of elements that involve an individual's mental image of oneself
Mental Healthcare—P45.0
Actions taken to promote emotional well-being
   Mental Health History—P45.1
   Actions performed to obtain information about past or present emotional well-being
   Mental Health Promotion—P45.2
   Actions performed to encourage or further emotional well-being
   Mental Health Screening—P45.3
   Actions performed to systematically examine emotional well-being
   Mental Health Treatment—P45.4
   Actions performed to support protocols used to treat emotional problems

Q. Sensory Component

Cluster of elements that involve the senses, including pain
Pain Control—Q47.0
Actions performed to support responses to injury or damage
   Acute Pain Control—Q47.1
   Actions performed to control physical suffering, hurting, or distress
   Chronic Pain Control—Q47.2
   Actions performed to control physical suffering, hurting, or distress that continues longer than expected
Comfort Care—Q48.0
Actions performed to enhance or improve well-being
Ear Care—Q49.0
Actions performed to support ear problems
   Hearing Aid Care—Q49.1
   Actions performed to control the use of a hearing aid
   Wax Removal—Q49.2
   Actions performed to remove cerumen from the ear
Eye Care—Q50.0
Actions performed to support eye problems
   Cataract Care—Q50.1
   Actions performed to control cataract conditions
   Vision Care—Q50.2
   Actions performed to control vision problems

R. Skin Integrity Component

Cluster of elements that involve the mucous membrane, corneal, integumentary, or subcutaneous structures of the body
Pressure Ulcer Care—R51.0
Actions performed to prevent, detect, and treat skin integrity breakdown caused by pressure

(Continued)

TABLE 8.11 ■ Clinical Care Classification of 201 Nursing Interventions, Version 2.5: Coded with Definitions and Classified by 21 Care Components[1,2] (*Continued*)

Pressure Ulcer Stage 1 Care—R51.1
Actions performed to prevent, detect, and treat stage 1 skin breakdown
Pressure Ulcer Stage 2 Care—R51.2
Actions performed to prevent, detect, and treat stage 2 skin breakdown
Pressure Ulcer Stage 3 Care—R51.3
Actions performed to prevent, detect, and treat stage 3 skin breakdown
Pressure Ulcer Stage 4 Care—R51.4
Actions performed to prevent, detect, and treat stage 4 skin breakdown
Mouth Care—R53.0
Actions performed to support oral cavity problems
Denture Care—R53.1
Actions performed to control the use of artificial teeth
Skin Care—R54.0
Actions to control the integument/skin
Skin Breakdown Control—R54.1
Actions performed to support integument/skin problems
Wound Care—R55.0
Actions performed to support open skin areas
Drainage Tube Care—R55.1
Actions performed to support wound drainage from body tubes
Dressing Change—R55.2
Actions performed to remove and replace a new bandage on a wound
Incision Care—R55.3
Actions performed to support a surgical wound
Burn Care—R81.0
Actions performed to support burned areas of the body

S. Tissue Perfusion Component

Cluster of elements that involve the oxygenation of tissues, including the circulatory and vascular systems
Foot Care—S56.0
Actions performed to support foot problems
Perineal Care—S57.0
Actions performed to support perineal problems
Edema Control—S69.0
Actions performed to control excess fluid in tissue
Circulatory Care—S70.0
Actions performed to support the circulation of the blood (blood vessels)
Vascular System Care—S82.0
Actions performed to control problems of the vascular system

T. Urinary Elimination Component

Cluster of elements that involve the genitourinary system
Bladder Care—T58.0
Actions performed to control urinary drainage problems
Bladder Instillation—T58.1
Actions performed to pour liquid through a catheter into the bladder
Bladder Training—T58.2
Actions performed to provide instruction on the care of urinary drainage
Dialysis Care—T59.0
Actions performed to support the removal of waste products from the body
Hemodialysis Care—T59.1
Actions performed to support the mechanical removal of waste products from the blood
Peritoneal Dialysis Care—T59.2
Actions performed to support the osmotic removal of waste products from the blood

TABLE 8.11 ■ *(Continued)*

Urinary Catheter Care—T60.0
Actions performed to control the use of a urinary catheter
    Urinary Catheter Insertion—T60.1
    Actions performed to place a urinary catheter into the bladder
    Urinary Catheter Irrigation—T60.2
    Actions performed to flush a urinary catheter
Urinary Incontinence Care—T72.0
Actions performed to control the inability to retain and/or involuntary retain urine
Renal Care—T73.0
Actions performed to control problems pertaining to the kidney
Bladder Ostomy Care—T83.0
Actions performed to maintain the artificial opening to remove urine
    Bladder Ostomy Irrigation—T83.1
    Actions performed to flush or wash out the artificial opening to remove urine

U.   Life Cycle Component

Cluster of elements that involve the life span of individuals
Reproductive Care—U74.0
Actions performed to support the production of an offspring/child
    Fertility Care—U74.1
    Actions performed to increase the chance of conception of an offspring/child
    Infertility Care—U74.2
    Actions performed to promote conception by the infertile client of an offspring/child
    Contraception Care—U74.3
    Actions performed to prevent conception of an offspring/child
Perinatal Care—U75.0
Actions performed to support the period before, during, and immediately after the creation of an offspring/child
    Pregnancy Care—U75.1
    Actions performed to support the gestation period of the formation of an offspring/child (being with child)
    Labor Care—U75.2
    Actions performed to support the bringing forth of an offspring/child
    Delivery Care—U75.3
    Actions performed to support the expulsion of an offspring/child at birth
    Postpartum Care—U75.4
    Actions performed to support the period immediately after the delivery of an offspring/child
Growth and Development Care—U76.0
Actions performed to support age-specific normal growth standards and/or development skills

[1] Clinical Care Classification (CCC) System, Version 2.5 (previously known as: (a) Clinical Care Classification (CCC) System, Version 2.0, Copyright © 2004; and (b) Home Healthcare Classification (HHCC) System, Version 1.0, Copyright © 1994] pending Copyright © 2012 by Virginia K. Saba. EdD, RN, FAAN, FACMI, LL, may be used ONLY with written Permission by Dr. Virginia K. Saba. (Permission Form available from website <http://www.sabacare.com>)

[2] Revised 1992, 1994, 2004, 2006, and 2011.

TABLE 8.12 ■ Clinical Care Classification of 201 Nursing Interventions, Version 2.5: Coded Alphabetically with Definitions[1,2]

O43.1   Activities of Daily Living
Personal activities to maintain oneself

A01.0   Activity Care
Actions performed to carry out physiological and psychological daily activities

Q47.1   Acute Pain Control
Actions performed to control physical suffering, hurting, or distress

G17.1   Adult Day Center
Actions performed to direct the provision of a day program for adults in a specific location

N40.2   Alcohol Abuse Control
Actions performed to avoid, minimize, or control the use of distilled liquors

I26.0   Allergic Reaction Control
Actions performed to reduce symptoms or precautions to reduce allergies

A03.1   Ambulation Therapy
Actions performed to promote walking

F79.3   Arterial Catheter Care
Actions performed to support the use of an arterial infusion site

A03.2   Assistive Device Therapy
Actions performed to support the use of products to aid in caring for oneself

A61.0   Bedbound Care
Actions performed to support an individual confined to bed

D10.0   Behavior Care
Actions performed to support observable responses to internal and external stimuli

E14.1   Bereavement Support
Actions performed to provide comfort to the family/friends of the person who died

G19.1   Bill of Rights
Statements related to entitlement during an episode of illness

T58.0   Bladder Care
Actions performed to control urinary drainage problems

T58.1   Bladder Instillation
Actions performed to pour liquid into a catheter

T83.0   Bladder Ostomy Care
Actions performed to maintain the artificial opening to remove urine

T83.1   Bladder Ostomy Irrigation
Actions performed to flush or wash out the artificial opening to remove urine

T58.2   Bladder Training
Actions performed to provide instruction on the care of urinary drainage problems

K33.1   Blood Pressure
Actions performed to measure the diastolic and systolic pressure of the blood

K32.1   Blood Specimen Care
Actions performed to collect and/or examine a sample of blood

B06.0   Bowel Care
Actions performed to control or restore the functioning of the bowel

B07.0   Bowel Ostomy Care
Actions performed to maintain the artificial opening that removes bowel waste products

B07.1   Bowel Ostomy Irrigation
Actions performed to flush or wash out the artificial opening that removes bowel waste products

B06.1   Bowel Training
Actions performed to provide instruction on bowel elimination conditions

J66.0   Breastfeeding Support
Actions performed to support nourishment of an infant at the breast

L36.1   Breathing Exercises
Actions performed to provide therapy on respiratory or lung exertion

R81.0   Burn Care
Actions performed to support burned areas of the body

TABLE 8.12 ▨ (*Continued*)

C08.0   Cardiac Care
Actions performed to control changes in the heart or blood vessels

C08.1   Cardiac Rehabilitation
Actions performed to restore cardiac health

A02.1   Cast Care
Actions performed to control a rigid dressing

Q50.1   Cataract Care
Actions performed to control cataract conditions

H22.0   Chemotherapy Care
Actions performed to control and monitor antineoplastic agents

L36.2   Chest Physiotherapy
Exercises to provide postural drainage of lungs

Q47.2   Chronic Pain Control
Actions performed to control physical suffering, hurting, or distress that continues longer than expected

S70.0   Circulatory Care
Actions performed to support the circulation of the blood (blood vessels)

K31.4   Clinical Measurements
Actions performed to conduct procedures to evaluate somatic events

Q48.0   Comfort Care
Actions performed to enhance or improve well-being

M38.0   Communication Care
Actions performed to exchange verbal/nonverbal and/or translation of information

G17.0   Community Special Services
Actions performed to provide advice or information about special community services

G18.0   Compliance Care
Actions performed to encourage adherence to care regimen

G18.1   Compliance with Diet
Actions performed to encourage adherence to diet/food intake

G18.2   Compliance with Fluid Volume
Actions performed to encourage adherence to therapeutic intake of liquids

G18.3   Compliance with Medical Regimen
Actions performed to encourage adherence to physician's/provider's treatment plan

G18.4   Compliance with Medication Regimen
Actions performed to encourage adherence to follow prescribed course of medicinal substances

G18.5   Compliance with Safety Precautions
Actions performed to encourage adherence with measures to protect self or others from injury, danger, or loss

G18.6   Compliance with Therapeutic Regimen
Actions performed to encourage adherence with the plan of care

U74.3   Contraception Care
Actions performed to prevent conception of an offspring/child

E12.1   Coping Support
Actions performed to sustain a person dealing with responsibilities, problems, or difficulties

E12.0   Counseling Service
Actions performed to provide advice or instruction to help another

E12.3   Crisis Therapy
Actions performed to sustain a person dealing with a condition, event, or radical change in status

U75.3   Delivery Care
Actions performed to support the expulsion of an offspring/child at birth

R53.1   Denture Care
Actions performed to control the use of artificial teeth

(*Continued*)

TABLE 8.12 ▦ Clinical Care Classification of 201 Nursing Interventions, Version 2.5: Coded Alphabetically with Definitions[1,2] (*Continued*)

I27.0   Diabetic Care
Actions performed to control diabetic conditions

T59.0   Dialysis Care
Actions performed to support the removal of waste products from the body

B06.4   Diarrhea Care
Actions performed to control the abnormal frequency and fluidity of feces

B06.2   Disimpaction
Actions performed to manually remove feces

A77.0   Diversional Care
Actions performed to support interest in leisure activities or play

R55.1   Drainage Tube Care
Actions performed to support wound drainage from body tubes

R55.2   Dressing Change
Actions performed to remove and replace new bandage(s) on a wound

N40.3   Drug Abuse Control
Actions performed to avoid, minimize, or control the use of any habit-forming medication

E14.2   Dying/Death Measures
Actions performed to support the dying process

Q49.0   Ear Care
Actions performed to support ear problems

S69.0   Edema Control
Actions performed to control excess fluid in tissue

N41.0   Emergency Care
Actions performed to support a sudden or unexpected occurrence

E13.0   Emotional Support
Actions performed to sustain a positive affective state

B06.3   Enema
Actions performed to give fluid rectally

A01.2   Energy Conservation
Actions performed to preserve energy

J29.5   Enteral Feeding
Actions performed to provide nourishment through a gastrointestinal route

J28.0   Enteral Tube Care
Actions performed to control the use of an enteral drainage tube

J28.1   Enteral Tube Insertion
Actions performed in the placement of an enteral drainage tube

J28.2   Enteral Tube Irrigation
Actions performed to flush or wash out an enteral tube

N42.1   Environmental Safety
Precautions recommended to prevent or reduce environmental injury

N42.2   Equipment Safety
Precautions recommended to prevent or reduce equipment injury

Q50.0   Eye Care
Actions performed to support eye problems

M39.3   Family Process Analysis
Actions performed to support the change and/or modification of a related group

J29.2   Feeding Technique
Actions performed to provide special measures to provide nourishment

U74.1   Fertility Care
Actions performed to increase the chance of conception of an offspring/child

F15.0   Fluid Therapy
Actions performed to provide liquid volume intake

TABLE 8.12 ■ (*Continued*)

S56.0   Foot Care
Actions performed to support foot problems

A02.0   Fracture Care
Actions performed to control broken bones

E14.3   Funeral Arrangements
Actions performed to direct the preparation measures for burial

B62.0   Gastric Care
Actions performed to control changes in the stomach or intestines

U76.0   Growth and Development Care
Actions performed to support age-specific normal growth standards and/or development skills

G21.1   Health Aide Service
Actions performed to support care services by a health aide

K31.1   Health History
Actions performed to obtain information about past illness and health status

K31.2   Health Promotion
Actions performed to encourage behaviors to enhance health state

Q49.1   Hearing Aid Care
Actions performed to control the use of a hearing aid

T59.1   Hemodialysis Care
Actions performed to support the mechanical removal of waste products from the blood

F79.0   Hemodynamic Care
Actions performed to support the movement of solutions through the blood

M39.1   Home Situation Analysis
Analysis of living environment

G17.2   Hospice
Actions performed to support the provision of offering and/or providing care for terminally ill persons

F15.1   Hydration Control
Actions performed to control the state of fluid balance

A02.2   Immobilizer Care
Actions performed to control a splint, cast, or prescribed bed rest

I65.0   Immunologic Care
Actions performed to protect against a particular disease

R55.3   Incision Care
Actions performed to support a surgical wound

N42.3   Individual Safety
Precautions to reduce individual injury

K30.0   Infection Control
Actions performed to contain a communicable illness

U74.2   Infertility Care
Actions performed to promote conception by an infertile client of an offspring/child

L36.3   Inhalation Therapy
Actions performed to support breathing treatments

H23.0   Injection Administration
Actions performed to dispense a medication by a hypodermic

O43.2   Instrumental Activities of Daily Living
Complex activities performed to support basic life skills

F15.3   Intake
Actions performed to measure the amount of fluid volume taken into the body

M39.2   Interpersonal Dynamics Analysis
Analysis of the driving forces in a relationship between people

(*Continued*)

TABLE 8.12 ■ Clinical Care Classification of 201 Nursing Interventions, Version 2.5: Coded Alphabetically with Definitions[1,2] (*Continued*)

F79.1	Intravenous Care	
	Actions performed to support the use of infusion equipment	
U75.2	Labor Care	
	Actions performed to support the bringing forth of an offspring/child	
G17.3	Meals on Wheels	
	Actions performed to direct the provision of a community program of delivering meals to the home	
G20.1	Medical Regimen Orders	
	Actions performed to support the physician's/provider's plan of treatment	
H24.1	Medication Actions	
	Actions performed to support and monitor the intended responses to prescribed drugs	
H24.0	Medication Care	
	Actions performed to support use of prescribed drugs or remedies regardless of route	
H24.2	Medication Prefill Preparation	
	Activities to ensure the continued supply of prescribed drugs	
H24.3	Medication Side Effects	
	Actions performed to control adverse untoward reactions or conditions to prescribed drugs	
H24.4	Medication Treatment	
	Actions performed to administer/give drugs or remedies regardless of route	
D64.0	Memory Loss Care	
	Actions performed to control a person's inability to recall ideas and/or events	
P45.0	Mental Healthcare	
	Actions taken to promote emotional well-being	
P45.1	Mental Health History	
	Actions performed to obtain information about past and present emotional well-being	
P45.2	Mental Health Promotion	
	Actions performed to encourage or further emotional well-being	
P45.3	Mental Health Screening	
	Actions performed to systematically examine emotional well-being	
P45.4	Mental Health Treatment	
	Actions performed to support protocols used to treat emotional problems	
A03.0	Mobility Therapy	
	Actions performed to advise and instruct on mobility deficits	
R53.0	Mouth Care	
	Actions performed to support oral cavity problems	
A05.0	Musculoskeletal Care	
	Actions performed to restore physical functioning	
B62.1	Nausea Care	
	Actions performed to control the distaste for food and desire to vomit	
D78.0	Neurological System Care	
	Actions performed to control problems of the neurological system	
G21.3	Nurse Specialist Service	
	Actions performed to obtain advice or instruction by advanced nurse specialists or nurse practitioners	
G19.2	Nursing Care Coordination	
	Actions performed to synthesize all plans of care	
G19.0	Nursing Contact	
	Actions performed to communicate with another nurse	
G19.3	Nursing Status Report	
	Actions performed to document patient condition by a nurse	
J29.0	Nutrition Care	
	Actions performed to support the intake of food and nutrients	

TABLE 8.12 ■ (*Continued*)

G21.4	Occupational Therapist Service
	Actions performed to provide advice or instruction by an occupational therapist
F15.4	Output
	Actions performed to measure the amount of fluid volume removed from the body
L35.0	Oxygen Therapy Care
	Actions performed to support the administration of oxygen treatment
C09.0	Pacemaker Care
	Actions performed to control the use of an electronic device that provides a normal heartbeat
Q47.0	Pain Control
	Actions performed to support responses to injury or damage
J29.6	Parental Feeding
	Actions performed to provide nourishment through intravenous or subcutaneous routes
U75.0	Perinatal Care
	Actions performed to support the period before, during, and immediately after the creation of an offspring/child
S57.0	Perineal Care
	Actions performed to support perineal problems
N80.0	Perioperative Injury Care
	Actions performed to support perioperative care requirements
T59.2	Peritoneal Dialysis Care
	Actions performed to support the osmotic removal of waste products from the blood
O43.0	Personal Care
	Actions performed to care for oneself
K31.3	Physical Examination
	Actions performed to observe somatic events
K31.0	Physical Healthcare
	Actions performed to support somatic problems
G21.5	Physical Therapist Service
	Actions performed to provide advice or instruction by a physical therapist
G20.0	Physician Contact
	Actions performed to communicate with a physician/provider
G20.2	Physician Status Report
	Actions performed to document patient condition by a physician/provider
A61.1	Positioning Therapy
	Process to support changes in body position
U75.4	Postpartum Care
	Actions performed to support the period immediately after delivery of an offspring/child
U75.1	Pregnancy Care
	Actions performed to support the gestation period of the formation of an offspring/child (being with child)
R51.0	Pressure Ulcer Care
	Actions performed to prevent, detect, and treat skin integrity breakdown caused by pressure
R51.1	Pressure Ulcer Stage 1 Care
	Actions performed to prevent stage 1 skin breakdown
R51.2	Pressure Ulcer Stage 2 Care
	Actions performed to prevent stage 2 skin breakdown
R51.3	Pressure Ulcer Stage 3 Care
	Actions performed to prevent stage 3 skin breakdown
R1.4	Pressure Ulcer Stage 4 Care
	Actions performed to prevent stage 4 skin breakdown

(*Continued*)

TABLE 8.12 ■ Clinical Care Classification of 201 Nursing Interventions, Version 2.5: Coded Alphabetically with Definitions[1,2] (*Continued*)

G21.0	Professional/Ancillary Services	
	Actions performed to support the duties performed by health team members	
M39.0	Psychosocial Care	
	Actions performed to support the study of psychological and social factors	
L36.0	Pulmonary Care	
	Actions performed to support pulmonary hygiene	
K33.3	Pulse	
	Actions performed to measure rhythmic beats of the heart	
H25.0	Radiation Therapy Care	
	Actions performed to control and monitor radiation therapy	
A05.1	Range of Motion	
	Actions performed to provide active or passive exercises to maintain joint function	
D11.0	Reality Orientation	
	Actions performed to promote the ability to locate oneself in environment	
J29.3	Regular Diet	
	Actions performed to support the ingestion of food and nutrients from established nutrition standards	
A05.2	Rehabilitation Exercise	
	Activities to promote physical functioning	
T73.0	Renal Care	
	Actions performed to control problems pertaining to the kidney	
U74.0	Reproductive Care	
	Actions performed to support the production of an offspring/child	
K33.4	Respiration	
	Actions performed to measure the function of breathing	
G21.7	Respiratory Therapist Service	
	Actions performed to provide advice or instruction by a respiratory therapist	
N42.0	Safety Precautions	
	Actions performed to advance measures to avoid injury, danger, or harm	
M39.4	Sexual Behavior Analysis	
	Actions performed to support the change and/or modification of a person's sexual response	
R54.1	Skin Breakdown Control	
	Actions performed to support integument/skin problems	
R54.0	Skin Care	
	Actions performed to control the integument/skin	
A04.0	Sleep Pattern Control	
	Actions performed to support the sleep/wake cycle	
M39.5	Social Network Analysis	
	Actions performed to improve the quantity or quality of personal relationships	
G21.2	Social Worker Service	
	Actions performed to provide advice or instruction by a social worker	
J29.4	Special Diet	
	Actions performed to support the ingestion of food and nutrients prescribed for a specific purpose	
K32.0	Specimen Analysis	
	Actions performed to direct the collection and/or examination of a bodily specimen	
G21.6	Speech Therapist Service	
	Actions performed to provide advice or instruction by a speech therapist	
E13.1	Spiritual Comfort	
	Actions performed to console, restore, or promote spiritual health	
K32.5	Sputum Specimen Care	
	Actions performed to collect and/or examine a sample of sputum	
K32.2	Stool Specimen Care	
	Actions performed to collect and/or examine a sample of feces	

TABLE 8.12 ▨ (*Continued*)

E12.2 Stress Control
Actions performed to support the physiological response of the body to a stimulus
N40.0 Substance Abuse Control
Actions performed to control substances to avoid, detect, or minimize harm

K33.2 Temperature
Actions performed to measure body temperature
E14.0 Terminal Care
Actions performed in the period surrounding death
N40.1 Tobacco Abuse Control
Actions performed to avoid, minimize, or control the use of tobacco products
L37.0 Tracheostomy Care
Actions performed to support a tracheostomy
A03.3 Transfer Care
Actions performed to assist in moving from one place to another

T60.0 Urinary Catheter Care
Actions performed to control the use of a urinary catheter
T60.1 Urinary Catheter Insertion
Actions performed to place a urinary catheter in bladder
T60.2 Urinary Catheter irrigation
Actions performed to flush out a urinary catheter
T72.0 Urinary Incontinence Care
Actions performed to control the inability to retain and/or involuntary retain urine
K32.3 Urine Specimen Care
Actions performed to collect and/or examine a sample of urine
K30.1 Universal Precautions
Practices to prevent spread of infection and infectious diseases

S82.0 Vascular System Care
Actions performed to control problems of the vascular system
F79.2 Venous Catheter Care
Actions performed to support the use of a venous infusion site
L36.4 Ventilator Care
Actions performed to control and monitor the use of a ventilator
N68.0 Violence Control
Actions performed to control behaviors that may cause harm to oneself or others
Q50.2 Vision Care
Actions performed to control vision problems
K33.0 Vital Signs
Actions performed to measure temperature, pulse, respirations, and blood pressure

D63.0 Wandering Control
Actions performed to control abnormal movability
Q49.2 Wax Removal
Actions performed to remove cerumen from the ear
J67.0 Weight Control
Actions performed to control obesity or debilitation
R55.0 Wound Care
Actions performed to support open skin areas

[1] Clinical Care Classification (CCC) System, Version 2.5 (previously known as: (a) Clinical Care Classification (CCC) System, Version 2.0, Copyright © 2004; and (b) Home Healthcare Classification (HHCC) System, Version 1.0, Copyright © 1994] pending Copyright © 2012 by Virginia K. Saba. EdD, RN, FAAN, FACMI, LL, may be used ONLY with written Permission by Dr. Virginia K. Saba. (Permission Form available from website <http://www.sabacare.com>)

[2] Revised 1992, 1994, 2004, 2006, and 2011.

TABLE 8.13 ■ Clinical Care Classification of 201 Nursing Interventions, Version 2.5: Listed Alphabetically by Code Numbers[1,2]

Activities of Daily Living	O43.1
Activity Care	A01.0
Acute Pain Control	Q47.1
Adult Day Center	G17.1
Alcohol Abuse Control	N40.2
Allergic Reaction Analysis	I26.0
Ambulation Therapy	A03.1
Arterial Catheter Care	F79.3
Assistive Device Therapy	A03.2
Bedbound Care	A61.0
Behavior Care	D10.0
Bereavement Support	E14.1
Bill of Rights	G19.1
Bladder Care	T58.0
Bladder Instillation	T58.1
Bladder Ostomy Care	T83.0
Bladder Ostomy Irrigation	T83.1
Bladder Training	T58.2
Blood Pressure	K33.1
Blood Specimen Care	K32.1
Bowel Care	B06.0
Bowel Ostomy Care	B07.0
Bowel Ostomy Irrigation	B07.1
Bowel Training	B06.1
Breastfeeding Support	J66.0
Breathing Exercises	L36.1
Burn Care	R81.0
Cardiac Care	C08.0
Cardiac Rehabilitation	C08.1
Cast Care	A02.1
Cataract Care	Q50.1
Chemotherapy Care	H22.0
Chest Physiotherapy	L36.2
Chronic Pain Control	Q47.2
Circulatory Care	S70.0
Clinical Measurements	K31.4
Comfort Care	Q48.0
Communication Care	M38.0
Community Special Services	G17.0
Compliance Care	G18.0
Compliance with Diet	G18.1
Compliance with Fluid Volume	G18.2
Compliance with Medical Regimen	G18.3
Compliance with Medication Regimen	G18.4
Compliance with Safety Precautions	G18.5
Compliance with Therapeutic Regimen	G18.6
Contraception Care	U74.3
Coping Support	E12.1
Counseling Services	E12.0
Crisis Therapy	E12.3

TABLE 8.13 ■ (*Continued*)

Delivery Care U75.3
Denture Care R53.1
Diabetic Care I27.0
Dialysis Care T59.0
Diarrhea Care B06.4
Disimpaction B06.2
Diversional Care A77.0
Drainage Tube Care R55.1
Dressing Change R55.2
Drug Abuse Control N40.3
Dying/Death Measures E14.2

Ear Care Q49.0
Edema Control S69.0
Emergency Care N41.0
Emotional Support E13.0
Enema B06.3
Energy Conservation A01.2
Enteral Feeding J29.5
Enteral Tube Care J28.0
Enteral Tube Insertion J28.1
Enteral Tube Irrigation J28.2
Environmental Safety N42.1
Equipment Safety N42.2
Eye Care Q50.0

Family Process Analysis M39.3
Feeding Technique J29.2
Fertility Care U74.1
Fluid Therapy F15.0
Foot Care S56.0
Fracture Care A02.0
Funeral Arrangements E14.3

Gastric Care B62.0
Growth and Development Care U76.0

Health Aide Service G21.1
Health History K31.1
Health Promotion K31.2
Hearing Aid Care Q49.1
Hemodialysis Care T59.1
Hemodynamic Care F79.0
Home situation Analysis M39.1
Hospice G17.2
Hydration Control F15.1

Immobilizer Care A02.2
Immunologic Care I65.0
Incision Care R55.3
Individual Safety N42.3
Infection Control K30.0
Infertility Care U74.2

(*Continued*)

TABLE 8.13 ■ Clinical Care Classification of 201 Nursing Interventions, Version 2.5: Listed Alphabetically by Code Numbers[1,2] (*Continued*)

Inhalation Therapy	L36.3
Injection Administration	H23.0
Instrumental Activities of Daily living	O43.2
Intake	F15.3
Interpersonal Dynamics Analysis	M39.2
Intravenous Care	F79.1
Labor Care	U75.2
Meals on Wheels	G17.3
Medical Regimen Orders	G20.1
Medication Actions	H24.1
Medication Care	H24.0
Medication Prefill Preparation	H24.2
Medication Side Effects	H24.3
Medication Treatment	H24.4
Memory Loss Care	D64.0
Mental Healthcare	P45.0
Mental Health History	P45.1
Mental Health Promotion	P45.2
Mental Health Screening	P45.3
Mental Health Treatment	P45.4
Mobility Therapy	A03.0
Mouth Care	R53.0
Musculoskeletal Care	A05.0
Nausea Care	B62.1
Neurological System Care	D78.0
Nurse Specialist Service	G21.3
Nursing Care Coordination	G19.2
Nursing Contact	G19.0
Nursing Status Report	G19.3
Nutrition Care	J29.0
Occupational Therapist Service	G21.4
Output	F15.4
Oxygen Therapy Care	L35.0
Pacemaker Care	C09.0
Pain Control	Q47.0
Parental Feeding	J29.6
Perinatal Care	U75.0
Perineal Care	S57.0
Perioperative Injury Care	N80.0
Peritoneal Dialysis Care	T59.2
Personal Care	O43.0
Physical Examination	K31.3
Physical Healthcare	K31.0
Physical Therapist Services	G21.5
Physician Contact	G20.0
Physician Status Report	G20.2

TABLE 8.13 ▦ (*Continued*)

Positioning Therapy A61.1
Postpartum Care U75.4
Pregnancy Care U75.1
Pressure Ulcer Care R51.0
Pressure Ulcer Stage 1 Care..R51.1
Pressure Ulcer Stage 2 Care R51.2
Pressure Ulcer Stage 3 Care..R51.3
Pressure Ulcer Stage 4 Care..R51.4
Professional/Ancillary Services... G21.0
Psychosocial Care M39.0
Pulmonary Care L36.0
Pulse K33.3

Radiation Therapy Care.. H25.0
Range of Motion..A05.1
Reality Orientation..D11.0
Regular Diet J29.3
Rehabilitation Exercise A05.2
Renal Care...T73.0
Reproductive Care U74.0
Respiration...K33.4
Respiratory Therapist Service G21.7

Safety Precautions N42.0
Sexual Behavior Analysis..M39.4
Skin Breakdown Control R54.1
Skin Care..R54.0
Sleep Pattern Control...A04.0
Social Network Analysis...M39.5
Social Worker Service G21.2
Special Diet.. J29.4
Specimen Care..K32.0
Speech Therapist Service G21.6
Spiritual Comfort... E13.1
Sputum Specimen Care...K32.5
Stool Specimen Care K32.2
Stress Control E12.2
Substance Abuse Control N40.0

Temperature..K33.2
Terminal Care E14.0
Tobacco Abuse Control... N40.1
Tracheostomy Care... L37.0
Transfer Care A03.3

Universal Precautions...K30.1
Urinary Catheter Care..T60.0
Urinary Catheter Insertion T60.1
Urinary Catheter Irrigation T60.2
Urinary Incontinence Care T72.0
Urine Specimen Care K23.3

(*Continued*)

TABLE 8.13 ■ Clinical Care Classification of 201 Nursing Interventions, Version 2.5: Listed Alphabetically by Code Numbers[1,2] (*Continued*)

Vascular System Care	S82.0
Venous Catheter Care	F79.2
Ventilator Care	L36.4
Violence Control	N68.0
Vision Care	Q50.2
Vital Signs	K33.0
Wandering Control	D63.0
Wax Removal	Q49.2
Weight Control	J67.0
Wound Care	R55.0

[1] Clinical Care Classification (CCC) System, Version 2.5 (previously known as: (a) Clinical Care Classification (CCC) System, Version 2.0, Copyright © 2004; and (b) Home Healthcare Classification (HHCC) System, Version 1.0, Copyright © 1994] pending Copyright © 2012 by Virginia K. Saba. EdD, RN, FAAN, FACMI, LL, may be used ONLY with written Permission by Dr. Virginia K. Saba. (Permission Form available from website <http://www.sabacare.com>)

[2] Revised 1992, 1994, 2004, 2006, and 2011.

TABLE 8.14 ▦ Clinical Care Classification of 201 Nursing Interventions, Version 2.5: Coded with Definitions and Four Action Types and Classified by 21 Care Components[1,2]

Assess/monitor   *Collect and analyze data on the health status*
Care/perform   *Perform a therapeutic action*
Teach/instruct   *Provide knowledge and skill*
Manage/refer   *Coordinate care process*

A.   Activity Component

Cluster of elements that involve the use of energy in carrying out musculoskeletal and bodily actions
Activity Care—A01.0
Activities performed to carry out physiological or psychological daily activities
A01.0.1   Assess Activity Care
A01.0.2   Perform Activity Care
A01.0.3   Teach Activity Care
A01.0.4   Manage Activity Care
　Energy Conservation—A01.2
　Actions performed to preserve energy
　A01.2.1   Assess Energy Conservation
　A01.2.2   Perform Energy Conservation
　A01.2.3   Teach Energy Conservation
　A01.2.4   Manage Energy Conservation
Fracture Care—A02.0
Actions performed to control broken bones
A02.0.1   Assess Fracture Care
A02.0.2   Perform Fracture Care
A02.0.3   Teach Fracture Care
A02.0.4   Manage Fracture Care
　Cast Care—A02.1
　Actions performed to control a rigid dressing
　A02.1.1   Assess Cast Care
　A02.1.2   Perform Cast Care
　A02.1.3   Teach Cast Care
　A02.1.4   Manage Cast Care
　Immobilizer Care—A02.2
　Actions performed to control a splint, cast, or prescribed bed rest
　A02.2.1   Assess Immobilizer Care
　A02.2.2   Perform Immobilizer Care
　A02.2.3   Teach Immobilizer Care
　A02.2.4   Manage Immobilizer Care
Mobility Therapy—A03.0
Actions performed to advise and instruct on mobility deficits
A03.0.1   Assess Mobility Therapy
A03.0.2   Perform Mobility Therapy
A03.0.3   Teach Mobility Therapy
A03.0.4   Manage Mobility Therapy
　Ambulation Therapy—A03.1
　Actions performed to promote walking
　A03.1.1   Assess Ambulation Therapy
　A03.1.2   Perform Ambulation Therapy
　A03.1.3   Teach Ambulation Therapy
　A03.1.4   Manage Ambulation Therapy

(Continued)

TABLE 8.14 ■ Clinical Care Classification of 201 Nursing Interventions, Version 2.5: Coded with Definitions and Four Action Types and Classified by 21 Care Components[1,2] (*Continued*)

Assistive Device Therapy—A03.2
Actions performed to support the use of products to aid in caring for oneself
A03.2.1   Assess Assistive Device Therapy
A03.2.2   Perform Assistive Device Therapy
A03.2.3   Teach Assistive Device Therapy
A03.2.4   Manage Assistive Device Therapy

Transfer Care—A03.3
Actions performed to assist in moving from one place to another
A03.3.1   Assess Transfer Care
A03.3.2   Perform Transfer Care
A03.3.3   Teach Transfer Care
A03.3.4   Manage Transfer Care

Sleep Pattern Control—A04.0
Actions performed to support the sleep/wake cycle
A04.0.1   Assess Sleep Pattern Control
A04.0.2   Perform Sleep Pattern Control
A04.0.3   Teach Sleep Pattern Control
A04.0.4   Manage Sleep Pattern Control

Musculoskeletal Care—A05.0
Actions performed to restore physical functioning
A05.0.1   Assess Rehabilitation Care
A05.0.2   Perform Rehabilitation Care
A05.0.3   Teach Rehabilitation Care
A05.0.4   Manage Rehabilitation Care

Range of Motion—A05.1
Actions performed to provide active and passive exercises to maintain joint function
A05.1.1   Assess Range of Motion
A05.1.2   Perform Range of Motion
A05.1.3   Teach Range of Motion
A05.1.4   Manage Range of Motion

Rehabilitation Exercise—A05.2
Actions performed to promote physical functioning
A05.2.1   Assess Rehabilitation Exercise
A05.2.2   Perform Rehabilitation Exercise
A05.2.3   Teach Rehabilitation Exercise
A05.2.4   Manage Rehabilitation Exercise

Bedbound Care—A61.0
Actions performed to support an individual confined to bed
A61.0.1   Assess Bedbound Care
A61.0.2   Perform Bedbound Care
A61.0.3   Teach Bedbound Care
A61.0.4   Manage Bedbound Care

Positioning Therapy—A61.1
Process to support changes in body positioning
A61.1.1   Assess Positioning Therapy
A61.1.2   Perform Positioning Therapy
A61.1.3   Teach Positioning Therapy
A61.1.4   Manage Positioning Therapy

Diversional Care—A77.0
Actions performed to support interest in leisure activities or play
A77.0.1   Assess Diversional Care
A77.0.2   Perform Diversional Care
A77.0.3   Teach Diversional Care
A77.0.4   Manage Diversional Care

TABLE 8.14 ■ (*Continued*)

B. Bowel/Gastric Component

Cluster of elements that involve the gastrointestinal system
Bowel Care—B06.0
Actions performed to control and restore the functioning of the bowel
B06.0.1   Assess Bowel Care
B06.0.2   Perform Bowel Care
B06.0.3   Teach Bowel Care
B06.0.4   Manage Bowel Care

   Bowel Training—B06.1
   Actions performed to provide instruction on bowel elimination conditions
   B06.1.1   Assess Bowel Training
   B06.1.2   Perform Bowel Training
   B06.1.3   Teach Bowel Training
   B06.1.4   Manage Bowel Training

   Disimpaction—B06.2
   Actions performed to manually remove feces
   B06.2.1   Assess Disimpaction
   B06.2.2   Perform Disimpaction
   B06.2.3   Teach Disimpaction
   B06.2.4   Manage Disimpaction

   Enema—B06.3
   Actions performed to give fluid rectally
   B06.3.1   Assess Enema
   B06.3.2   Perform Enema
   B06.3.3   Teach Enema
   B06.3.4   Manage Enema

   Diarrhea Care—B06.4
   Actions performed to control the abnormal frequency and fluidity of feces
   B06.4.1   Assess Diarrhea Care
   B06.4.2   Perform Diarrhea Care
   B06.4.3   Teach Diarrhea Care
   B06.4.4   Manage Diarrhea Care

Bowel Ostomy Care—B07.0
Actions performed to maintain the artificial opening that removes bowel waste products
B07.0.1   Assess Bowel Ostomy Care
B07.0.2   Perform Bowel Ostomy Care
B07.0.3   Teach Bowel Ostomy Care
B07.0.4   Manage Bowel Ostomy Care

   Bowel Ostomy Irrigation—B07.1
   Actions performed to flush or wash out the artificial opening that removes bowel waste products
   B07.1.1   Assess Bowel Ostomy Irrigation
   B07.1.2   Perform Bowel Ostomy Irrigation
   B07.1.3   Teach Bowel Ostomy Irrigation
   B07.1.4   Manage Bowel Ostomy Irrigation

Gastric Care—B62.0
Actions performed to control changes in the stomach and intestines
B62.0.1   Assess Gastric Care
B62.0.2   Perform Gastric Care
B62.0.3   Teach Gastric Care
B62.0.4   Manage Gastric Care

   Nausea Care—B62.1
   Actions performed to control the distaste for food and desire to vomit
   B62.1.1   Assess Nausea Care
   B62.1.2   Perform Nausea Care
   B62.1.3   Teach Nausea Care
   B62.1.4   Manage Nausea Care

(*Continued*)

TABLE 8.14 ■ Clinical Care Classification of 201 Nursing Interventions, Version 2.5: Coded with Definitions and Four Action Types and Classified by 21 Care Components[1,2] (*Continued*)

C. Cardiac Component

Cluster of elements that involve the heart and blood vessels
Cardiac Care—C08.0
Actions performed to control changes in the heart or blood vessels
C08.0.1   Assess Cardiac Care
C08.0.2   Perform Cardiac Care
C08.0.3   Teach Cardiac Care
C08.0.4   Manage Cardiac Care

   Cardiac Rehabilitation—C08.1
   Actions performed to restore cardiac health
   C08.1.1   Assess Cardiac Rehabilitation
   C08.1.2   Perform Cardiac Rehabilitation
   C08.1.3   Teach Cardiac Rehabilitation
   C08.1.4   Manage Cardiac Rehabilitation

Pacemaker Care—C09.0
Actions performed to control the use of an electronic device that provides a normal heartbeat
C09.0.1   Assess Pacemaker Care
C09.0.2   Perform Pacemaker Care
C09.0.3   Teach Pacemaker Care
C09.0.4   Manage Pacemaker Care

D. Cognitive/Neuro Component

Cluster of elements that involve the cognitive, mental, cerebral, and neurological processes
Behavior Care—D10.0
Actions performed to support observable responses to internal and external stimuli
D10.0.1   Assess Behavior Care
D10.0.2   Perform Behavior Care
D10.0.3   Teach Behavior Care
D10.0.4   Manage Behavior Care

Reality Orientation—D11.0
Actions performed to promote the ability to locate oneself in an environment
D11.0.1   Assess Reality Orientation
D11.0.2   Perform Reality Orientation
D11.0.3   Teach Reality Orientation
D11.0.4   Manage Reality Orientation

Wandering Control—D63.0
Actions performed to control abnormal movability
D63.0.1   Assess Wandering Control
D63.0.2   Perform Wandering Control
D63.0.3   Teach Wandering Control
D63.0.4   Manage Wandering Control

Memory Loss Care—D64.0
Actions performed to control a person's inability to recall ideas and/or events
D64.0.1   Assess Memory Loss Care
D64.0.2   Perform Memory Loss Care
D64.0.3   Teach Memory Loss Care
D64.0.4   Manage Memory Loss Care

Neurological System Care—D78.0
Actions performed to control problems of the neurological system
D78.0.1   Assess Neurological System Care
D78.0.2   Perform Neurological System Care
D78.0.3   Teach Neurological System Care
D78.0.4   Manage Neurological System Care

TABLE 8.14 ▩ (*Continued*)

E.   Coping Component

Cluster of elements that involve the ability to deal with responsibilities, problems, or difficulties
Counseling Service—E12.0
Actions performed to provide advice or instruction to help another
E12.0.1   Assess Counseling Service
E12.0.2   Perform Counseling Service
E12.0.3   Teach Counseling Service
E12.0.4   Manage Counseling Service
  Coping Support—E12.1
  Actions performed to sustain a person dealing with responsibilities, problems, or difficulties
  E12.1.1   Assess Coping Support
  E12.1.2   Perform Coping Support
  E12.1.3   Teach Coping Support
  E12.1.4   Manage Coping Support
  Stress Control—E12.2
  Actions performed to support the physiological response of the body to a stimulus
  E12.2.1   Assess Stress Control
  E12.2.2   Perform Stress Control
  E12.2.3   Teach Stress Control
  E12.2.4   Manage Stress Control
  Crisis Therapy—E12.3
  Actions performed to sustain a person dealing with a condition, event, or radical change in status
  E12.3.1   Assess Crisis Therapy
  E12.3.2   Perform Crisis Therapy
  E12.3.3   Teach Crisis Therapy
  E12.3.4   Manage Crisis Therapy
Emotional Support—E13.0
Actions performed to maintain a positive affective state
E13.0.1   Assess Emotional Support
E13.0.2   Perform Emotional Support
E13.0.3   Teach Emotional Support
E13.0.4   Manage Emotional Support
  Spiritual Comfort—E13.1
  Actions performed to console, restore, or promote spiritual health
  E13.1.1   Assess Spiritual Comfort
  E13.1.2   Perform Spiritual Comfort
  E13.1.3   Teach Spiritual Comfort
  E13.1.4   Manage Spiritual Comfort
Terminal Care—E14.0
Actions performed in the period surrounding death
E14.0.1   Assess Terminal Care
E14.0.2   Perform Terminal Care
E14.0.3   Teach Terminal Care
E14.0.4   Manage Terminal Care
  Bereavement Support—E14.1
  Actions performed to provide comfort to the family/friends of the person who died
  E14.1.1   Assess Bereavement Support
  E14.1.2   Perform Bereavement Support
  E14.1.3   Teach Bereavement Support
  E14.1.4   Manage Bereavement Support

(Continued)

TABLE 8.14 ■ Clinical Care Classification of 201 Nursing Interventions, Version 2.5: Coded with Definitions and Four Action Types and Classified by 21 Care Components[1,2] (*Continued*)

Dying/Death Measures—E14.2
Actions performed to support the dying process
E14.2.1   Assess Dying/Death Measures
E14.2.2   Perform Dying/Death Measures
E14.2.3   Teach Dying/Death Measures
E14.2.4   Manage Dying/Death Measures

Funeral Arrangements—E14.3
Actions performed to direct the preparation measures for burial
E14.3.1   Assess Funeral Arrangements
E14.3.2   Perform Funeral Arrangements
E14.3.3   Teach Funeral Arrangements
E14.3.4   Manage Funeral Arrangements

F.   Fluid Volume Component

Cluster of elements that involve liquid consumption
Fluid Therapy—F15.0
Actions performed to provide liquid volume intake
F15.0.1   Assess Fluid Therapy
F15.0.2   Perform Fluid Therapy
F15.0.3   Teach Fluid Therapy
F15.0.4   Manage Fluid Therapy

Hydration Control—F15.1
Actions performed to control the state of fluid balance
F15.1.1   Assess Hydration Control
F15.1.2   Perform Hydration Control
F15.1.3   Teach Hydration Control
F15.1.4   Manage Hydration Control

Intake—F15.3
Actions performed to measure the amount of fluid volume taken into the body
F15.3.1   Assess Intake
F15.3.2   Perform Intake
F15.3.3   Teach Intake
F15.3.4   Manage Intake

Output—F15.4
Actions performed to measure the amount of fluid volume removed from the body
F15.4.1   Assess Output
F15.4.2   Perform Output
F15.4.3   Teach Output
F15.4.4   Manage Output

Hemodynamic Care—F79.0
Actions performed to support the movement of solutions through the blood
F79.0.1   Assess Hemodynamic Care
F79.0.2   Perform Hemodynamic Care
F79.0.3   Teach Hemodynamic Care
F79.0.4   Manage Hemodynamic Care

Intravenous Care—F79.1
Actions performed to support the use of infusion equipment
F79.1.1   Assess Intravenous Care
F79.1.2   Perform Intravenous Care
F79.1.3   Teach Intravenous Care
F79.1.4   Manage Intravenous Care

Venous Catheter Care—F79.2
Actions performed to support the use of a venous infusion site

TABLE 8.14 ■ (*Continued*)

F79.2.1   Assess Venous Catheter Care
F79.2.2   Perform Venous Catheter Care
F79.2.3   Teach Venous Catheter Care
F79.2.4   Manage Venous Catheter Care

Arterial Catheter Care—F79.3
Actions performed to support the use of an arterial infusion site
F79.3.1   Assess Arterial Catheter Care
F79.3.2   Perform Arterial Catheter Care
F79.3.3   Teach Arterial Catheter Care
F79.3.4   Manage Arterial Catheter Care

G.   Health Behavior Component

Cluster of elements that involve actions to sustain, maintain, or regain health
Community Special Services—G17.0
Actions performed to provide advice or information about special community services
G17.0.1   Assess Community Special Services
G17.0.2   Perform Community Special Services
G17.0.3   Teach Community Special Services
G17.0.4   Manage Community Special Services

Adult Day Center—G17.1
Actions performed to direct the provision of a day program for adults in a specific location
G17.1.1   Assess Adult Day Center
G17.1.2   Perform Adult Day Center
G17.1.3   Teach Adult Day Center
G17.1.4   Manage Adult Day Center

Hospice—G17.2
Actions performed to support the provision of offering and/or providing care for terminally ill persons
G17.2.1   Assess Hospice
G17.2.2   Perform Hospice
G17.2.3   Teach Hospice
G17.2.4   Manage Hospice

Meals on Wheels—G17.3
Actions performed to direct the provision of a community program of delivering meals to the home
G17.3.1   Assess Meals on Wheels
G17.3.2   Perform Meals on Wheels
G17.3.3   Teach Meals on Wheels
G17.3.4   Manage Meals on Wheels

Compliance Care—G18.0
Actions performed to encourage adherence to care regimen
G18.0.1   Assess Compliance Care
G18.0.2   Perform Compliance Care
G18.0.3   Teach Compliance Care
G18.0.4   Manage Compliance Care

Compliance with Diet—G18.1
Actions performed to encourage adherence to diet/food intake
G18.1.1   Assess Compliance with Diet
G18.1.2   Perform Compliance with Diet
G18.1.3   Teach Compliance with Diet
G18.1.4   Manage Compliance with Diet

(*Continued*)

TABLE 8.14 ■ Clinical Care Classification of 201 Nursing Interventions, Version 2.5: Coded with Definitions and Four Action Types and Classified by 21 Care Components[1,2] (*Continued*)

Compliance with Fluid Volume—G18.2

Actions performed to encourage adherence to therapeutic intake of liquids

G18.2.1 Assess Compliance with Fluid Volume
G18.2.2 Perform Compliance with Fluid Volume
G18.2.3 Teach Compliance with Fluid Volume
G18.2.4 Manage Compliance with Fluid Volume

Compliance with Medical Regimen—G18.3

Actions performed to encourage adherence to physician's/provider's treatment plan

G18.3.1 Assess Compliance with Medical Regimen
G18.3.2 Perform Compliance with Medical Regimen
G18.3.3 Teach Compliance with Medical Regimen
G18.3.4 Manage Compliance with Medical Regimen

Compliance with Medication Regimen—G18.4

Actions performed to encourage adherence to prescribed course of medicinal substances

G18.4.1 Assess Compliance with Medication Regimen
G18.4.2 Perform Compliance with Medication Regimen
G18.4.3 Teach Compliance with Medication Regimen
G18.4.4 Manage Compliance with Medication Regimen

Compliance with Safety Precaution—G18.5

Actions performed to encourage adherence with measures to protect self or others from injury, danger, or loss

G18.5.1 Assess Compliance with Safety Precautions
G18.5.2 Perform Compliance with Safety Precautions
G18.5.3 Teach Compliance with Safety Precautions
G18.5.4 Manage Compliance with Safety Precautions

Compliance with Therapeutic Regimen—G18.6

Actions performed to encourage adherence with the plan of care

G18.6.1 Assess Compliance with Therapeutic Regimen
G18.6.2 Perform Compliance with Therapeutic Regimen
G18.6.3 Teach Compliance with Therapeutic Regimen
G18.6.4 Manage Compliance with Therapeutic Regimen

Nursing Contact—G19.0

Actions performed to communicate with another nurse

G19.0.1 Assess Nursing Contact
G19.0.2 Perform Nursing Contact
G19.0.3 Teach Nursing Contact
G19.0.4 Manage Nursing Contact

Bill of Rights—G19.1

Statements related to entitlements during an episode of illness

G19.1.1 Assess Bill of Rights
G19.1.2 Perform Bill of Rights
G19.1.3 Teach Bill of Rights
G19.1.4 Manage Bill of Rights

Nursing Care Coordination—G19.2

Actions performed to synthesize all plans of care by a nurse

G19.2.1 Assess Nursing Care Coordination
G19.2.2 Perform Nursing Care Coordination
G19.2.3 Teach Nursing Care Coordination
G19.2.4 Manage Nursing Care Coordination

Nursing Status Report—G19.3

Actions performed to document patient condition by a nurse

G19.3.1 Assess Nursing Status Report
G19.3.2 Perform Nursing Status Report
G19.3.3 Teach Nursing Status Report
G19.3.4 Manage Nursing Status Report

TABLE 8.14 ▓ (*Continued*)

Physician Contact—G20.0

Actions performed to communicate with a physician/provider

G20.0.1　Assess Physician Contact
G20.0.2　Perform Physician Contact
G20.0.3　Teach Physician Contact
G20.0.4　Manage Physician Contact

　Medical Regimen Orders—G20.1

　Actions performed to support the physician's/provider's plan of treatment

　G20.1.1　Assess Medical Regimen Orders
　G20.1.2　Perform Medical Regimen Orders
　G20.1.3　Teach Medical Regimen Orders
　G20.1.4　Manage Medical Regimen Orders

　Physician Status Report—G20.2

　Actions performed to document patient condition by a physician/provider

　G20.2.1　Assess Physician Status Report
　G20.2.2　Perform Physician Status Report
　G20.2.3　Teach Physician Status Report
　G20.2.4　Manage Physician Status Report

Professional/Ancillary Services—G21.0

Actions performed to support the duties performed by health team members

G21.0.1　Assess Professional/Ancillary Services
G21.0.2　Perform Professional/Ancillary Services
G21.0.3　Teach Professional/Ancillary Services
G21.0.4　Manage Professional/Ancillary Services

　Health Aide Service—G21.1

　Actions performed to support care services by a health aide

　G21.1.1　Assess Health Aide Service
　G21.1.2　Perform Health Aide Service
　G21.1.3　Teach Health Aide Service
　G21.1.4　Manage Health Aide Service

　Social Worker Service—G21.2

　Actions performed to provide advice or instruction by a social worker

　G21.2.1　Assess Social Worker Service
　G21.2.2　Perform Social Worker Service
　G21.2.3　Teach Social Worker Service
　G21.2.4　Manage Social Worker Service

　Nurse Specialist Service—G21.3

　Actions performed to provide advice or instruction by an advanced practice nurse or nurse practitioner

　G21.3.1　Assess Nurse Specialist Service
　G21.3.2　Perform Nurse Specialist Service
　G21.3.3　Teach Nurse Specialist Service
　G21.3.4　Manage Nurse Specialist Service

　Occupational Therapist Service—G21.4

　Actions performed to provide advice or instruction by an occupational therapist

　G21.4.1　Assess Occupational Therapist Service
　G21.4.2　Perform Occupational Therapist Service
　G21.4.3　Teach Occupational Therapist Service
　G21.4.4　Manage Occupational Therapist Service

　Physical Therapist Service—G21.5

　Actions performed to provide advice or instruction by a physical therapist

　G21.5.1　Assess Physical Therapist Service
　G21.5.2　Perform Physical Therapist Service
　G21.5.3　Teach Physical Therapist Service
　G21.5.4　Manage Physical Therapist Service

(Continued)

TABLE 8.14 ■ Clinical Care Classification of 201 Nursing Interventions, Version 2.5: Coded with Definitions and Four Action Types and Classified by 21 Care Components[1,2] (*Continued*)

Speech Therapist Service—G21.6
Actions performed to provide advice or instruction by a speech therapist
G21.6.1   Assess Speech Therapist Service
G21.6.2   Perform Speech Therapist Service
G21.6.3   Teach Speech Therapist Service
G21.6.4   Manage Speech Therapist Service

Respiratory Therapist Service—G21.7
Actions performed to provide advice or instruction by a respiratory therapist
G21.7.1   Assess Respiratory Therapist Service
G21.7.2   Perform Respiratory Therapist Service
G21.7.3   Teach Respiratory Therapist Service
G21.7.4   Manage Respiratory Therapist Service

H.   Medication Component

Cluster of elements that involve medicinal substances
Chemotherapy Care—H22.0
Actions performed to control and monitor antineoplastic agents
H22.0.1   Assess Chemotherapy Care
H22.0.2   Perform Chemotherapy Care
H22.0.3   Teach Chemotherapy Care
H22.0.4   Manage Chemotherapy Care

Injection Administration—H23.0
Actions performed to dispense medication by a hypodermic
H23.0.1   Assess Injection Administration
H23.0.2   Perform Injection Administration
H23.0.3   Teach Injection Administration
H23.0.4   Manage Injection Administration

Medication Care—H24.0
Actions performed to support use of prescribed drugs or remedies regardless of route
H24.0.1   Assess Medication Care
H24.0.2   Perform Medication Care
H24.0.3   Teach Medication Care
H24.0.4   Manage Medication Care

Medication Actions—H24.1
Actions performed to support and monitor the intended responses to prescribed drugs
H24.1.1   Assess Medication Actions
H24.1.2   Perform Medication Actions
H24.1.3   Teach Medication Actions
H24.1.4   Manage Medication Actions

Medication Prefill Preparation—H24.2
Actions performed to ensure the continued supply of prescribed drugs
H24.2.1   Assess Medication Prefill Preparation
H24.2.2   Perform Medication Prefill Preparation
H24.2.3   Teach Medication Prefill Preparation
H24.2.4   Manage Medication Prefill Preparation

Medication Side Effects—H24.3
Actions performed to control adverse untoward reactions or conditions to prescribed drugs
H24.3.1   Assess Medication Side Effects
H24.3.2   Perform Medication Side Effects
H24.3.3   Teach Medication Side Effects
H24.3.4   Manage Medication Side Effects

TABLE 8.14 ■ (*Continued*)

Medication Treatment—H23.4
Actions performed to administer/give drugs or remedies regardless of route
H24.4.1   Assess Medication Treatment
H24.4.2   Perform Medication Treatment
H24.4.3   Teach Medication Treatment
H24.4.4   Manage Medication Treatment
Radiation Therapy Care—H25.0
Actions performed to control and monitor radiation therapy
H25.0.1   Assess Radiation Therapy Care
H25.0.2   Perform Radiation Therapy Care
H25.0.3   Teach Radiation Therapy Care
H25.0.4   Manage Radiation Therapy Care

I.   Metabolic Component

Cluster of elements that involve the endocrine and immunologic processes
Allergic Reaction Care—I26.0
Actions performed to reduce symptoms or precautions to reduce allergies
I26.0.1   Assess Allergic Reaction Care
I26.0.2   Perform Allergic Reaction Care
I26.0.3   Teach Allergic Reaction Care
I26.0.4   Manage Allergic Reaction Care
Diabetic Care—I27.0
Actions performed to support the control of diabetic conditions
I27.0.1   Assess Diabetic Care
I27.0.2   Perform Diabetic Care
I27.0.3   Teach Diabetic Care
I27.0.4   Manage Diabetic Care
Immunologic Care—I65.0
Actions preformed to protect against a particular disease
I65.0.1   Assess Immunologic Care
I65.0.2   Perform Immunologic Care
I65.0.3   Teach Immunologic Care
I65.0.4   Manage Immunologic Care

J.   Nutritional Component

Cluster of elements that involve the intake of food and nutrients
Enteral Tube Care—J28.0
Actions performed to control the use of an enteral drainage tube
J28.0.1 Assess Enteral Tube Care
J28.0.2 Perform Enteral Tube Care
J28.0.3 Teach Enteral Tube Care
J28.0.4 Manage Enteral Tube Care
Enteral Tube Insertion—J28.1
Actions performed to support the placement of an enteral drainage tube
J28.1.1 Assess Enteral Tube Insertion
J28.1.2 Perform Enteral Tube Insertion
J28.1.3 Teach Enteral Tube Insertion
J28.1.4 Manage Enteral Tube Insertion
Enteral Tube Irrigation—J28.2
Actions performed to flush or wash out an enteral tube
J28.2.1 Assess Enteral Tube Irrigation
J28.2.2 Perform Enteral Tube Irrigation
J28.2.3 Teach Enteral Tube Irrigation
J28.2.4 Manage Enteral Tube Irrigation

(*Continued*)

TABLE 8.14 ■ Clinical Care Classification of 201 Nursing Interventions, Version 2.5: Coded with Definitions and Four Action Types and Classified by 21 Care Components[1,2] (*Continued*)

Nutrition Care—J29.0
Actions performed to support the intake of food and nutrients
J29.0.1   Assess Nutrition Care
J29.0.2   Perform Nutrition Care
J29.0.3   Teach Nutrition Care
J29.0.4   Manage Nutrition Care

Feeding Technique—J29.2
Actions performed to provide special measures to provide nourishment
J29.2.1   Assess Feeding Technique
J29.2.2   Perform Feeding Technique
J29.2.3   Teach Feeding Technique
J29.2.4   Manage Feeding Technique

Regular Diet—J29.3
Actions performed to support the ingestion of food and nutrients from established nutrition standards
J29.3.1   Assess Regular Diet
J29.3.2   Perform Regular Diet
J29.3.3   Teach Regular Diet
J29.3.4   Manage Regular Diet

Special Diet—J29.4
Actions performed to support the ingestion of food and nutrients prescribed for a specific purpose
J29.4.1   Assess Special Diet
J29.4.2   Perform Special Diet
J29.4.3   Teach Special Diet
J29.4.4   Manage Special Diet

Enteral Feeding—J29.5
Actions performed to provide nourishment through a gastrointestinal route
J29.5.1   Assess Enteral Feeding
J29.5.2   Perform Enteral Feeding
J29.5.3   Teach Enteral Feeding
J29.5.4   Manage Enteral Feeding

Parenteral Feeding—J29.6
Actions performed to provide nourishment through intravenous or subcutaneous routes
J29.6.1   Assess Parenteral Feeding
J29.6.2   Perform Parenteral Feeding
J29.6.3   Teach Parenteral Feeding
J29.6.4   Manage Parenteral Feeding

Breastfeeding Support—J66.0
Actions performed to provide nourishment of an infant at the breast
J66.0.1   Assess Breastfeeding Support
J66.0.2   Perform Breastfeeding Support
J66.0.3   Teach Breastfeeding Support
J66.0.4   Manage Breastfeeding Support

Weight Control—J67.0
Actions performed to control obesity or debilitation
J67.0.1   Assess Weight Control
J67.0.2   Perform Weight Control
J67.0.3   Teach Weight Control
J67.0.4   Manage Weight Control

TABLE 8.14 ▦ (*Continued*)

K. Physical Regulation Component

Cluster of elements that involve bodily processes

Infection Control—K30.0

Actions performed to contain a communicable disease

K30.0.1   Assess Infection Control

K30.0.2   Perform Infection Control

K30.0.3   Teach Infection Control

K30.0.4   Manage Infection Control

   Universal Precautions—K30.1

   Practices to prevent the spread of infections and infectious diseases

   K30.1.1   Assess Universal Precautions

   K30.1.2   Perform Universal Precautions

   K30.1.3   Teach Universal Precautions

   K30.1.4   Manage Universal Precautions

Physical Healthcare—K31.0

Actions performed to support somatic problems

K31.0.1   Assess Physical Healthcare

K31.0.2   Perform Physical Healthcare

K31.0.3   Teach Physical Healthcare

K31.0.4   Manage Physical Healthcare

   Health History—K31.1

   Actions performed to obtain information about past illness and health status

   K31.1.1   Assess Health History

   K31.1.2   Perform Health History

   K31.1.3   Teach Health History

   K31.1.4   Manage Health History

   Health Promotion—K31.2

   Actions performed to encourage behaviors to enhance health state

   K31.2.1   Assess Health Promotion

   K31.2.2   Perform Health Promotion

   K31.2.3   Teach Health Promotion

   K31.2.4   Manage Health Promotion

   Physical Examination—K31.3

   Actions performed to observe somatic events

   K31.3.1   Assess Physical Examination

   K31.3.2   Perform Physical Examination

   K31.3.3   Teach Physical Examination

   K31.3.4   Manage Physical Examination

   Clinical Measurements—K31.4

   Actions performed to conduct procedures to evaluate somatic events

   K31.4.1   Assess Clinical Measurements

   K31.4.2   Perform Clinical Measurements

   K31.4.3   Teach Clinical Measurements

   K31.4.4   Manage Clinical Measurements

Specimen Care—K32.0

Actions performed to direct the collection and/or the examination of a bodily specimen

K32.0.1   Assess Specimen Care

K32.0.2   Perform Specimen Care

K32.0.3   Teach Specimen Care

K32.0.4   Manage Specimen Care

   Blood Specimen Care—K32.1

   Actions performed to collect and/or examine a sample of blood

   K32.1.1   Assess Blood Specimen Care

   K32.1.2   Perform Blood Specimen Care

   K32.1.3   Teach Blood Specimen Care

   K32.1.4   Manage Blood Specimen Care

(*Continued*)

TABLE 8.14 ▦ Clinical Care Classification of 201 Nursing Interventions, Version 2.5: Coded with Definitions and Four Action Types and Classified by 21 Care Components[1,2]   (*Continued*)

Stool Specimen Care—K32.2
Actions performed to collect and/or examine a sample of feces
K32.2.1   Assess Stool Specimen Care
K32.2.2   Perform Stool Specimen Care
K32.2.3   Teach Stool Specimen Care
K32.2.4   Manage Stool Specimen Care

Urine Specimen Care—K32.3
Actions performed to collect and/or examine a sample of urine
K32.3.1   Assess Urine Specimen Care
K32.3.2   Perform Urine Specimen Care
K32.3.3   Teach Urine Specimen Care
K32.3.4   Manage Urine Specimen Care

Sputum Specimen Care—K32.5
Actions performed to collect and/or examine a sample of sputum
K32.5.1   Assess Sputum Specimen Care
K32.5.2   Perform Sputum Specimen Care
K32.5.3   Teach Sputum Specimen Care
K32.5.4   Manage Sputum Specimen Care

Vital Signs—K33.0
Actions performed to measure temperature, pulse, respiration, and blood pressure
K33.0.1   Assess Vital Signs
K33.0.2   Perform Vital Signs
K33.0.3   Teach Vital Signs
K33.0.4   Manage Vital Signs

Blood Pressure—K33.1
Actions performed to measure the diastolic and systolic pressure of the blood
K33.1.1   Assess Blood Pressure
K33.1.2   Perform Blood Pressure
K33.1.3   Teach Blood Pressure
K33.1.4   Manage Blood Pressure

Temperature—K33.2
Actions performed to measure the body temperature
K33.2.1   Assess Temperature
K33.2.2   Perform Temperature
K33.2.3   Teach Temperature
K33.2.4   Manage Temperature

Pulse—K33.3
Actions performed to measure rhythmic beats of the heart
K33.3.1   Assess Pulse
K33.3.2   Perform Pulse
K33 3.3   Teach Pulse
K33.3.4   Manage Pulse

Respiration—K33.4
Actions performed to measure the function of breathing
K33.4.1   Assess Respiration
K33.4.2   Perform Respiration
K33.4.3   Teach Respiration
K33 4.4   Manage Respiration

L.   Respiratory Component

Cluster of elements that involve breathing and the pulmonary system
Oxygen Therapy Care—L35.0
Actions performed to support the administration of oxygen treatment
L35.0.1   Assess Oxygen Therapy Care
L35.0.2   Perform Oxygen Therapy Care
L35.0.3   Teach Oxygen Therapy Care
L35.0.4   Manage Oxygen Therapy Care

TABLE 8.14 ■ (*Continued*)

Pulmonary Care—L36.0
Actions performed to support pulmonary hygiene
L36.0.1   Assess Pulmonary Care
L36.0.2   Perform Pulmonary Care
L36.0.3   Teach Pulmonary Care
L36.0.4   Manage Pulmonary Care

    Breathing Exercises—L36.1
    Actions performed to provide therapy on respiratory or lung exertion
    L36.1.1   Assess Breathing Exercises
    L36.1.2   Perform Breathing Exercises
    L36.1.3   Teach Breathing Exercises
    L36.1.4   Manage Breathing Exercises

    Chest Physiotherapy—L36.2
    Actions performed to provide exercises for postural drainage of lungs
    L36.2.1   Assess Chest Physiotherapy
    L36.2.2   Perform Chest Physiotherapy
    L36.2.3   Teach Chest Physiotherapy
    L36.2.4   Manage Chest Physiotherapy

    Inhalation Therapy—L36.3
    Actions performed to support breathing treatments
    L36.3.1   Assess Inhalation Therapy
    L36.3.2   Perform Inhalation Therapy
    L36.3.3   Teach Inhalation Therapy
    L36.3.4   Manage Inhalation Therapy

    Ventilator Care—L36.4
    Actions performed to control and monitor the use of a ventilator
    L36.4.1   Assess Ventilator Care
    L36.4.2   Perform Ventilator Care
    L36.4.3   Teach Ventilator Care
    L36.4.4   Manage Ventilator Care

Tracheostomy Care—L37.0
Actions performed to support a tracheostomy
L37.0.1   Assess Tracheostomy Care
L37.0.2   Perform Tracheostomy Care
L37.0.3   Teach Tracheostomy Care
L37.0.4   Manage Tracheostomy Care

M.   Role Relationship Component

Cluster of elements involving interpersonal, work, social, family, and sexual interactions

Communication Care—M38.0
Actions performed to exchange verbal/nonverbal and/or translation of information
M38.0.1   Assess Communication Care
M38.0.2   Perform Communication Care
M38.0.3   Teach Communication Care
M38.0.4   Manage Communication Care

Psychosocial Care—M39.0
Actions performed to support the study of psychological and social factors
M39.0.1   Assess Psychosocial Care
M39.0.2   Perform Psychosocial Care
M39.0.3   Teach Psychosocial Care
M39.0.4   Manage Psychosocial Care

    Home Situation Analysis—M39.1
    Actions performed to analyze the living environment
    M39.1.1   Assess Home Situation Analysis
    M39.1.2   Perform Home Situation Analysis
    M39.1.3   Teach Home Situation Analysis
    M39.1.4   Manage Home Situation Analysis

(*Continued*)

TABLE 8.14 ▨ Clinical Care Classification of 201 Nursing Interventions, Version 2.5: Coded with Definitions and Four Action Types and Classified by 21 Care Components[1,2] (*Continued*)

Interpersonal Dynamics Analysis—M39.2
Actions performed to support the analysis of the driving forces in a relationship between people
M39.2.1   Assess Interpersonal Dynamics Analysis
M39.2.2   Perform Interpersonal Dynamics Analysis
M39.2.3   Teach Interpersonal Dynamics Analysis
M39.4.4   Manage Interpersonal Dynamics Analysis

Family Process Analysis—M39.3
Actions performed to support the change and/or modification of a related group
M39.3.1   Assess Family Process Analysis
M39.3.2   Perform Family Process Analysis
M39.3.3   Teach Family Process Analysis
M39.3.4   Manage Family Process Analysis

Sexual Behavior Analysis—M39.4
Actions performed to support the change and/or modification of a person's sexual response
M39.4.1   Assess Sexual Behavior Analysis
M39.4.2   Perform Sexual Behavior Analysis
M39.4.3   Teach Sexual Behavior Analysis
M39.4.4   Manage Sexual Behavior Analysis

Social Network Analysis—M39.5
Actions performed to improve the quantity or quality of personal relationships
M39.5.1   Assess Social Network Analysis
M39.5.2   Perform Social Network Analysis
M39.5.3   Teach Social Network Analysis
M39.5.4   Manage Social Network Analysis

N.   Safety Component

Cluster of elements that involve prevention of injury, danger, loss, or abuse
Substance Abuse Control—N40.0
Actions performed to control substances to avoid, detect, or minimize harm
N40.0.1   Assess Substance Abuse Control
N40.0.2   Perform Substance Abuse Control
N40.0.3   Teach Substance Abuse Control
N40.0.4   Manage Substance Abuse Control

Tobacco Abuse Control—N40.1
Actions performed to avoid, minimize, or control the use of tobacco
N40.1.1   Assess Tobacco Abuse Control
N40.1.2   Perform Tobacco Abuse Control
N40.1.3   Teach Tobacco Abuse Control
N40.1.4   Manage Tobacco Abuse Control

Alcohol Abuse Control—N40.2
Actions performed to avoid, minimize, or control the use of distilled liquors
N40.2.1   Assess Alcohol Abuse Control
N40.2.2   Perform Alcohol Abuse Control
N40.2.3   Teach Alcohol Abuse Control
N40.2.4   Manage Alcohol Abuse Control

Drug Abuse Control—N40.3
Actions performed to avoid, minimize, or control the use of any habit-forming medication
N40.3.1   Assess Drug Abuse Control
N40.3.2   Perform Drug Abuse Control
N40.3.3   Teach Drug Abuse Control
N40.3.4   Manage Drug Abuse Control

TABLE 8.14 ▦ (*Continued*)

Emergency Care—N41.0
Actions performed to support a sudden or unexpected occurrence
N41.0.1   Assess Emergency Care
N41.0.2   Perform Emergency Care
N41.0.3   Teach Emergency Care
N41.0.4   Manage Emergency Care

Safety Precautions—N42.0
Actions performed to advance measures to avoid danger or harm
N42.0.1   Assess Safety Precautions
N42.0.2   Perform Safety Precautions
N42.0.3   Teach Safety Precautions
N42.0.4   Manage Safety Precautions

   Environmental Safety—N42.1
   Precautions recommended to prevent or reduce environmental injury
   N42.1.1   Assess Environmental Safety
   N42.1.2   Perform Environmental Safety
   N42.1.3   Teach Environmental Safety
   N42.1.4   Manage Environmental Safety

   Equipment Safety—N42.2
   Precautions recommended to prevent or reduce equipment injury
   N42.2.1   Assess Equipment Safety
   N42.2.2   Perform Equipment Safety
   N42.2.3   Teach Equipment Safety
   N42.2.4   Manage Equipment Safety

   Individual Safety—N42.3
   Precautions to reduce individual injury
   N42.3.1   Assess Individual Safety
   N42.3.2   Perform Individual Safety
   N42.3.3   Teach Individual Safety
   N42.4.4   Manage Individual Safety

Violence Control—N68.0
Actions performed to control behaviors that may cause harm to oneself or others
N68.0.1   Assess Violence Control
N68.0.2   Perform Violence Control
N68.0.3   Teach Violence Control
N68.0.4   Manage Violence Control

Perioperative Injury Care—N80.0
Actions performed to support perioperative care requirements
N80.0.1   Assess Perioperative Injury Care
N80.0.2   Perform Perioperative Injury Care
N80.0.3   Teach Perioperative Injury Care
N80.0.4   Manage Perioperative Injury Care

O.   Self-Care Component

Cluster of elements that involve the ability to carry out activities to maintain oneself
Personal Care—O43.0
actions performed to care for oneself
O43.0.1   Assess Personal Care
O43.0.2   Perform Personal Care
O43.0.3   Teach Personal Care
O43.0.4   Manage Personal Care

   Activities of Daily Living—O43.1
   Actions performed to support personal activities to maintain oneself
   O43.1.1   Assess Activities of Daily Living
   O43.1.2   Perform Activities of Daily Living
   O43.1.3   Teach Activities of Daily Living
   O43.1.4   Manage Activities of Daily Living

(*Continued*)

TABLE 8.14 ■ Clinical Care Classification of 201 Nursing Interventions, Version 2.5: Coded with Definitions and Four Action Types and Classified by 21 Care Components[1,2] (*Continued*)

Instrumental Activities of Daily Living—O43.2
Complex activities performed to support basic life skills
O43.2.1   Assess Instrumental Activities of Daily Living
O43.2.2   Perform Instrumental Activities of Daily Living
O43.2.3   Teach Instrumental Activities of Daily Living
O43.2.4   Manage Instrumental Activities of Daily Living

P.   Self-Concept Component

Cluster of elements that involve an individual's mental image of oneself
Mental Healthcare—P45.0
Actions taken to promote emotional well-being
P45.0.1   Assess Mental Healthcare
P45.0.2   Perform Mental Healthcare
P45.0.3   Teach Mental Healthcare
P45.0.4   Manage Mental Healthcare

Mental Health History—P45.1
Actions performed to obtain information about past or present emotional well-being
P45.1.1   Assess Mental Health History
P45.1.2   Perform Mental Health History
P45.1.3   Teach Mental Health History
P45.1.4   Manage Mental Health History

Mental Health Promotion—P45.2
Actions performed to encourage or further emotional well-being
P45.2.1   Assess Mental Health Promotion
P45.2.2   Perform Mental Health Promotion
P45.2.3   Teach Mental Health Promotion
P45.2.4   Manage Mental Health Promotion

Mental Health Screening—P45.3
Actions performed to systematically examine emotional well-being
P45.3.1   Assess Mental Health Screening
P45.3.2   Perform Mental Health Screening
P45.3.3   Teach Mental Health Screening
P45.3.4   Manage Mental Health Screening

Mental Health Treatment—P45.4
Actions performed to support protocols used to treat emotional problems
P45.4.1   Assess Mental Health Treatment
P45.4.2   Perform Mental Health Treatment
P45.4.3   Teach Mental Health Treatment
P45.4.4   Manage Mental Health Treatment

Q.   Sensory Component

Cluster of elements that involve the senses, including pain
Pain Control—Q47.0
Actions performed to support responses to injury or damage
Q47.0.1   Assess Pain Control
Q47.0.2   Perform Pain Control
Q47.0.3   Teach Pain Control
Q47.0.4   Manage Pain Control

Acute Pain Control—Q47.1
Actions performed to control physical suffering, hurting, or distress
Q47.1.1   Assess Acute Pain Control
Q47.1.2   Perform Acute Pain Control
Q47.1.3   Teach Acute Pain Control
Q47.1.4   Manage Acute Pain Control

TABLE 8.14 ▪ (*Continued*)

Chronic Pain Control—Q47.2
Actions performed to control physical suffering, hurting, or distress that continues longer than expected
Q47.2.1   Assess Chronic Pain Control
Q47.2.2   Perform Chronic Pain Control
Q47.2.3   Teach Chronic Pain Control
Q47.2.4   Manage Chronic Pain Control
Comfort Care—Q48.0
Actions performed to enhance or improve well-being
Q48.0.1   Assess Comfort Care
Q48.0.2   Perform Comfort Care
Q48.0.3   Teach Comfort Care
Q48.0.4   Manage Comfort Care
Ear Care—Q49.0
Actions performed to support ear problems
Q49.0.1   Assess Ear Care
Q49.0.2   Perform Ear Care
Q49.0.3   Teach Ear Care
Q49.0.4   Manage Ear Care
   Hearing Aid Care—Q49.1
   Actions performed to control the use of a hearing aid
   Q49.1.1   Assess Hearing Aid Care
   Q49.1.2   Perform Hearing Aid Care
   Q49.1.3   Teach Hearing Aid Care
   Q49.1.4   Manage Hearing Aid Care
   Wax Removal—Q49.2
   Actions performed to remove cerumen from ear
   Q49.2.1   Assess Wax Removal
   Q49.2.2   Perform Wax Removal
   Q49.2.3   Teach Wax Removal
   Q49.2.4   Manage Wax Removal
Eye Care—Q50.0
Actions performed to support eye problems
Q50.0.1   Assess Eye Care
Q50.0.2   Perform Eye Care
Q50.0.3   Teach Eye Care
Q50.0.4   Manage Eye Care
   Cataract Care—Q50.1
   Actions performed to control cataract conditions
   Q50.1.1   Assess Cataract Care
   Q50.1.2   Perform Cataract Care
   Q50.1.3   Teach Cataract Care
   Q50.1.4   Manage Cataract Care
   Vision Care—Q50.2
   Actions performed to control vision problems
   Q50.2.1   Assess Vision Care
   Q50.2.2   Perform Vision Care
   Q50.2.3   Teach Vision Care
   Q50.2.4   Manage Vision Care

R.   Skin Integrity Component

Cluster of elements that involve the mucous membrane, corneal, integumentary, or subcutaneous structures of the body
Pressure Ulcer Care—R51.0
Actions performed to prevent, detect, and treat skin integrity breakdown caused by pressure
R51.0.1   Assess Pressure Ulcer Care
R51.0.2   Perform Pressure Ulcer Care

(Continued)

TABLE 8.14 ▧ Clinical Care Classification of 201 Nursing Interventions, Version 2.5: Coded with Definitions and Four Action Types and Classified by 21 Care Components[1,2] (*Continued*)

R51.0.3 Teach Pressure Ulcer Care
R51.0.4 Manage Pressure Ulcer Care

Pressure Ulcer Stage 1 Care—R51.1

Actions performed to prevent, detect, and treat stage 1 skin breakdown

R51.1.1 Assess Pressure Ulcer Stage 1 Care
R51.1.2 Perform Pressure Ulcer Stage 1 Care
R51.1.3 Teach Pressure Ulcer Stage 1 Care
R51.1.4 Manage Pressure Ulcer Stage 1 Care

Pressure Ulcer Stage 2 Care—R51.2

Actions performed to prevent, detect, and treat stage 2 skin breakdown

R51.2.1 Assess Pressure Ulcer Stage 2 Care
R51.2.2 Perform Pressure Ulcer Stage 2 Care
R51.2.3 Teach Pressure Ulcer Stage 2 Care
R51.2.4 Manage Pressure Ulcer Stage 2 Care

Pressure Ulcer Stage 3 Care—R51.3

Actions performed to prevent, detect, and treat stage 3 skin breakdown

R51.3.1 Assess Pressure Ulcer Stage 3 Care
R51.3.2 Perform Pressure Ulcer Stage 3 Care
R51.3.3 Teach Pressure Ulcer Stage 3 Care
R51.3.4 Manage Pressure Ulcer Stage 3 Care

Pressure Ulcer Stage 4 Care—R51.4

Actions performed to prevent, detect, and treat stage 4 skin breakdown

R51.4.1 Assess Pressure Ulcer Stage 4 Care
R51.4.2 Perform Pressure Ulcer Stage 4 Care
R51.4.3 Teach Pressure Ulcer Stage 4 Care
R51.4.4 Manage Pressure Ulcer Stage 4 Care

Mouth Care—R53.0

Actions performed to support oral cavity problems

R53.0.1 Assess Mouth Care
R53.0.2 Perform Mouth Care
R53.0.3 Teach Mouth Care
R53.0.4 Manage Mouth Care

Denture Care—R53.1

Actions performed to control the use of artificial teeth

R53.1.1 Assess Denture Care
R53.1.2 Perform Denture Care
R53.1.3 Teach Denture Care
R53.1.4 Manage Denture Care

Skin Care—R54.0

Actions to control the integument/skin

R54.0.1 Assess Skin Care
R54.0.2 Perform Skin Care
R54.0.3 Teach Skin Care
R54.0.4 Manage Skin Care

Skin Breakdown Control—R54.1

Actions performed to support integument/skin problems

R54.1.1 Assess Skin Breakdown Control
R54.1.2 Perform Skin Breakdown Control
R54.1.3 Teach Skin Breakdown Control
R54.1.4 Manage Skin Breakdown Control

Wound Care—R55.0

Actions performed to support open skin areas

R55.0.1 Assess Wound Care
R55.0.2 Perform Wound Care
R55.0.3 Teach Wound Care
R55.0.4 Manage Wound Care

TABLE 8.14 ▨ (*Continued*)

Drainage Tube Care—R55.1
Actions performed to support wound drainage from body tubes
R55.1.1 Assess Drainage Tube Care
R55.1.2 Perform Drainage Tube Care
R55.1.3 Teach Drainage Tube Care
R55.1.4 Manage Drainage Tube Care

Dressing Change—R55.2
Actions performed to remove and replace a new bandage on a wound
R55.2.1 Assess Dressing Change
R55.2.2 Perform Dressing Change
R55.2.3 Teach Dressing Change
R55.2.4 Manage Dressing Change

Incision Care—R55.3
Actions performed to support a surgical wound
R55.3.1 Assess Incision Care
R55.3.2 Perform Incision Care
R55.3.3 Teach Incision Care
R55.3.4 Manage Incision Care

Burn Care—R81.0
Actions performed to support burned areas of the body
R81.0.1 Assess Burn Care
R81.0.2 Perform Burn Care
R81.0.3 Teach Burn Care
R81.0.4 Manage Burn Care

S. Tissue Perfusion Component

Cluster of elements that involve the oxygenation of tissues, including the circulatory and vascular systems

Foot Care—S56.0
Actions performed to support foot problems
S56.0.1 Assess Foot Care
S56.0.2 Perform Foot Care
S56.0.3 Teach Foot Care
S56.0.4 Manage Foot Care

Perineal Care—S57.0
Actions performed to support perineal problems
S57.0.1 Assess Perineal Care
S57.0.2 Perform Perineal Care
S57.0.3 Teach Perineal Care
S57.0.4 Manage Perineal Care

Edema Control—S69.0
Actions performed to control excess fluid in tissue
S69.0.1 Assess Edema Control
S69.0.2 Perform Edema Control
S69.0.3 Teach Edema Control
S69.0.4 Manage Edema Control

Circulatory Care—S70.0
Actions performed to support the circulation of the blood (blood vessels)
S70.0.1 Assess Circulatory Care
S70.0.2 Perform Circulatory Care
S70.0.3 Teach Circulatory Care
S70.0.4 Manage Circulatory Care

Vascular System Care—S82.0
Actions performed to control problems of the vascular system
S82.0.1 Assess Vascular System Care

(*Continued*)

TABLE 8.14 ■ Clinical Care Classification of 201 Nursing Interventions, Version 2.5: Coded with Definitions and Four Action Types and Classified by 21 Care Components[1,2] (*Continued*)

S82.0.2   Perform Vascular System Care
S82.0.3   Teach Vascular System Care
S82.0.4   Manage Vascular System Care

T.   Urinary Elimination Component

Cluster of elements that involve the genitourinary system
Bladder Care—T58.0
Actions performed to control urinary drainage problems
T58.0.1   Assess Bladder Care
T58.0.2   Perform Bladder Care
T58.0.3   Teach Bladder Care
T58.0.4   Manage Bladder Care

Bladder Instillation—T58.1
Actions performed to pour liquid through a catheter into the bladder
T58.1.1   Assess Bladder Instillation
T58.1.2   Perform Bladder Instillation
T58.1.3   Teach Bladder Instillation
T58.1.4   Manage Bladder Instillation

Bladder Training—T58.2
Actions performed to provide instruction on the care of urinary drainage
T58.2.1   Assess Bladder Training
T58.2.2   Perform Bladder Training
T58.2.3   Teach Bladder Training
T58.2.4   Manage Bladder Training

Dialysis Care—T59.0
Actions performed to support the removal of waste products from the body
T59.0.1   Assess Dialysis Care
T59.0.2   Perform Dialysis Care
T59.0.3   Teach Dialysis Care
T59.0.4   Manage Dialysis Care

Hemodialysis Care—T59.1
Actions performed to support the mechanical removal of waste products from the blood
T59.1.1   Assess Hemodialysis Care
T59.1.2   Perform Hemodialysis Care
T59.1.3   Teach Hemodialysis Care
T59.1.4   Manage Hemodialysis Care

Peritoneal Dialysis Care—T59.2
Actions performed to support the osmotic removal of waste products from the blood
T59.2.1   Assess Peritoneal Dialysis Care
T59.2.2   Perform Peritoneal Dialysis Care
T59.2.3   Teach Peritoneal Dialysis Care
T59.2.4   Manage Peritoneal Dialysis Care

Urinary Catheter Care—T60.0
Actions performed to control the use of a urinary catheter
T60.0.1   Assess Urinary Catheter Care
T60.0.2   Perform Urinary Catheter Care
T60.0.3   Teach Urinary Catheter Care
T60.0.4   Manage Urinary Catheter Care

Urinary Catheter Insertion—T60.1
Actions performed to place a urinary catheter in the bladder
T60.1.1   Assess Urinary Catheter Insertion
T60.1.2   Perform Urinary Catheter Insertion
T60.1.3   Teach Urinary Catheter Insertion
T60.1.4   Manage Urinary Catheter Insertion

TABLE 8.14 ■ *(Continued)*

Urinary Catheter Irrigation—T60.2

Actions performed to flush a urinary catheter

T60.2.1 Assess Urinary Catheter Irrigation

T60.2.2 Perform Urinary Catheter Irrigation

T60.2.3 Teach Urinary Catheter Irrigation

T60.2.4 Manage Urinary Catheter Irrigation

Urinary Incontinence Care—T72.0

Actions performed to control the inability to retain and/or involuntary retain urine

T72.0.1 Assess Urinary Incontinence Care

T72.0.2 Perform Urinary Incontinence Care

T72.0.3 Teach Urinary Incontinence Care

T72.0.4 Manage Urinary Incontinence Care

Renal Care—T73.0

Actions performed to control problems pertaining to the kidney

T73.0.1 Assess Renal Care

T73.0.2 Perform Renal Care

T73.0.3 Teach Renal Care

T73.0.4 Manage Renal Care

Bladder Ostomy Care—T83.0

Actions performed to maintain the artificial opening to remove urine

T83.0.1 Assess Bladder Ostomy Care

T83.0.2 Perform Bladder Ostomy Care

T83.0.3 Teach Bladder Ostomy Care

T83.0.4 Manage Bladder Ostomy Care

Bladder Ostomy Irrigation—T83.1

Actions performed to flush or wash out the artificial opening to remove urine

T83.1.1 Assess Bladder Ostomy Irrigation

T83.1.2 Perform Bladder Ostomy Irrigation

T83.1.3 Teach Bladder Ostomy Irrigation

T83.1.4 Manage Bladder Ostomy Irrigation

U. Life Cycle Component

Cluster of elements that involve the life span of individuals

Reproductive Care—U74.0

Actions performed to support the production of an offspring/child

U74.0.1 Assess Reproductive Care

U74.0.2 Perform Reproductive Care

U74.0.3 Teach Reproductive Care

U74.0.4 Manage Reproductive Care

Fertility Care—U74.1

Actions performed to increase the chance of conception of an offspring/child

U74.1.1 Assess Fertility Care

U74.1.2 Perform Fertility Care

U74.1.3 Teach Fertility Care

U74.1.4 Manage Fertility Care

Infertility Care—U74.2

Actions performed to promote conception by the infertile client of an offspring/child

U74.2.1 Assess Infertility Care

U74.2.2 Perform Infertility Care

U74.2.3 Teach Infertility Care

U74.2.4 Manage Infertility Care

Contraception Care—U74.3

Actions performed to prevent conception of an offspring/child

U74.3.1 Assess Contraception Care

U74.3.2 Perform Contraception Care

U74.3.3 Teach Contraception Care

U74.3.4 Manage Contraception Care

(Continued)

TABLE 8.14 ■ Clinical Care Classification of 201 Nursing Interventions, Version 2.5: Coded with Definitions and Four Action Types and Classified by 21 Care Components[1,2] (*Continued*)

Perinatal Care—U75.0
Actions performed to support the period before, during, and immediately after the creation of an offspring/child
U75.0.1   Assess Perinatal Care
U75.0.2   Perform Perinatal Care
U75.0.3   Teach Perinatal Care
U75.0.4   Manage Perinatal Care

Pregnancy Care—U75.1
Actions performed to support the gestation period of the formation of an offspring/child (being with child)
U75.1.1   Assess Pregnancy Care
U75.1.2   Perform Pregnancy Care
U75.1.3   Teach Pregnancy Care
U75.1.4   Manage Pregnancy Care

Labor Care—U75.2
Actions performed to support the bringing forth of an offspring/child
U75.2.1   Assess Labor Care
U75.2.2   Perform Labor Care
U75.2.3   Teach Labor Care
U75.2.4   Manage Labor Care

Delivery Care—U75.3
Actions performed to support the expulsion of an offspring/child at birth
U75.3.1   Assess Delivery Care
U75.3.2   Perform Delivery Care
U75.3.3   Teach Delivery Care
U75.3.4   Manage Delivery Care

Postpartum Care—U75.4
Actions performed to support the period immediately after the delivery of an offspring/child
U75.4.1   Assess Postpartum Care
U75.4.2   Perform Postpartum Care
U75.4.3   Teach Postpartum Care
U75.4.4   Manage Postpartum Care

Growth and Development Care—U76.0
Actions performed to support age-specific normal growth standards and/or development skills
U76.0.1   Assess Growth and Development Care
U76.0.2   Perform Growth and Development Care
U76.0.3   Teach Growth and Development Care
U76.0.4   Manage Growth and Development Care

[1] Clinical Care Classification (CCC) System, Version 2.5 (previously known as: (a) Clinical Care Classification (CCC) System, Version 2.0, Copyright © 2004; and (b) Home Healthcare Classification (HHCC) System, Version 1.0, Copyright © 1994] pending Copyright © 2012 by Virginia K. Saba. EdD, RN, FAAN, FACMI, LL, may be used ONLY with written Permission by Dr. Virginia K. Saba. (Permission Form available from website <http://www.sabacare.com>)

[2] Revised 1992, 1994, 2004, 2006, and 2011.

TABLE 8.15 ▪ Clinical Care Classification System, Version 2.5: CCC of Nursing Diagnoses and Outcomes and CCC of Nursing Interventions/Actions with Definitions Classified by 21 Care Components[1,2]

Care Components (A–U)	Nursing Diagnoses and Outcomes	Nursing Interventions/Actions
Coding structure consists of five alphanumeric digits First—A to U: **CCCs** Second/third—major category Fourth—subcategory Fifth—qualifier	**Expected Outcomes and Actual Outcomes** To improve (.1) or improved (.1) To stabilize (.2) or stabilized (.2) Deterioration (.3) or deteriorated (.3) *Example expected outcome: activity alteration improve—A01.0.1* *Example actual outcome: activity alteration improved—A01.0.1*	**Nursing Intervention—Action Types** Assess or monitor (.1) Perform or care (.2) Teach or instruct (.3) Manage or refer (.4) Example: *perform activity care: A01.0.2*
A. Activity Component *Cluster of elements that involve the use of energy in carrying out musculoskeletal and bodily actions*	**Activity Alteration—A01.0** *Change in or modification of energy used by the body* **Activity Intolerance—A01.1** *Incapacity to carry out physiological or psychological daily activities* **Activity Intolerance Risk—A01.2** *Increased chance of an incapacity to carry out physiological or psychological daily activities* **Diversional Activity Deficit—A01.3** *Lack of interest or engagement in leisure activities* **Fatigue—A01.4** *Exhaustion that interferes with physical and mental activities* **Physical Mobility Impairment—A01.5** *Diminished ability to perform independent movement* **Sleep Pattern Disturbance—A01.6** *Imbalance in the normal sleep/wake cycle* **Sleep Deprivation—A01.7** *Lack of a normal sleep/wake cycle* **Musculoskeletal Alteration—A02.0** *Change in or modification of the muscles, bones, or support structures*	**Activity Care—A01.0** *Activities performed to carry out physiological or psychological daily activities* **Energy Conservation—A01.2** *Actions performed to preserve energy* **Fracture Care —A02.0** *Actions performed to control broken bones* **Cast Care—A02.1** *Actions performed to control a rigid dressing* **Immobilizer Care—A02.2** *Actions performed to control a splint, cast, or prescribed bed rest* **Mobility Therapy—A03.0** *Actions performed to advise and instruct on mobility deficits* **Ambulation Therapy—A03.1** *Actions performed to promote walking* **Assistive Device Therapy—A03.2** *Actions performed to support the use of products to aid in caring for oneself* **Transfer Care—A03.3** *Actions performed to assist in moving from one place to another* **Sleep Pattern Control—A04.0** *Actions performed to support the sleep/wake cycle* **Musculoskeletal Care—A05.0** *Actions performed to restore physical functioning* **Range of Motion—A05.1** *Actions performed to provide active and passive exercises to maintain joint function* **Rehabilitation Exercise—A05.2** *Actions performed to promote physical functioning* **Bedbound Care—A61.0** *Actions performed to support an individual confined to bed* **Positioning Therapy—A61.1** *Process to support changes in body positioning* **Diversional Care—A77.0** *Actions performed to support interest in leisure activities or play*

(Continued)

TABLE 8.15 ■ Clinical Care Classification (CCC) System, Version 2.5: CCC of Nursing Diagnoses and Outcomes and CCC of Nursing Interventions/Actions with Definitions Classified by 21 Care Components[1,2] (*Continued*)

Care Components (A–U)	Nursing Diagnoses and Outcomes	Nursing Interventions/Actions
B. Bowel/Gastric Component *Cluster of elements that involve the gastrointestinal system*	**Bowel Elimination Alteration—B03.0** *Change in or modification of the gastrointestinal system* **Bowel Incontinence—B03.1** *Involuntary defecation* **Diarrhea—B03.3** *Abnormal frequency and fluidity of feces* **Fecal Impaction—B03.4** *Feces wedged in intestines* **Perceived Constipation—B03.5** *Impression of infrequent or difficult passage of hard, dry feces without cause* **Constipation—B03.6** *Difficult passage of hard, dry feces* **Gastrointestinal Alteration—B04.0** *Change in or modification of the stomach or intestines* **Nausea—B04.1** *Distaste for food/fluids and an urge to vomit* **Vomiting—B04.2** *Expulsion of stomach contents through the mouth*	**Bowel Care—B06.0** *Actions performed to control and restore the functioning of the bowel* **Bowel Training—B06.1** *Actions performed to provide instruction on bowel elimination conditions* **Disimpaction—B06.2** *Actions performed to manually remove feces* **Enema—B06.3** *Actions performed to give fluid rectally* **Diarrhea Care—B06.4** *Actions performed to control the abnormal frequency and fluidity of feces* **Bowel Ostomy Care—B07.0** *Actions performed to maintain the artificial opening that removes bowel waste products* **Bowel Ostomy Irrigation—B07.1** *Actions performed to flush or wash out the artificial opening that removes bowel waste products* **Gastric Care—B62.0** *Actions performed to control changes in the stomach and intestines* **Nausea Care—B62.1** *Actions performed to control the distaste for food and desire to vomit*
C. Cardiac Component *Cluster of elements that involve the heart and blood vessels*	**Cardiac Output Alteration—C05.0** *Change in or modification of the pumping action of the heart* **Cardiovascular Alteration—C06.0** *Change in or modification of the heart or blood vessels* **Blood Pressure Alteration—C06.1** *Change in or modification of the systolic or diastolic pressure* **Bleeding Risk—C06.2** *Increased chance of loss of blood volume*	**Cardiac Care—C08.0** *Actions performed to control changes in the heart or blood vessels* **Cardiac Rehabilitation—C08.1** *Actions performed to restore cardiac health* **Pacemaker Care—C09.0** *Actions performed to control the use of an electronic device that provides a normal heartbeat*
D. Cognitive/Neuro Component *Cluster of elements involving the cognitive, mental, cerebral, and neurological processes*	**Cerebral Alteration—D07.0** *Change in or modification of mental processes* **Confusion—D07.1** *State of being disoriented (mixed up)* **Knowledge Deficit—D08.0** *Lack of information, understanding, or comprehension* **Knowledge Deficit of Diagnostic Test—D08.1** *Lack of information on test(s) to identify disease or assess health condition* **Knowledge Deficit of Dietary Regimen—D08.2** *Lack of information on the prescribed diet/food intake*	**Behavior Care—D10.0** *Actions performed to support observable responses to internal and external stimuli* **Reality Orientation—D11.0** *Actions performed to promote the ability to locate oneself in an environment* **Wandering Control—D63.0** *Actions performed to control abnormal movability* **Memory Loss Care—D64.0** *Actions performed to control a person's inability to recall ideas and/or events* **Neurological System Care—D78.0** *Actions performed to control problems of the neurological system*

TABLE 8.15 ■ (*Continued*)

Care Components (A–U)	Nursing Diagnoses and Outcomes	Nursing Interventions/Actions
	Knowledge Deficit of Disease Process—D08.3 *Lack of information on the morbidity, course, or treatment of the health condition* **Knowledge Deficit of Fluid Volume— D08.4** *Lack of information on fluid volume intake requirements* **Knowledge Deficit of Medication Regimen—D08.5** *Lack of information on prescribed regulated course of medicinal substances* **Knowledge Deficit of Safety Precautions—D08.6** *Lack of information on measures to prevent injury, danger, or loss* **Knowledge Deficit of Therapeutic Regimen—D08.7** *Lack of information on regulated course of treating disease* **Thought Process Alteration—D09.0** *Change in or modification of thought and cognitive processes* **Memory Impairment—D09.1** *Diminished ability or inability to recall past events*	
E. Coping Component *Cluster of elements that involve the ability to deal with responsibilities, problems, or difficulties*	**Dying Process—E10.0** *Physical and behavioral responses associated with death* **Community Coping Impairment—E52.0** *Inadequate community response to problems or difficulties* **Family Coping Impairment—E11.0** *Inadequate family response to problems or difficulties* **Disabled Family Coping—E11.2** *Inability of family to function optimally* **Individual Coping Impairment—E12.0** *Inadequate personal response to problems or difficulties* **Adjustment Impairment—E12.1** *Inadequate adjustment to condition or change in health status* **Decisional Conflict—E12.2** *Struggle related to determining a course of action* **Defensive Coping—E12.3** *Self-protective strategies to guard against threats to self* **Denial—E12.4** *Attempt to reduce anxiety by refusal to accept thoughts, feelings, or facts*	**Counseling Service—E12.0** *Actions performed to provide advice or instruction to help another* **Coping Support—E12.1** *Actions performed to sustain a person dealing with responsibilities, problems, or difficulties* **Stress Control—E12.2** *Actions performed to support the physiological response of the body to a stimulus* **Crisis Therapy—E12.3** *Actions performed to sustain a person dealing with a condition, event, or radical change in status* **Emotional Support—E13.0** *Actions performed to maintain a positive affective state* **Spiritual Comfort—E13.1** *Actions performed to console, restore, or promote spiritual health* **Terminal Care—E14.0** *Actions performed in the period surrounding death* **Bereavement Support—E14.1** *Actions performed to provide comfort to the family/friends of the person who died*

(*Continued*)

TABLE 8.15 ■ Clinical Care Classification (CCC) System, Version 2.5: CCC of Nursing Diagnoses and Outcomes and CCC of Nursing Interventions/Actions with Definitions Classified by 21 Care Components[1,2] (*Continued*)

Care Components (A–U)	Nursing Diagnoses and Outcomes	Nursing Interventions/Actions
	Posttrauma Response—E13.0 *Sustained behavior related to a traumatic event* **Rape Trauma Syndrome—E13.1** *Group of symptoms related to a forced sexual act* **Spiritual State Alteration—E14.0** *Change in or modification of the spirit or soul* **Spiritual Distress—E14.1** *Anguish related to the spirit or soul* **Grieving—E53.0** *Feeling of great sorrow* **Anticipatory Grieving—E53.1** *Feeling great sorrow before the event or loss* **Dysfunctional Grieving—E53.2** *Prolonged feeling of great sorrow*	**Dying/Death Measures—E14.2** *Actions performed to support the dying process* **Funeral Arrangements—E14.3** *Actions performed to direct the preparation for burial*
F. Fluid Volume Component *Cluster of elements that involve liquid consumption*	**Fluid Volume Alteration—F15.0** *Change in or modification of bodily fluid* **Fluid Volume Deficit—F15.1** *Dehydration or fluid loss* **Fluid Volume Deficit Risk—F15.2** *Increased chance of dehydration or fluid loss* **Fluid Volume Excess—F15.3** *Fluid retention, overload, or edema* **Fluid Volume Excess Risk—F15.4** *Increased chance of fluid retention, overload, or edema* **Electrolyte Imbalance—F62.0** *Higher or lower body electrolyte levels*	**Fluid Therapy—F15.0** *Actions performed to provide liquid volume intake* **Hydration Control—F15.1** *Actions performed to control the state of fluid balance* **Intake—F15.3** *Actions performed to measure the amount of fluid volume taken into the body* **Output—F15.4** *Actions performed to measure the amount of fluid volume removed from the body.* **Hemodynamic Care—F79.0** *Actions performed to support the movement of solutions through the blood* **Intravenous Care—F79.1** *Actions performed to support the use of infusion equipment* **Venous Catheter Care—F79.2** *Actions performed to support the use of a venous infusion site* **Arterial Catheter Care—F79.3** *Actions performed to support the use of an arterial infusion site*
G. Health Behavior Component *Cluster of elements that involve actions to sustain, maintain, or regain health*	**Health Maintenance Alteration—G17.0** *Change in or modification of ability to manage health-related needs.* **Failure to Thrive—G17.1** *Inability to grow and develop normally* **Health-Seeking Behavior Alteration—G18.0** *Change in or modification of actions needed to improve health state* **Home Maintenance Alteration—G19.0** *Inability to sustain a safe, healthy environment*	**Community Special Services—G17.0** *Actions performed to provide advice or information about special community services* **Adult Day Center—G17.1** *Actions performed to direct the provision of a day program for adults in a specific location* **Hospice—G17.2** *Actions performed to support the provision of offering and/or providing care for terminally ill persons*

TABLE 8.15 ■ (*Continued*)

Care Components (A–U)	Nursing Diagnoses and Outcomes	Nursing Interventions/Actions
	Noncompliance—G20.0 *Failure to follow therapeutic recommendations* **Noncompliance of Diagnostic Test—G20.1** *Failure to follow therapeutic recommendations on tests to identify disease or assess health condition* **Noncompliance of Dietary Regimen—G20.2** *Failure to follow the prescribed diet/food intake* **Noncompliance of Fluid Volume—G20.3** *Failure to follow fluid volume intake requirements* **Noncompliance of Medication Regimen—G20.4** *Failure to follow prescribed regulated course of medicinal substances* **Noncompliance of Safety Precautions—G20.5** *Failure to follow measures to prevent injury, danger, or loss* **Noncompliance of Therapeutic Regimen—G20.6** *Failure to follow regulated course of treating disease or health condition*	**Meals on Wheels—G17.3** *Actions performed to direct the provision of a community program of delivering meals to the home* **Compliance Care—G18.0** *Actions performed to encourage adherence to care regimen* **Compliance with Diet—G18.1** *Actions performed to encourage adherence to diet/food intake* **Compliance with Fluid Volume—G18.2** *Actions performed to encourage adherence to therapeutic intake of liquids* **Compliance with Medical Regimen—G18.3** *Actions performed to encourage adherence to physician's/provider's treatment plan* **Compliance with Medication Regimen—G18.4** *Actions performed to encourage adherence to prescribed course of medicinal substances* **Compliance with Safety Precaution—G18.5** *Actions performed to encourage adherence with measures to protect self or others from injury, danger, or loss* **Compliance with Therapeutic Regimen—G18.6** *Actions performed to encourage adherence with plan of care* **Nursing Contact—G19.0** *Actions performed to communicate with another nurse* **Bill of Rights—G19.1** *Statements related to entitlements during an episode of illness* **Nursing Care Coordination—G19.2** *Actions performed to synthesize all plans of care by a nurse* **Nursing Status Report—G19.3** *Actions performed to document patient condition by a nurse* **Physician Contact—G20.0** *Actions performed to communicate with a physician/provider* **Medical Regimen Orders—G20.1** *Actions performed to support the physician's/provider's plan of treatment* **Physician Status Report—G20.2** *Actions performed to document patient condition by a physician/provider* **Professional/Ancillary Services—G21.0** *Actions performed to support the duties performed by health team members*

TABLE 8.15 ▧ Clinical Care Classification (CCC) System, Version 2.5: CCC of Nursing Diagnoses and Outcomes and CCC of Nursing Interventions/Actions with Definitions Classified by 21 Care Components[1,2] (*Continued*)

Care Components (A–U)	Nursing Diagnoses and Outcomes	Nursing Interventions/Actions
		Health Aide Service—G21.1 *Actions performed to support care services by a health aide* **Social Worker Service—G21.2** *Actions performed to provide advice or instruction by a social worker* **Nurse Specialist Service—G21.3** *Actions performed to provide advice or instruction by an advanced practice nurse or nurse practitioner* **Occupational Therapist Service—G21.4** *Actions performed to provide advice or instruction by an occupational therapist* **Physical Therapist Service—G21.5** *Actions performed to provide advice or instruction by a physical therapist* **Speech Therapist Service—G21.6** *Actions performed to provide advice or instruction by a speech therapist* **Respiratory Therapist Service—G21.7** *Actions performed to provide advice or instruction by a respiratory therapist*
H. Medication Component *Cluster of elements that involve medicinal substances*	**Medication Risk—H21.0** *Increased chance of negative response to medicinal substances* **Polypharmacy—H21.1** *Use of two or more drugs together*	**Chemotherapy Care—H22.0** *Actions performed to control and monitor antineoplastic agents* **Injection Administration—H23.0** *Actions performed to dispense medication by a hypodermic* **Medication Care—H24.0** *Actions performed to support use of prescribed drugs or remedies regardless of route* **Medication Actions—H24.1** *Actions performed to support and monitor the intended responses to prescribed drugs* **Medication Prefill Preparation—H24.2** *Actions performed to ensure the continued supply of prescribed drugs* **Medication Side Effects—H24.3** *Actions performed to control adverse untoward reactions or conditions to prescribed drugs* **Medication Treatment—H24.4** *Actions performed to administer/give drugs or remedies regardless of route* **Radiation Therapy Care—H25.0** *Actions performed to control and monitor radiation therapy*
I. Metabolic Component *Cluster of elements that involve the endocrine and immunologic processes*	**Endocrine Alteration—I22.0** *Change in or modification of internal secretions or hormones* **Immunologic Alteration—I23.0** *Change in or modification of the immune system*	**Allergic Reaction Care—I26.0** *Actions performed to reduce symptoms or precautions to reduce allergies* **Diabetic Care—I27.0** *Actions performed to support the control of diabetic conditions*

TABLE 8.15 ■ (*Continued*)

Care Components (A–U)	Nursing Diagnoses and Outcomes	Nursing Interventions/Actions
		Immunologic Care—I65.0 *Actions performed to protect against a particular disease*
J. Nutritional Component *Cluster of elements that involve the intake of food and nutrients*	**Nutrition Alteration—J24.0** *Change in or modification of food and nutrients* **Body Nutrition Deficit—J24.1** *Less than adequate intake or absorption of food or nutrients* **Body Nutrition Deficit Risk—J24.2** *Increased chance of less than adequate intake or absorption of food or nutrients* **Body Nutrition Excess—J24.3** *More than adequate intake or absorption of food or nutrients* **Body Nutrition Excess Risk—J24.4** *Increased chance of more than adequate intake or absorption of food or nutrients* **Swallowing Impairment—J24.5** *Inability to move food from mouth to stomach* **Infant Feeding Pattern Impairment—J54.0** *Imbalance in the normal feeding habits of an infant* **Breastfeeding Impairment—J55.0** *Diminished ability to nourish infant at the breast*	**Enteral Tube Care—J28.0** *Actions performed to control the use of an enteral drainage tube* **Enteral Tube Insertion—J28.1** *Actions performed to support the placement of an enteral drainage tube* **Enteral Tube Irrigation—J28.2** *Actions performed to flush or wash out an enteral tube* **Nutrition Care—J29.0** *Actions performed to support the intake of food and nutrients* **Feeding Technique—J29.2** *Actions performed to provide special measures to provide nourishment* **Regular Diet—J29.3** *Actions performed to support the ingestion of food and nutrients from established nutrition standards* **Special Diet—J29.4** *Actions performed to support the ingestion of food and nutrients prescribed for a specific purpose* **Enteral Feeding—J29.5** *Actions performed to provide nourishment through a gastrointestinal route* **Parenteral Feeding—J29.6** *Actions performed to provide nourishment through intravenous or subcutaneous routes* **Breastfeeding Support—J66.0** *Actions performed to provide nourishment of an infant at the breast* **Weight Control—J67.0** *Actions performed to control obesity or debilitation*
K. Physical Regulation Component *Cluster of elements that involve bodily processes*	**Physical Regulation Alteration—K25.0** *Change in or modification of somatic control* **Autonomic Dysreflexia—K25.1** *Life-threatening inhibited sympathetic response to noxious stimuli in a person with a spinal cord injury at or above T7* **Hyperthermia—K25.2** *Abnormally high body temperature* **Hypothermia—K25.3** *Abnormally low body temperature* **Thermoregulation Impairment—K25.4** *Fluctuation of temperature between hypothermia and hyperthermia*	**Infection Control—K30.0** *Actions performed to contain a communicable disease* **Universal Precautions—K30.1** *Practices to prevent the spread of infections and infectious diseases* **Physical Healthcare—K31.0** *Actions performed to support somatic problems* **Health History—K31.1** *Actions performed to obtain information about past illness and health status* **Health Promotion—K31.2** *Actions performed to encourage behaviors to enhance health state*

(*Continued*)

TABLE 8.15 ■ Clinical Care Classification (CCC) System, Version 2.5: CCC of Nursing Diagnoses and Outcomes and CCC of Nursing Interventions/Actions with Definitions Classified by 21 Care Components[1,2] (*Continued*)

Care Components (A–U)	Nursing Diagnoses and Outcomes	Nursing Interventions/Actions
	Infection Risk—K25.5 *Increased chance of contamination with disease-producing germs* **Infection—K25.6** *Contamination with disease-producing germs* **Intracranial Adaptive Capacity Impairment —K25.7** *Intracranial fluid volumes are compromised*	**Physical Examination—K31.3** *Actions performed to observe somatic events* **Clinical Measurements—K31.4** *Actions performed to conduct procedures to evaluate somatic events* **Specimen Care—K32.0** *Actions performed to direct the collection and/ or the examination of a bodily specimen* **Blood Specimen Care—K32.1** *Actions performed to collect and/or examine a sample of blood* **Stool Specimen Care—K32.2** *Actions performed to collect and/or examine a sample of feces* **Urine Specimen Care—K32.3** *Actions performed to collect and/or examine a sample of urine* **Sputum Specimen Care—K32.5** *Actions performed to collect and/or examine a sample of sputum* **Vital Signs—K33.0** *Actions performed to measure temperature, pulse, respiration, and blood pressure* **Blood Pressure—K33.1** *Actions performed to measure the diastolic and systolic pressure of the blood* **Temperature—K33.2** *Actions performed to measure the body temperature* **Pulse—K33.3** *Actions performed to measure rhythmic beats of the heart* **Respiration—K33.4** *Actions performed to measure the function of breathing*
L. Respiratory Component *Cluster of elements that involve breathing and the pulmonary system*	**Respiration Alteration—L26.0** *Change in or modification of the breathing function* **Airway Clearance Impairment—L26.1** *Inability to clear secretions/obstructions in airway* **Breathing Pattern Impairment—L26.2** *Inadequate inhalation or exhalation* **Gas Exchange Impairment—L26.3** *Imbalance of oxygen and carbon dioxide transfer between lung and vascular system* **Ventilatory Weaning Impairment—L56.0** *Inability to tolerate decreased levels of ventilator support*	**Oxygen Therapy Care—L35.0** *Actions performed to support the administration of oxygen treatment* **Pulmonary Care—L36.0** *Actions performed to support pulmonary hygiene* **Breathing Exercises—L36.1** *Actions performed to provide therapy on respiratory or lung exertion* **Chest Physiotherapy—L36.2** *Actions performed to provide exercises for postural drainage of lungs* **Inhalation Therapy—L36.3** *Actions performed to support breathing treatments* **Ventilator Care—L36.4** *Actions performed to control and monitor the use of a ventilator* **Tracheostomy Care—L37.0** *Actions performed to support a tracheostomy*

TABLE 8.15 ■ (*Continued*)

Care Components (A–U)	Nursing Diagnoses and Outcomes	Nursing Interventions/Actions

M. Role Relationship Component
Cluster of elements involving interpersonal work, social, family, and sexual interactions
	Role Performance Alteration—M27.0
	Change in or modification of carrying out responsibilities
	  Parental Role Conflict—M27.1
	  Struggle with parental position and responsibilities
	  Parenting Alteration—M27.2
	  Change in or modification of nurturing figure's ability to promote growth
	  Sexual Dysfunction—M27.3
	  Deleterious change in sexual response
	  Caregiver Role Strain—M27.4
	  Excessive tension of one who gives physical or emotional care and support to another person or patient
	Communication Impairment—M28.0
	Diminished ability to exchange thoughts, opinions, or information
	  Verbal Impairment—M28.1
	  Diminished ability to exchange thoughts, opinions, or information through speech
	Family Process Alteration—M29.0
	Change in or modification of usual functioning of a related group
	Sexuality Pattern Alteration—M31.0
	Change in or modification of a person's sexual response
	Socialization Alteration—M32.0
	Change in or modification of personal identity
	  Social Interaction Alteration—M32.1
	  Change in or modification of inadequate quantity or quality of personal relations
	  Social Isolation—M32.2
	  State of aloneness, lack of interaction with others
	  Relocation Stress Syndrome—M32.3
	  Excessive tension from moving to a new location
		Communication Care—M38.0
		Actions performed to exchange verbal/ nonverbal and/or translation information
		Psychosocial Care—M39.0
		Actions performed to support the study of psychological and social factors
		  Home Situation Analysis—M39.1
		  Actions performed to analyze the living environment
		  Interpersonal Dynamics Analysis— M39.2
		  Actions performed to support the analysis of the driving forces in a relationship between people
		  Family Process Analysis—M39.3
		  Actions performed to support the change and/or modification of a related group
		  Sexual Behavior Analysis—M39.4
		  Actions performed to support the change and/or modification of a person's sexual response
		  Social Network Analysis—M39.5
		  Actions performed to improve the quantity or quality of personal relationships

N. Safety Component
Cluster of elements that involve prevention of injury, danger, loss, or abuse
	Injury Risk—N33.0
	Increased chance of danger or loss
	  Aspiration Risk—N33.1
	  Increased chance of material into trachea–bronchial passage.
	  Disuse Syndrome—N33.2
	  Group of symptoms related to effects of immobility
	  Poisoning Risk—N33.3
	  Exposure to or ingestion of dangerous products
	  Suffocation Risk—N33.4
	  Increased chance of inadequate air for breathing
		Substance Abuse Control—N40.0
		Actions performed to control substances to avoid, detect, or minimize harm
		  Tobacco Abuse Control—N40.1
		  Actions performed to avoid, minimize, or control the use of tobacco
		  Alcohol Abuse Control—N40.2
		  Actions performed to avoid, minimize, orcontrol the use of distilled liquors
		  Drug Abuse Control—N40.3
		  Actions performed to avoid, minimize, or control the use of any habit-forming medication

(*Continued*)

TABLE 8.15 ■ Clinical Care Classification (CCC) System, Version 2.5: CCC of Nursing Diagnoses and Outcomes and CCC of Nursing Interventions/Actions with Definitions Classified by 21 Care Components[1,2] (*Continued*)

Care Components (A–U)	Nursing Diagnoses and Outcomes	Nursing Interventions/Actions
	Trauma Risk—N33.5 *Increased chance of accidental tissue processes* **Fall Risk—N33.6** *Increased chance of conditions that result in falls* **Violence Risk—N34.0** *Increased chance of harming self or others* **Suicide Risk—N34.1** *Increased chance of taking one's life intentionally* **Self-Mutilation Risk—N34.2** *Increased chance of destroying a limb or essential part of the body* **Perioperative Injury Risk—N57.0** *Increased chance of injury during the operative processes* **Perioperative Positioning Injury— N57.1** *Damages from operative process positioning* **Surgical Recovery Delay—N57.2** *Slow or delayed recovery from a surgical procedure* **Substance Abuse—N58.0** *Excessive use of harmful bodily materials* **Tobacco Abuse—N58.1** *Excessive use of tobacco products* **Alcohol Abuse—N58.2** *Excessive use of distilled liquors* **Drug Abuse—N58.3** *Excessive use of habit-forming medications*	**Emergency Care—N41.0** *Actions performed to support a sudden or unexpected occurrence* **Safety Precautions—N42.0** *Actions performed to advance measures to avoid danger or harm* **Environmental Safety—N42.1** *Precautions recommended to prevent or reduce environmental injury* **Equipment Safety—N42.2** *Precautions recommended to prevent or reduce equipment injury* **Individual Safety—N42.3** *Precautions to reduce individual injury* **Violence Control—N68.0** *Actions performed to control behaviors that may cause harm to oneself or others* **Perioperative Injury Care—N80.0** *Actions performed to support perioperative care requirements*
O. Self-Care Component *Cluster of elements that involve the ability to carry out activities to maintain oneself*	**Bathing/Hygiene Deficit—O35.0** *Impaired ability to cleanse oneself* **Dressing/Grooming Deficit—O36.0** *Inability to clothe and groom oneself* **Feeding Deficit—O37.0** *Impaired ability to feed oneself* **Self-Care Deficit—O38.0** *Impaired ability to maintain oneself* **Activities of Daily Living Alteration— O38.1** *Change in or modification of ability to maintain oneself* **Instrumental Activities of Daily Living Alteration—O38.2** *Change in or modification of more complex activities than those needed to maintain oneself* **Toileting Deficit—O39.0** *Impaired ability to urinate or defecate for oneself*	**Personal Care—O43.0** *Actions performed to care for oneself* **Activities of Daily Living—O43.1** *Actions performed to support personal activities to maintain oneself* **Instrumental Activities of Daily Living— O43.2** *Complex activities performed to support basic life skills*

TABLE 8.15 ■ (*Continued*)

Care Components (A–U)	Nursing Diagnoses and Outcomes	Nursing Interventions/Actions
P. Self-Concept Component *Cluster of elements that involve an individual's mental image of oneself*	**Anxiety—P40.0** *Feeling of distress or apprehension whose source is unknown* **Fear—P41.0** *Feeling of dread or distress whose cause can be identified* **Meaningfulness Alteration—P42.0** *Change in or modification of the ability to see the significance, purpose, or value in something* 　**Hopelessness—P42.1** 　*Feeling of despair or futility and passive involvement* 　**Powerlessness—P42.2** 　*Feeling of helplessness or inability to act* **Self-Concept Alteration—P43.0** *Change in or modification of ability to maintain one's image of self* 　**Body Image Disturbance—P43.1** 　*Imbalance in the perception of the way one's body looks* 　**Personal Identity Disturbance—P43.2** 　*Imbalance in the ability to distinguish between the self and the nonself* 　**Chronic Low Self-Esteem Disturbance—P43.3** 　*Persistent negative evaluation of oneself* 　**Situational Self-Esteem Disturbance—P43.4** 　*Negative evaluation of oneself in response to a loss or change*	**Mental Healthcare—P45.0** *Actions taken to promote emotional well-being* 　**Mental Health History—P45.1** 　*Actions performed to obtain information about past or present emotional well-being* 　**Mental Health Promotion—P45.2** 　*Actions performed to encourage or further emotional well-being* 　**Mental Health Screening—P45.3** 　*Actions performed to systematically examine emotional well-being* 　**Mental Health Treatment—P45.4** 　*Actions performed to support protocols used to treat emotional problems*
Q. Sensory Component *Cluster of elements that involve the senses, including pain*	**Sensory Perceptual Alteration—Q44.0** *Change in or modification of the response to stimuli* 　**Auditory Alteration—Q44.1** 　*Change in or modification of diminished ability to hear* 　**Gustatory Alteration—Q44.2** 　*Change in or modification of diminished ability to taste* 　**Kinesthetic Alteration—Q44.3** 　*Change in or modification of diminished balance* 　**Olfactory Alteration—Q44.4** 　*Change in or modification of diminished ability to smell* 　**Tactile Alteration—Q44.5** 　*Change in or modification of diminished ability to feel* 　**Unilateral Neglect—Q44.6** 　*Lack of awareness of one side of the body* 　**Visual Alteration—Q44.7** 　*Change in or modification of diminished ability to see*	**Pain Control—Q47.0** *Actions performed to support responses to injury or damage* 　**Acute Pain Control—Q47.1** 　*Actions performed to control physical suffering, hurting, or distress* 　**Chronic Pain Control—Q47.2** 　*Actions performed to control physical suffering, hurting, or distress that continues longer than expected* **Comfort Care—Q48.0** *Actions performed to enhance or improve well-being* **Ear Care—Q49.0** *Actions performed to support ear problems* 　**Hearing Aid Care—Q49.1** 　*Actions performed to control the use of a hearing aid* 　**Wax Removal—Q49.2** 　*Actions performed to remove cerumen from ear* **Eye Care—Q50.0** *Actions performed to support eye problems*

(*Continued*)

TABLE 8.15 ■ Clinical Care Classification (CCC) System, Version 2.5: CCC of Nursing Diagnoses and Outcomes and CCC of Nursing Interventions/Actions with Definitions Classified by 21 Care Components[1,2] (*Continued*)

Care Components (A–U)	Nursing Diagnoses and Outcomes	Nursing Interventions/Actions
	Comfort Alteration—Q45.0 *Change in or modification of sensation that is distressing* **Pain—Q63.0** *Physical suffering or distress; to hurt* **Acute Pain—Q63.1** *Severe pain of limited duration* **Chronic Pain—Q63.2** *Pain that persists over time*	**Cataract Care—Q50.1** *Actions performed to control cataract conditions* **Vision Care—Q50.2** *Actions performed to control vision problems*
R. Skin Integrity Component *Cluster of elements that involve the mucous membrane, corneal, integumentary, or subcutaneous structures of the body*	**Skin Integrity Alteration—R46.0** *Change in or modification of skin conditions* **Oral Mucous Membrane Impairment—R46.1** *Diminished ability to maintain the tissues of the oral cavity* **Skin Integrity Impairment—R46.2** *Decreased ability to maintain the integument* **Skin Integrity Impairment Risk—R46.3** *Increased chance of skin breakdown* **Skin Incision—R46.4** *Cutting of the integument/skin* **Latex Allergy Response—R46.5** *Pathological reaction to latex products* **Peripheral Alteration—R47.0** *Change in or modification of neurovascularization of the extremities*	**Pressure Ulcer Care—R51.0** *Actions performed to prevent, detect, and treat skin integrity breakdown caused by pressure* **Pressure Ulcer Stage 1 Care—R51.1** *Actions performed to prevent, detect, and treat stage 1 skin breakdown* **Pressure Ulcer Stage 2 Care—R51.2** *Actions performed to prevent, detect, and treat stage 2 skin breakdown* **Pressure Ulcer Stage 3 Care—R51.3** *Actions performed to prevent, detect, and treat stage 3 skin breakdown* **Pressure Ulcer Stage 4 Care—R51.4** *Actions performed to prevent, detect, and treat stage 4 skin breakdown* **Mouth Care—R53.0** *Actions performed to support oral cavity problems* **Denture Care—R53.1** *Actions performed to control the use of artificial teeth* **Skin Care—R54.0** *Actions to control the integument/skin* **Skin Breakdown Control—R54.1** *Actions performed to support tissue integrity problems* **Wound Care—R55.0** *Actions performed to support open skin areas* **Drainage Tube Care—R55.1** *Actions performed to support wound drainage from body tubes* **Dressing Change—R55.2** *Actions performed to remove and replace a new bandage on a wound* **Incision Care—R55.3** *Actions performed to support a surgical wound* **Burn Care—R81.0** *Actions performed to support burned areas of the body*

TABLE 8.15 ■ (*Continued*)

Care Components (A–U)	Nursing Diagnoses and Outcomes	Nursing Interventions/Actions
S. Tissue Perfusion Component *Cluster of elements that involve the oxygenation of tissues, including the circulatory and vascular systems*	**Tissue Perfusion Alteration—S48.0** *Change in or modification of the oxygenation of tissues*	**Foot Care—S56.0** *Actions performed to support foot problems* **Perineal Care—S57.0** *Actions performed to support perineal problems* **Edema Control—S69.0** *Actions performed to control excess fluid in tissue* **Circulatory Care—S70.0** *Actions performed to support the circulation of the blood (blood vessels)* **Vascular System Care—S82.0** *Actions performed to control problems of the vascular system*

T. Urinary Elimination Component
Cluster of elements that involve the genitourinary systems
	Urinary Elimination Alteration—T49.0
	Change in or modification of excretion of the waste matter of the kidneys
	  Functional Urinary Incontinence—T49.1
	  Involuntary, unpredictable passage of urine
	  Reflex Urinary Incontinence—T49.2
	  Involuntary passage of urine occurring at predictable intervals
	  Stress Urinary Incontinence—T49.3
	  Loss of urine occurring with increased abdominal pressure
	  Urge Urinary Incontinence—T49.5
	  Involuntary passage of urine following a sense of urgency to void
	  Urinary Retention—T49.6
	  Incomplete emptying of the bladder
	Renal Alteration—T50.0
	Change in or modification of kidney function
		Bladder Care—T58.0
		Actions performed to control urinary drainage problems
		  Bladder Instillation—T58.1
		  Actions performed to pour liquid through a catheter into the bladder
		  Bladder Training—T58.2
		  Actions performed to provide instruction on the care of urinary drainage
		Dialysis Care—T59.0
		Actions performed to support the removal of waste products from the body
		  Hemodialysis Care—T59.1
		  Actions performed to support the mechanical removal of waste products from the blood
		  Peritoneal Dialysis Care—T59.2
		  Actions performed to support the osmotic removal of waste products from the blood
		Urinary Catheter Care—T60.0
		Actions performed to control the use of a urinary catheter
		  Urinary Catheter Insertion—T60.1
		  Actions performed to place a urinary catheter in bladder
		  Urinary Catheter Irrigation—T60.2
		  Actions performed to flush a urinary catheter
		Urinary Incontinence Care—T72.0
		Actions performed to control the inability to retain and/or involuntarily retain urine
		Renal Care—T73.0
		Actions performed to control problems pertaining to the kidney
		Bladder Ostomy Care—T83.0
		Actions performed to maintain the artificial opening to remove urine
		  Bladder Ostomy Irrigation—T83.1
		  Actions performed to flush and wash out the artificial opening to remove urine

(*Continued*)

TABLE 8.15 ■ Clinical Care Classification (CCC) System, Version 2.5: CCC of Nursing Diagnoses and Outcomes and CCC of Nursing Interventions/Actions with Definitions Classified by 21 Care Components[1,2] *(Continued)*

Care Components (A–U)	Nursing Diagnoses and Outcomes	Nursing Interventions/Actions
U. Life Cycle Component *Cluster of elements that involve the life span of individuals*	**Reproductive Risk—U59.0** *Increased chance of harm in the process of replicating or giving rise to an offspring/child* **Fertility Risk—U59.1** *Increased chance of conception to develop an offspring/child* **Infertility Risk—U59.2** *Decreased chance of conception to develop an offspring/child* **Contraception Risk—U59.3** *Increased chance of harm preventing the conception of an offspring/child* **Perinatal Risk—U60.0** *Increased chance of harm before, during, and immediately after the creation of an offspring/child* **Pregnancy Risk—U60.1** *Increased chance of harm during the gestational period of the formation of an offspring/child* **Labor Risk—U60.2** *Increased chance of harm during the period supporting the bringing forth of an offspring/child* **Delivery Risk—U60.3** *Increased chance of harm during the period supporting the expulsion of an offspring/child* **Postpartum Risk—U60.4** *Increased chance of harm during the period immediately following the delivery of an offspring/child* **Growth and Development Alteration— U61.0** *Change in or modification of age-specific normal growth standards and/or developmental skills*	**Reproductive Care—U74.0** *Actions performed to support the production of an offspring/child* **Fertility Care—U74.1** *Actions performed to increase the chance of conception of an offspring/child.* **Infertility Care—U74.2** *Actions performed to promote conception by the infertile client of an offspring/child* **Contraception Care—U74.3** *Actions performed to prevent conception of an offspring/child* **Perinatal Care—U75.0** *Actions performed to support the period before, during, and immediately after the creation of an offspring/child* **Pregnancy Care—U75.1** *Actions performed to support the gestation period of the formation of an offspring/ child (being with child)* **Labor Care—U75.2** *Actions performed to support the bringing forth of an offspring/child* **Delivery Care—U75.3** *Actions performed to support the expulsion of an offspring/child at birth* **Postpartum Care—U75.4** *Actions performed to support the period immediately after the delivery of an offspring/child* **Growth and Development Care—U76.0** *Actions performed to support age-specific normal growth standards and/or developmental skills*

[1] Clinical Care Classification (CCC) System, Version 2.5 (previously known as: (a) Clinical Care Classification (CCC) System, Version 2.0, Copyright © 2004; and (b) Home Healthcare Classification (HHCC) System, Version 1.0, Copyright © 1994] pending Copyright © 2012 by Virginia K. Saba. EdD, RN, FAAN, FACMI, LL, may be used ONLY with written Permission by Dr. Virginia K. Saba. (Permission Form available from website <http://www.sabacare.com>)

[2] Revised 1992, 1994, 2004, 2006, and 2011.

CLINICAL CARE CLASSIFICATION (CCC) SYSTEM, VERSION 2.5: CARE COMPONENTS, NURSING DIAGNOSES, AND NURSING INTERVENTIONS REVISIONS FROM CLINICAL CARE CLASSIFICATION (CCC) SYSTEM, VERSION 2.0

● **Summary Changes in Version 2.5**

CCC Care Components = 21 classes
    1 revised name
    2 revised definitions

CCC Diagnoses = 176 concepts
    4 new concepts
    10 retired concepts
    16 revised definitions

CCC Interventions = 201 concepts
    14 new concepts
    11 retired concepts
    25 revised definitions

Approved February 11, 2011, by the CCC System National Scientific Advisory Board and published as the Clinical Care Classification System, Version 2.5, Fall 2011.

Virginia K. Saba Copyright: 2004, 2006, 2012

● **Revision Guide**

ADD code = single entry represents NEW OR REVISED CODE NUMBER (UPPERCASE)

ADD term = single entry represents NEW OR REVISED TERM (UPPERCASE)

ADD definition = single entry represents NEW OR REVISED DEFINITION (UPPERCASE)

ADD code/term = single entry represents NEW CODE/TERM (UPPERCASE)

ADD code/term/definition = single entry Represents NEW CODE/TERM/DEFINITION (UPPERCASE)

DELETE code = single entry represents retired code (lowercase)

DELETE term = single entry represents retired term (lowercase)

DELETE definition = singe entry represents retired definition (lowercase)

DELETE code/term = single entry represents retired code/term (lowercase)

DELETE code/term/definition = single entry represents retired code/term/definition (lowercase)

TABLE A.1 ■ Clinical Care Classification (CCC) System Care Components, Version 2.5: Revisions From CCC System, Version 2.0

DELETE term	C—Cognitive Component
ADD term	C—Cognitive/Neuro Component
DELETE definition	C—Cognitive/Neuro Component: Cluster of elements that involve the mental and cerebral processes
ADD definition	C—Cognitive/Neuro Component: Cluster of elements that involve the cognitive, mental, cerebral, and neurological processes
DELETE definition	S—Tissue Perfusion: Cluster of elements that involve the oxygenation of tissues, including the circulatory and neurovascular systems
ADD definition	S—Tissue Perfusion: Cluster of elements that involve the oxygenation of tissues, including the circulatory and vascular systems

TABLE A.2 ■ Clinical Care Classification (CCC) System of Nursing Diagnoses, Version 2.5: Revisions From CCC System Version 2.0

ADD code/term/definition	B04.2—Vomiting: Expulsion of stomach contents through the mouth
DELETE code	B51—Nausea: Distaste for fool/fluids and an urge to vomit
ADD code	B04.1—Nausea: Distaste for food/fluid and an urge to vomit
DELETE code/term/ definition	B03.2—Colonic Constipation: Infrequent or difficult passage of hard, dry, feces
DELETE definition	B03.5—Perceived Constipation: Belief and treatment of infrequent or difficult passage of hard, dry feces without cause
ADD definition	B03.5—Perceived Constipation: Impression of infrequent or difficult passage of hard, dry feces without cause
DELETE term/definition	B03.6—Unspecified Constipation: Other form of abnormal feces
ADD term/definition	B03.6—Constipation: Difficult passage of hard, dry, feces
ADD code/term/definition	C06.2—Bleeding Risk: Increased chance of loss of blood volume
DELETE definition	D07.0—Cerebral Alteration: Change in or modification of thought process or mentation
ADD definition	D07.0—Cerebral Alteration: Change in or modification of mental pricesses
DELETE definition	D08.2—Knowledge Deficit of Dietary Regimen: Lack of information on the prescribed food/fluid intake
ADD definition	D08.2—Knowledge Deficit of Dietary Regimen: Lack of information on the prescribed diet/food intake
DELETE definition	D09.0—Thought Process Alteration: Change in or modification of cognitive processes
ADD Definition	D09.0—Thought Process Alteration: Change in or modification of thought and cognitive processes

(Continued)

TABLE A.2 ■ (*Continued*)

DELETE code/term/ definition	E11.1—Compromised Family Coping: Inability of family to function optimally
DELETE definition	E11.2—Disabled Family Coping: Dysfunctional ability of family to function
ADD definition	E11.2—Disabled Family Coping: Inability of family to function optimally
DELETE definition	F15.1—Fluid Volume Deficit: Dehydration
ADD definition	F15.1—Fluid Volume Deficit: Dehydration or fluid loss
DELETE definition	F15.2—Fluid Volume Deficit Risk: Dehydration
ADD definition	F15.1—Fluid Volume Deficit Risk: Dehydration or fluid loss
ADD code/term/definition	F62.0—Electrolyte Imbalance: Higher or lower body electrolyte levels
DELETE definition	G20.2—Noncompliance of Dietary Regimen: Failure to follow the prescribed food or fluid intake
ADD definition	G20.2—Noncompliance of Dietary Regimen: Failure to follow the prescribed diet/food intake
DELETE code/term/ definition	I23.1—Protection Alteration: Change in or modification of the ability to guard against internal and external treats to the body
DELETE term/definition	K25.6—Unspecified Infection: Unknown contamination with disease-producing germs
ADD term/definition	K25.6—Infection: Contamination with disease-producing germs
ADD code/term/definition	N33.6—Fall Risk: Increased chance of conditions that results in falls
DELETE definition	Q44.3—Kinesthetic Alteration: Change in or modification of diminished ability to move
ADD definition	Q44.3—Kinesthetic Alteration: Change in or modification of diminished balance
DELETE code/term/ definition	Q45.3—Unspecified Pain: Pain that is difficult to pinpoint
ADD code/term/definition	Q63.0—Pain: Physical suffering or distress, to hurt
DELETE code/definition	Q45.1—Acute Pain: Physical suffering or distress; to hurt
ADD code/definition	Q63.1—Acute Pain: Severe pain of limited duration
DELETE code/definition	Q45.2—Chronic Pain: Pain that continues for longer than expected
DELETE definition	Q44.3—Peripheral Alteration: Change in or modification of vascularization of the extremities
ADD definition	Q44.3—Peripheral Alteration: Change in or modification of neurovascularization of the extremities
ADD code/definition	Q63.2—Chronic Pain: Pain that persists over time
DELETE code/term/ definition	T49.4—Total Urinary Incontinence: Continuous and unpredictable loss of urine
DELETE definition	U61.0—Growth and Development Alteration: Change in or modification of growth standards and/or developmental skills for an individual's age

(*Continued*)

TABLE A.2 ▤ Clinical Care Classification (CCC) System of Nursing Diagnoses, Version 2.5: Revisions From CCC System Version 2.0 (*Continued*)

ADD definition	U61.0—Growth and Development Alteration: Change in or modification of age-specific normal growth standards and/or developmental skills
DELETE code/term/ definition	U61.1—Newborn Behavior Alteration: Change in or modification of normal standards of performing developmental skills and behavior of a typical newborn the first 30 days of life
DELETE code/term/ definition	U61.2—Infant Behavior Alteration: Change in or modification of normal standards of performing developmental skills and behavior of a typical infant from 31 days through 11 months of age
DELETE code/term/ definition	U61.3—Child Behavior Alteration: Change in or modification of normal standards of performing developmental skills and behavior of a typical child from 1 year through 11 years of age
DELETE code/term/ definition	U61.4—Adolescent Behavior Alteration: Change in or modification of normal standards of performing developmental skills and behavior of a typical adolescent from 12 years through 20 years of age
DELETE code/term/ definition	U61.5—Adult Behavior Alteration: Change in or modification of normal standards of performing developmental skills and behavior of a typical adult from 21 years through 64 years of age
DELETE code/term/ definition	U61.6—Older Adult Behavior Alteration: Change in or modification of normal standards of performing developmental skills and behavior of a typical older adult 65 years of age and over

TABLE A.3 ▤ Clinical Care Classification (CCC) System of Nursing Interventions, Version 2.5: Revisions From CCC System, Version 2.0

ADD code/term/definition	A77.0—Diversional Care: Actions performed to support interest in leisure activities or play
DELETE definition	B06.3—Enema: Actions performed to administer fluid rectally
ADD definition	B06.3—Enema: Actions performed to give fluid rectally
DELETE term/definition	B07.0—Ostomy Care: Actions performed to control the artificial opening that removes waste
ADD term/definition	B07.0—Bowel Ostomy Care: Actions performed to maintain the artificial opening that removes bowel waste
DELETE term/definition	B07.1—Bowel Ostomy Irrigation: Actions performed to flush or wash an ostomy
ADD term/definition	B07.1—Bowel Ostomy Irrigation: Actions performed to flush or wash out the artificial opening that removes bowel waste
ADD code/term/definition	D78.0—Neurological System Care: Actions performed to control problems of the neurological system
DELETE code/term/ definition	F15.3—Intake/Output: Actions performed to measure the amount of fluid/food and excretion of waste

(Continued)

TABLE A.3 ▨ (*Continued*)

ADD code/term/definition	F15.3—Intake: Actions performed to measure the amount of fluid volume taken into the body
ADD code/term/definition	F15.4—Output: Actions performed to measure the amount of fluid volume removed from the body
DELETE code/term/ definition	F16—Infusion Care: Actions performed to support solutions given through the vein
ADD code/term/definition	F79.0—Hemodynamic Care: Actions performed to support the movement of solutions through the blood
DELETE code/definition	F16.2—Intravenous Care: Actions performed to administer an infusion through a vein
ADD code/definition	F79.1—Intravenous Care: Actions performed to support the use of infusion equipment
DELETE code/definition	F16.2—Venous Catheter Care: Actions performed to control the use of infusion equipment
ADD code/definition	F79.2—Venous Catheter Care: Actions performed to support the use of a venous infusion site
ADD code/term/definition	F79.3—Arterial Catheter Care: Actions performed to support the use of an arterial infusion site
DELETE definition	G18—Compliance Care: Actions performed to encourage conformity in therapeutic regimen
ADD definition	G18.0—Compliance Care: Actions performed to encourage adherence in care regimen
DELETE definition	G18.1—Compliance with Diet: Actions performed to encourage conformity to food or fluid intake in therapeutic regimen
ADD definition	G18.1—Compliance with Diet: Actions performed to encourage adherence to diet/food intake
DELETE definition	G18.2—Compliance with Fluid Volume: Actions performed to encourage conformity to therapeutic intake of fluids
ADD definition	G18.2—Compliance with Fluid Volume: Actions performed to encourage adherence to therapeutic intake of fluids
DELETE definition	G18.3—Compliance with Medical Regimen: Actions performed to encourage conformity to physician's treatment plan
ADD definition	G18.3—Compliance with Medical Regimen: Actions performed to encourage adherence to physician's/ provider's treatment plan
DELETE definition	G18.4—Compliance with Medication Regimen: Actions performed to encourage conformity to follow prescribed course of medicinal substances
ADD definition	G18.4—Compliance with Medication Regimen: Actions performed to encourage adherence to follow prescribed course of medicinal substances
DELETE definition	G18.5—Compliance with Safety Precautions: Actions performed to encourage conformity with measures to protect self or others from injury, danger, or loss

(*Continued*)

TABLE A.3 ▪ (*Continued*)

ADD definition	G18.5—Compliance with Safety Precautions: Actions performed to encourage adherence with measures to protect self or others from injury, danger, or loss
DELETE definition	G18.6—Compliance with Therapeutic Regimen: Actions performed to encourage conformity with health team's plan of care
ADD definition	G18.5—Compliance with Therapeutic Regimen: Actions performed to encourage adherence with plan of care
DELETE definition	G20—Physician Contact: Actions performed to communicate with a physician
ADD definition	G20.0—Physician Contact: Actions performed to communicate with a physician/provider
DELETE definition	G20.1—Medical Regimen Orders: Actions performed to support the physician's plan of treatment
ADD definition	G20.1—Medical Regimen Orders: Actions performed to support the physician's/provider's plan of treatment
DELETE definition	G20.2—Physician Status Report: Actions performed to document patient's condition by a physician
ADD definition	G20.2—Physician Status Report: Actions performed to document patient's condition by a physician/provider
DELETE term/definition	G21.1—Home Health Aide: Actions performed to support the services by a home health aide
ADD term/definition	G21.1—Health Aide: Actions performed to support the services by a health aide
DELETE term/definition	G21.2—Medical Social Worker: Actions performed to provide advice or instructions by a medical social worker
ADD term/definition	G21.2—Social Worker: Actions performed to provide advice or instructions by a social worker
ADD code/term/definition	G21.7—Respiratory Therapist Service: Actions performed to provide advice or instruction by a respiratory therapist
DELETE code/term/ definition	H23.1—Insulin Injection: Actions performed to administer a hypodermic administration of insulin
DELETE code/term/ definition	H23.2—Vitamin B_{12} Injection: Actions performed to administer a hypodermic administration of vitamin B_{12}
DELETE definition	H24—Medication Care: Actions performed to direct the dispensing of prescribed drugs or remedies regardless of route
ADD definition	H24.0—Medication Care: Actions performed to support the use of prescribed drugs or remedies regardless of route
DELETE definition	H24.1—Medication Action: Actions performed to support and monitor the use of medicinal substances
ADD definition	H24.1—Medication Action: Actions performed to support and monitor the intended responses to prescribed drugs
DELETE definition	H24.3—Medication Side Effects: Actions performed to control untoward reactions or conditions to prescribed drugs

(*Continued*)

TABLE A.3 ▪ (*Continued*)

ADD definition	H24.3—Medication Side Effects: Actions performed to control adverse untoward reactions or conditions to prescribed drugs
DELETE definition	H24.4—Medication Treatment: Actions performed to administer drugs or remedies regardless of route
ADD definition	H24.4—Medication Treatment: Actions performed to administer/give drugs or remedies regardless of route
DELETE definition	M38—Communication Care: Actions performed to exchange information
ADD definition	M38.0—Communication Care: Actions performed to exchange verbal/nonverbal and/or translation of information
ADD code/term/definition	N80.0—Perioperative Injury Care: Actions performed to support perioperative care requirements
DELETE definition	R55.1—Drainage Tube Care: Actions performed to support drainage from tubes
ADD definition	R55.1—Drainage Tube Care: Actions performed to support wound drainage from body tubes
ADD code/term/definition	R81.0—Burn Care: Actions performed to support burned areas of the body
DELETE code/term/ definition	S71—Neurovascular Care: Actions performed to control problems of the nerves and vascular system
ADD code/term/definition	S82.0—Vascular System Care: Actions performed to control problems of the vascular system
DELETE definition	T59—Dialysis Care: Actions performed to support dialysis treatments
ADD definition	T59.0—Dialysis Care: Actions performed to support the removal of waste products from the body
ADD code/term/definition	T59.1—Hemodialysis: Actions performed to support the mechanical removal of waste products from the blood
ADD code/term/definition	T59.2—Peritoneal Dialysis Care: Actions performed to support the osmotic removal of waste products from the blood
ADD code/term/definition	T83.0—Bladder Ostomy Care: Actions performed to maintain the artificial opening to remove urine
ADD code/term/definition	T83.1—Bladder Ostomy: Performed to flush or wash out the artificial opening to remove urine
DELETE definition	U76—Growth and Development Care: Actions performed to support age-specific normal growth standards and/or developmental skills and behavior of an individual age group
ADD definition	U76.0—Growth and Development Care: Actions performed to support age-specific normal growth standards and/or developmental skills
DELETE code/term/ definition	U76.1—Newborn Behavior Care: Actions performed to support normal standards of performing developmental skills and behavior of a typical newborn for the first 30 days of life

(Continued)

TABLE A.3 ◾ Clinical Care Classification (CCC) System of Nursing Interventions, Version 2.5: Revisions From CCC System, Version 2.0 (*Continued*)

DELETE code/term/ definition	U76.2—Infant Behavior Care: Actions performed to support normal standards of performing developmental skills and behavior of a typical infant 31 days through 11 months of age
DELETE code/term/ definition	U76.3—Child Behavior Care: Actions performed to support normal standards of performing developmental skills and behavior of a typical child 1 year through 11 years of age
DELETE code/term/ definition	U76.4—Adolescent Behavior Care: Actions performed to support normal standards of performing developmental skills and behavior of a typical adolescent 12 years through 20 years of age
DELETE code/term/ definition	U76.5—Adult Behavior Care: Actions performed to support normal standards of performing developmental skills and behavior of an adult 21 years through 64 years of age
DELETE code/term/ definition	U76.6—Older Adult Behavior Care: Actions performed to support normal standards of performing developmental skills and behavior of a typical older adult 65 years of age and over

Date	Highlights
2012, June	SabaCare Inc. forms a collaborative relationship between SabaCare Inc. and Clinical Care Classification (CCC) System with International Council of Nurses (ICN) and International Classification of Nursing Practice (ICNP).
2012, June	CCC System Version 2.5 mapped to ICNP for publication by ICN.
2012, June	Copyright Office Certificate of Registration (Pending). Clinical Care Classification (CCC) System Version 2.5.
2012, March	CCC System Version 2.5 uploaded on website, <http://www.clinicalcareclassification.com>
2012, January	CCC System updated on American Nurses Association (ANA). (January 17, 2012). List of *ANA Recognized Terminologies that Support Nursing Practice.* Silver Spring, MD: ANA. Retrieved on April 2, 2012. (http://nursingworld.org/npii/terminologies.html)
2011, November	CCC System Version 2.5 submitted to the National Library of Medicine for inclusion in Metathesaurus of the Unified Medical Language System (UMLS).
2011, September	CCC System Version 2.5 Registered by Health Level Seven (HL7) Object Identifier.
2011, August	CCC System Version 2.5 integrated into Systemized Nomenclature of Medical Clinical Terms (SNOMED CT), Chicago, IL.
2011, June	CCC System Version 2.5 finalized by CCC National Scientific Advisory Board for publication and distribution by SabaCare Inc. Arlington, VA.
2011	Clinical Care Classification (CCC) System Version 2.0 Wikipedia: http://en.wikipedia.org/wiki/Clinical_Care_Classification_System
2010, December	U.S. Patent and Trademark Office, Certification of Registration: Clinical Care Classification (CCC) System Logo (3019288) Combined Declaration of Use and Incontestability (update 11/29/2005).
2010	CCC System manual translated into German by Karl–Heinz Grimm and Jurgen Georg and published by HUBER Publishing into German.
2010	CCC System (Version 2.0) translated into Spanish by Professor Patricia Levi, RN, MPH, Escuela De Enfermeria Universidad De Guayaquil, Ciudadela Universitaria, Avenida Delta Guayaquil, Ecuador.
2010	Integrating the Healthcare Enterprise Patient Care Coordination Technical Committee selected the CCC System as the nursing terminology standard in the Reconciliation of Diagnoses, Allergies and Medications profile.

2009	Medicomp Systems selected and integrated the CCC System as the nursing terminology standard in the MEDCIN® Engine, a robust clinical knowledgebase in use throughout the world for the documentation of healthcare.
2008	Integrating the Healthcare Enterprise Patient Care Coordination Technical Committee selected the CCC System as the exemplar terminology standard in patient plan of care profile.
2007	Alliance for Nursing Informatics (ANI) press release: "CCC nursing terminology accepted by HHS." ANI announced that "a nationally endorsed nursing standard was selected by the Healthcare Information Technology Standards Panel and the American Health Information Community."
2007	The Office of the National Coordinator for Health Information Technology recommended the CCC System in the HITSP Biosurveillance Interoperability Specification (IS-02) to the HHS for the exchange of health data.
2007, January	The CCC System was accepted as a named National Nursing Terminology Standard and recognized by the Secretary of the U.S. Department of Health and Human Services (HHS) as submitted by the American Health Information Community.
2006	The HITSP approved the CCC System as the first nationwide nursing terminology standard for the exchange of electronic health record documentation in the Biosurveillance Technical Committee standards to support the early detection, situational awareness, and rapid response management across care delivery settings, including public health.
2006	CCC of Nursing Interventions (Version 2.0) integrated into ABC Codes for Complementary and Alternative Medicine and Conventional Nursing.
2006	CCC System (Version 2.0) *Mapped to* International Classification of Nursing Practice (ICNP), Geneva, Switzerland.
2005, October	CCC System (Version 2.0) registered by Health Level Seven (HL7) Object Identifier.
2005, October	CCC System (Version 2.0) mapped to Logical Observations, Identifiers, Names and Codes.
2005, December	U.S. Patent and Trademark Office Certificate of Registration: *Clinical Care Classification System* logo (Registration no. 3,019,288).
2005	FinCC named the National Nursing Classification Standard for documenting nursing practice in ALL Finnish hospitals.
2005	CCC System Manual translated into Portuguese by Dr. Heimar F. Marin, PhD, RN, FACMI, Professor and Director, Graduate Program in Health Informatics, Federal University of Sao Paulo, Brazil.
2004, October	U.S. Copyright Office Certificate of Registration: *Clinical Care Classification (CCC) System* (Registration no. 6-100-481).
2004, July	CCC System (Version 2.0) integrated into Systematized Nomenclature of Medical Clinical Terms (SNOMED CT), Chicago, IL.
2004, February	CCC System (Version 2.0) new name and version announced at the Health Information and Management System Society (HIMSS) meeting in Orlando, FL.

2004	CCC System (Version 2.0) indexed in the United States Health Information Knowledgebase (www.ushik.org), administered by the Agency for Healthcare Research and Quality.
2003, April	CCC System (Version 2.0) submitted to National Library of Medicine for inclusion into the Metathesaurus of the Unified Medical Language System (UMLS).
2003	CCC System (Version 2.0) indexed in Cumulative Index of Nursing and Allied Health Literature (CINAHL) Information Systems: *CINAHL 2004 Subject Heading List Thesaurus*, Glendale, CA.
2003, February	CCC terminology questionnaire submitted to Developers of Candidate Terminologies for Patient Medical Record Information (PMRI) Standards Panel, Subcommittee on Standards and Security, National Committee on Vital and Health Statistics (NCVHS), Washington, DC (in reference to PMRI, required by the Administration Simplification provision of the Health Insurance Portability and Accountability Act [HIPAA] of 1966, Pub. L. No. 104-191).
2003, January	CCC System (Version 2.0) updated on website: http://www.sabacare.com
2000, July	Home Health Care Classification (HHCC) System of Nursing Diagnoses and Nursing Interventions submitted to National Center for Health and Vital Statistics (NCHVS) for compliance to the *Uniform Data Standards for Patient Medical Record Information. Report to the Secretary of the US-DHHS*, as required by the Administration Simplification provision of the HIPAA of 1966, Pub. L. No. 104-191.
2000	HHCC of Nursing Diagnoses (Version 1.0) integrated into Systematized Nomenclature of Medical Reference Terms, Chicago, IL.
1999, May	Testimony entitled "Home Health Care Classification System (HHCC)" to Work Group on Computer-based Patient Records, National Committee on Vital and Health Statistics (HCVHS), Rockville, MD: AHCPR (in reference to the HIPAA of 1996, Pub. L. No. 104-191).
1999	HHCC of Nursing Diagnoses and Outcomes (Version 1.0) integrated into Logical Observations, Identifiers, Names and Codes.
1999	HHCC System (Version 1.0) registered by Health Level Seven.
1999/1998	"Home Health Care Classification (HHCC) of Nursing Diagnoses and Nursing Interventions" approved and published in ANSI HISB's *Inventory of Clinical Information Standards:* Washington, DC: ANSI.
1998, February	Testimony entitled "Home Health Care Classification (HHCC) of Nursing Diagnoses and Nursing Interventions" to the Safety Regulations and Electronic Dissemination of Billing Data Committee, American National Standards Institute—Healthcare Informatics Standards Board (ANSI HISB): Inventory of Clinical Information Standards: Template C: Code Sets. Washington, DC: DHHS (in reference to the HIPAA of 1996, Pub. L. No. 104-191).
1998	HHCC of Nursing Interventions (Version 1.0) integrated into ABC Codes for Complementary and Alternative Medicine and Conventional Nursing.

1998	First Commercial Website for HHCC System (Version 1.0): http://www.Sabacare.com
1997, May	Testimony entitled "Home Health Care Classification (HHCC) of Nursing Diagnoses and Nursing Interventions" to Developers of Coding and Classification Systems Panel, Subcommittee on Health Data Needs, Standards, and Security, NCVHS (in reference to the HIPAA of 1996, Pub. L. No. 104-191).
1995	HHCC of Nursing Interventions (Version 1.0) translated into Finnish (second translation).
1995	Initiated website at Georgetown University Dahlgren Medical Library, Washington, DC, for Home Health Care Classification: Nursing Diagnoses and Interventions: http://www.dml.georgetown.edu/research/hhcc
1995	HHCC of Nursing Diagnoses and HHCC of Nursing Interventions indexed in CINAHL Information Systems: *CINAHL 2004 Subject Heading List Thesaurus*, Glendale, CA.
1994	Published revised manual, *Home Health Care Classification Nursing Diagnoses and Interventions*: Washington, DC: Georgetown University Press.
1993	HHCC System (Version 1.0), title terms only, indexed in CINAHL Information Systems: *CINAHL 2004 Subject Heading List Thesaurus*, Glendale, CA.
1993	First publication of Manual: *Home Health Care Classification Nursing Diagnoses and Interventions*, Washington, DC: Georgetown University Press.
1993	HHCC System (Version 1.0) submitted to National Library of Medicine for inclusion into the Metathesaurus of the UMLS by the American Nurses Association (ANA).
1993, February	U.S. Copyright Office certificate of registration: *Classification of Home Health Nursing Diagnoses and Interventions* (registration no. 573-483).
1992, December	First integration of HHCC System (Version 1.0) in a nursing terminology database, by E. R. Gabrieli: *6-3-1-10 = Nursing Terminology* (V. Saba), Buffalo, NY: Gabrieli.
1992, November	First translation of the HHCC System (Version 1.0) into Dutch by Marlou de Fuiper, RN, MSN: "Diagnose en interventie" (in Classification of Home Health Care Nursing Diagnoses and Interventions). In L. Regeer (Ed.), *Verpleegkundige Diagnostiek in Nederland* (pp. 62–82), Amsterdam, the Netherlands: LEO Verpleegkundig Management.
1992, February	HHCC System (Version 1.0) recognized by the ANA Congress on Nursing Practice.
1991, November	HHCC System (Version 1.0) recognized by the ANA Steering Committee on Databases to Support Clinical Nursing Practice.
1991, June	First published article: Saba, V. K., O'Hare, P., Zuckerman, A. E., Boondas, J., Levine, E., and Oatway, D. M. A nursing intervention taxonomy for home healthcare. *Nursing and Health Care, 12*(6), 296–299.
1991, February	Final report, *Home Health Care Classification Project*, submitted to the Health Care Financing Administration. Report contained preliminary HHCC of Nursing Diagnoses and Interventions.

| 1988, May | Home Health Care Classification Project, Georgetown University, School of Nursing: "Develop and Demonstrate a Method for Classifying Home Health Patients to Predict Resource Requirements and to Measure Outcomes" funded by the Health Care Financing Administration (cooperative agreement no. 17-C-98983/3/01). |

The bibliography chapter consists of major articles written about the Clinical Care Classification (CCC) System since the CCC System was first published in *Nursing Outlook* in 1991. Many of the articles refer to the original name of the CCC System—the Home Health Care Classification (HHCC) System, Version 1.0. The HHCC was changed to the CCC System in 2003. The reason for the change was the applicability and usability of the CCC System framework and terminologies to ALL healthcare settings.

Many of the articles were published in nursing journals, conference proceedings, and other printed sources, such as online media. The articles were authored by experts involved in nursing languages, vocabularies, classifications, and terminologies, including Dr. Virginia K. Saba, EdD, RN, FAAN, FACMI. The articles included research studies, theses/dissertations, evaluation studies, and "vision" papers.

The CCC System has been studied extensively since 1991 (initial CCC System publication announcement) by several nursing informatics theorists, expert terminologists, and researchers who focused on the major nursing languages recognized by the American Nurses Association (ANA). Other CCC System research studies have focused on the CCC's characteristics and features and on the comparison of the CCC to the ANA-recognized classifications. Some CCC System research studies have highlighted the usability of the CCC System in different healthcare settings, such as hospitals, and for various patient conditions, such as: Depression, Postpartum Care, Human Immunodeficiency Virus (HIV) Care, Critical Care and others. Other research studies evaluated the capabilities of the CCC System in meeting the major Cimino (1998) criteria of a complete terminology for the EHR/HIT systems. Many nursing informatics and terminology experts indicated that the CCC System successfully provided a standardized framework for documenting the six steps/standards of the nursing process according to the *Scope and Standards of Nursing Practice* (ANA, 2010) and concluded that the CCC System could be used to improve quality; ensure safety; measure care outcomes; and determine care workload, resources, and cost.

A recent study by Mannino and Feeg (2011) demonstrated the use of the CCC System to teach students the value of electronic documentation of clinical practice and how to electronically document patient plans of care following the nursing process in an EHR. Other recent research by Dykes et al. (2011) explored the interoperability of the CCC System with SNOMED CT using the Unified Medical Language System (UMLS) Metathesaurus browser as a validation tool. Dr. Dykes determined that CCC concepts were interoperable with and mapped to SNOMED CT.

The bibliography represents a body of knowledge about the CCC System. This chapter provides background information on the scope of nursing terminology for interested informaticians/informaticists. The chapter clearly identifies the CCC System as a standardized national nursing terminology important for the documentation of clinical practice for nursing and allied health professions. The articles are listed in descending order, beginning with 2012.

● References

Cimino, T. T., (1998). Desiderata for controlled medical vocabularies in the twenty-first century. *Methods of Information in Medicine*, 37, 304–403.

Dykes, P. C., Da Damio, R. R., Goldsmith, D., Kim, H., Ohashi, K., & Saba, V. K., (2011). Leveraging standards to support patient-centric interdisciplinary plans of care. (2011). In S. Evans, C. Lehmann, &

W. Pratt (Eds.), *American Medical Informatics Association 2011 Proceedings* (pp. 356–363). Washington, DC: AMIA.

Mannino, J. E., & Feeg, V. D. (2011). Field-testing a PC electronic documentation system using the Clinical Care Classification© System with nursing students. *Journal of Healthcare Engineering, 2*(2). doi: 10.1260/2040-2295.2.2.223.

● Bibliography

2012

Saba, V. K. (2012). The Clinical Care Classification. In J. Fitzpatrick, & M. W. Kazer (Eds.), *The Encyclopedia of Nursing Research* (3rd ed.). New York, NY: Springer Publishing Company.

2011

Dykes, P. C., Da Damio, R. R., Goldsmith, D., Kim, H. E., Ohashi, K., & Saba, V. K. (2011). Leveraging standards to support patient-centric interdisciplinary plans of care. In S. Evans, C. Lehmann, & W. Pratt (Eds.). *American Medical Informatics Association 2011 Proceedings.* Washington, DC: AMIA.

Gartee, R., & Beale, S. (2011). *Electronic health records and nursing.* Upper Saddle River, NJ: Pearson/Prentice Hall.

Kim, H., Dykes, P. C., Thomas, D., Winfield, L. A., & Rocha, R. A. (2011). A closer look at nursing documentation on paper forms: Preparation for computerizing a nursing documentation system. *Computers in Biology and Medicine, 41*(4), 182–189.

Mannino, J. E., & Feeg, V. D. (2011). Field-testing a PC electronic documentation system using the Clinical Care Classification© System with nursing students. *Journal of Healthcare Engineering, 2*(2). doi: 10.1260/2040-2295.2.2.223.

Saba, V. K. (2012). Clinical Care Classification. In J. Fitzpatrick, & M. W. Kazer (Eds.), *Essentials of Nursing Research* (3rd ed.). New York, NY: Springer Publishing Company.

Saba, V. K. (2011). Appendix A: Clinical Care Classification (CCC) System Version 2.0: CCC of Nursing Diagnoses and Outcomes and the CCC of Nursing Interventions and Actions classified by 21 Care Components. In V. K. Saba & K. A. McCormick (Eds.), *Essentials of Nursing Informatics* (5th ed., pp. 777–795). New York, NY: McGraw–Hill Publishing.

Saba, V. K., Ensio, A., & Kinnunen, U. (2011). Nursing terminology and meaningful use. In K. Saranto (Ed.), *Ascendio: Eighth European Conference of the Association for Common European Nursing Diagnoses, Interventions, & Outcomes: Funchal, Madeira, 25–26 March 2011*, Dublin, Ireland: ASCENDIO-CD.

Saba, V. K., & McCormick, K. A. (2011). *Essentials of nursing informatics* (5th ed.). New York, NY: McGraw–Hill.

Saba, V. K., Moss, K., & Whittenburg, L. (2011). Overview of the Clinical Care Classification System: A National Nursing Standard. In V. K. Saba, & K. A. McCormick (Eds.), *Essentials of Nursing Informatics* (5th. ed., pp. 217–229). New York, NY: McGraw–Hill Publishing.

Whittenburg, L. (2011). *Postpartum nursing records: Utility of the Clinical Care Classification System,* Fairfax, VA: George Mason University, AAT 3455048.

2010

Moss, S. K., Moss, J., & Jylha, V. (2010). Medication counseling: Analysis of electronic documentation using the Clinical Care Classification System. *Studies in Health Technology and Informatics, 160*(Pt. 1), 284–8.

Saba, V. K. (2010). Clinical Care Classification (CCC) System: An overview. In M. D. Harris (Ed.), *Handbook of home health care administration* (5th ed., pp. 263–276). Sudbury, MA: Jones & Bartlett Publishing.

2009

Hao, A. T., Lin, C., Lu, S. & Lin, Z. (2009). Nursing terminology standards in Taiwan: Current situation and trends [Chinese]. *Journal of Nursing, 56* (3), 12–17.

Saba, V. K., & Enzio, A. (2009). Nursing documentation using CCC/FinCC Systems. In K. Saranto, P. F. Brennan, H. A. Park, W. Sermeus, A. Enzio, & M. Tallberg (Eds.), *NI 2009: Tenth International Congress on Nursing Informatics Proceedings: Nursing informatics—Connecting health and humans.* Helsinki, Finland: Finnish Nurses Association.

Saba, V. K., McCormick, K., Berg, C., Grobe, S., Newbold, S., & Skiba, D. (2009). Pioneers of innovation in education and transforming health care. In K. Saranto, P. F. Brennan, H. A. Park, W. Sermeus, A. Enzio, & M. Tallberg (Eds.), *NI 2009: Tenth International Congress on Nursing Informatics Proceedings: Nursing informatics—Connecting health and humans.* Helsinki, Finland: Finnish Nurses Association.

Whittenburg, L. (2009). Nursing point of care documentation for the evaluation of human quality. *Studies in Health Technology and Informatics, 146,* 713–4.

Whittenburg, L. (2009). Nursing terminology: Documentation of quality outcomes. *Journal of Healthcare Information Management, 23*(3), 51–55.

2008

Feeg, V. D., Saba, V. K., & Feeg, A. (2008). Testing of a bedside personal computer (PC) Clinical Care Classification System for nursing students using Microsoft Access. *Computers in Nursing, 26*(6), 339–349.

Matney, S. A., DaDamio, R., Couderc, C., Dlugos, M., Evans, J., Gianonne, G., Haskell, R., Hardiker, N., Coenen, A., & Saba, V. K. (2008). Translation and integration of CCC Nursing Diagnoses into ICNP. *Journal of the American Medical Informatics Association, 15*(6), 791–793.

Ozbolt, J. G., & Saba, V. K. (2008). A brief history of nursing informatics in the United States of America. *Nursing Outlook, 56*(5), 199–205. doi:10.1016.

Westra, B. L., Delaney, C. W., Konicek, D., & Keenan, G. (2006). Nursing standards to support the electronic health record. *Nursing Outlook, 56*(5), 258–266.

2007

Moss, J., Andison, M., & Sobko, H. (2007). An analysis of narrative nursing documentation in an otherwise structured intensive care clinical documentation system. In *AMIA 2007 Proceedings.* Washington, DC: AMIA.

Saba, V. K., & Taylor, S. L. (2007). Moving past theory: Use of a standardized, coded nursing terminology to enhance nursing visibility. *Computers, Informatics, Nursing, 25*(6), 324–333.

Whittenburg, L., & Saba, V. K. (2007). Sustainable health systems: Using metadata registries with nursing terminology. In *Medinfo 2007: Proceedings of the 12th World Congress on Health Informatics; Building sustainable health (medical) systems.* Amsterdam, Netherlands: IOS Press.

2006

Botsivaly, M., Spyropoulos, B., Koutsourakis, K., & Mertika, K. (2006). Enhancing continuity in care: An implementation of the ASTM E2369-05 standard specification for continuity of care record in a homecare application. In *AMIA 2006 Proceedings* (pp. 66–70). Washington, DC: AMIA.

Douglas, M. (2006). Clinical Care Classification (CCC) system manual: A guide to nursing documentation [book review]. *CARING Newsletter, 21*(4), 1–4.

Saba, V. K. (2006). Appendix: Clinical Care Classification (Version 2.0). Two terminologies: CCC of Nursing Diagnoses and CCC of Nursing Interventions classified by 21 care components. In V. K. Saba & K. A. McCormick (Eds.), *Essentials of Nursing Informatics* (4th ed., pp. 681–686). New York: McGraw–Hill.

Struk, C. M., Peters, D. A., & Saba, V. K. (2006). Community health applications. In V. K. Saba & K. A. McCormick. *Essentials of Nursing Informatics* (4th ed., pp. 391–412). New York: McGraw–Hill.

2005

Bakken, S., Holzemer, W. L., Portillo, C. J., Grimes, R., Welch, J., & Wantland, D. (2005). Utility of a standardized nursing terminology to evaluate dosage and tailoring of an HIV/AIDS adherence intervention. *Journal of Nursing Scholarship, 37*(3), 251–257.

Choi, J., Jenkins, M. L., Cimino, J. J., White, T. M., & Bakken, S. (2005). Toward semantic interoperability in home health care: Formally representing OASIS items for integration into a concept-oriented terminology. *Journal of the American Medical Informatics Association, 12*(4), 410–417.

Moss, J., Damrongsak, M., & Gallichio, K. (2005). Representing critical care data using the Clinical Care Classification. In C. P. Friedman, J. Ash, & P. Tarcy–Hornoch (Eds.), *Proceedings of the AMIA 2005 Annual Symposium* [CD-ROM] (pp. 545–549). Washington, DC: OmniPress, Omnipro-CD.

New version of Home Health Care Classification: Renamed as Clinical Care Classification. (2005). *ACENDIO Newsletter, 1*(15), 3.

Saba, V. K. (2005). Home Health Care Classification (HHCC) System: An overview. In M. D. Harris, (Ed.), *Handbook of home healthcare administration* (pp. 247–260). Sudbury, MA: Jones & Bartlett Publishing, Inc.

2004

Bakken, S., Cook, S. S., Curtis, L., Desjardins, K., Hyun, S., Jenkins, M., John, R., et al. (2004). Promoting patient safety through informatics-based nursing education. *International Journal of Medical Informatics, 73*(7–8), 581–589.

Kuntze, A. (2004). The evaluation of the Home Health Care Classification for its practical use in German-speaking countries. *PR-Internet fur die Pflege, 6*(11), 621–626.

Lee, N. J., Bakken, S., & Saba, V. K. (2004). Representing public health nursing information concepts with HHCC and NIC. In M. Fieschi, E. Coiera, & Y. C. J. Li (Eds.), *MEDINFO 2004* (pp. 525–529). Amsterdam, Netherlands: IOS Press.

Saba, V. K. (2004). Costing nursing care using the Clinical Care Classification Systems. In *Connecting the health care continuum: 14th Annual Summer Institute in Nursing Informatics, July 21–24, 2004* (p. 5). Baltimore, MD: University of Maryland, Summer Institute of Nursing.

Saba, V. K., & Arnold, J. M. (2004). Clinical care costing method for the Clinical Care Classification System. *International Journal of Nursing Terminologies and Classifications, 15*(3), 69–77.

Saba, V. K., & Arnold, J. M. (2004). A clinical care costing method. In M. Fieschi, E. Coiera, & Y. C. J. Li (Eds.), *MEDINFO 2004* (pp. 1372–1373). Amsterdam, Netherlands: IOS Press.

2003

Arnold, J. M., & Saba, V. K. (2003). Linking Home Health Care Classification System and ambulatory patient classification for nurse practitioner services. In H. Marin, E. Marques, E. Hovenga, & W. Goossen (Eds.), *NI-2003: Proceedings of the 8th International Congress in Nursing Informatics* (pp. 257–261). Rio de Janeiro, Brazil: e-Papers Services Editorials, Ltd.

Bakken, S., Cook, S. S., Curtis, L., Soupious, M., & Curran, C. (2003). Informatics competencies pre- and post-implementation of a Palm-based student clinical log and informatics for evidence-based practice curriculum. *Proceedings of the AMIA 2003 Annual Symposium* (pp. 41–45). Nashville, TN: Hanley & Belfus.

Bakken, S., Curran, C., Delaleu-McIntosh, J., Desjardins, K., Hyun, S., Jenkins, M., John, R., et al. (2003). Informatics for evidence-based nurse practitioner practice at the Columbia University School of Nursing. In H. F. Marin, E. P. Marques, E. Hovenga, & W. Goossen (Eds.), *NI 2003: Proceedings of the 8th International Congress on Nursing Informatics* (pp. 420–424). Rio De Janeiro, Brazil: e-Papers Servicos Editorials, Ltd.

Charters, K. G. (2003). Nursing informatics, outcomes, and quality improvement. *AACN Issues: Advanced Practice in Acute and Critical Care, 14*(3), 282–294.

Ensio, A., & Saranto, K. (2003). Finland: The Finnish classification of nursing interventions (FICNI)—Development and use in nursing documentation. In J. Clark (Ed.), *Naming nursing: Proceedings of the 1st ACENDIO Ireland/UK Conference held September 2003 in Swansea, Wales, UK* (pp. 191–195). Bern, Germany: Verlag Hans Huber.

Grim, K. (2003). The Home Health Care Classification System (German). *PR-Internet fur die Pflege, 5*(5), 12–20.

Hwang, J. I., Cimino, J. J., & Bakken, S. (2003). Integrating nursing diagnosis constructs into the Medical Entities Dictionary using the ISO Reference Terminology Model for Nursing Diagnosis. *Journal of the Medical Informatics Association, 10*, 382–388.

Irwin, R. G., & Saba, V. K. (2003). An electronic 3 care tracking system. In H. P. Marin, E. P. Marques, E. Hovenga, & W. Goossen (Eds.), *NI-2003: Proceedings of the 8th International Congress in Nursing Informatics* (pp. 124–125). Rio de Janeiro, Brazil: e-Papers Services Editorials, Ltd.

Junttila, J., Saranto, K., & Ensio, A. (2003). Nursing diagnosis in Finnish perioperative documentation. In H. F. Marin, E. P. Marques, E. Hovenga, & W. Gossen (Eds.), *NI 2003: Proceedings, 8th International Congress in Nursing Informatics* (p. 667). Rio de Janeiro, Brazil: e-Papers Services Editorials, Ltd.

Klein, W. T., & Bakken, S. (2003). Design and implementation of a student clinical log database and knowledge base. In H. F. Marin, E. P. Marques, E. Hovenga, & W. Goossen (Eds.), *NI 2003: Proceedings of the 8th International Congress on Nursing Informatics* (pp. 617–622). Rio De Janeiro, Brazil: e-Papers Servicos Editorials, Ltd.

Matney, S. (2003). Nursing terminology update. *On-Line Journal of Nursing Informatics, 7*(3), 8.

Moss, J., Coenen. A., & Mills, M. (2003). Evaluation of the draft international standard for a reference terminology model for nursing actions. *Journal of Biomedical Informatics, 36*, 271–278.

Saba, V. K. (2003). The Home Health Care Classification System (HHCC). In J. Clark (Ed.), *Naming nursing: Proceedings of the 1st ACENDIO Ireland/UK Conference held September 2003 in Swansea, Wales, UK* (pp. 131–138). Bern, Germany: Verlag Hans Huber.

2002

Hardiker, N. R., Bakken, S., Casey, A., & Hoy, D. (2002). Formal nursing terminology systems: Means to an end. *Journal of Biomedical Informatics, 35*, 298–305.

Hyun, S. J., & Park, H. S. (2002). Cross-mapping the ICNP with NANDA, HHCC, Omaha System and NIC for unified nursing language system development. *International Nursing Review, 49*(2), 99–110.

Saba, V. K. (2002). Nursing classifications: Home Health Care Classification System (HHCC): An overview. *Online Journal of Issues in Nursing.* Retrieved from http://www.nursingworld.org/ojin/tpct/tpc7_7.htm

Saba, V. K. (2002). Nursing information technology: Classifications and management. In J. Mantas, & A. Hasman (Eds.), *Textbook in health informatics: A nursing perspective* (pp. 21–44). Amsterdam, Netherlands: IOS Press.

Saba, V. K. (2002). Overview of Home Health Care Classification System (HHCC). In N. Oud (Ed.), *Acendio 2002: Proceedings of the Special Conference of the Association of Common European Nursing Diagnoses, Interventions and Outcomes in Vienna* (pp. 65–90). Bern: Verlag Hans Huber.

Schoneman, D. (2002). The intervention of surveillance across classification systems. *International Journal of Nursing Terminologies and Classifications, 13*(4), 137–147.

2001

Alfrink, V., Bakken, S., Coenen, A., McNeil, B., & Bickford, C. (2001). Standardized nursing vocabularies: A foundation for quality care. *Seminars in Oncology Nursing, 17*(1), 18–23.

Coenen, A., Marin, H., Park. H. A., & Bakken, S. (2001). Collaborative efforts for representing nursing concepts in computer-based systems. *Journal of the American Medical Informatics Association, 8*(3), 202–211.

Coenen, A., McNeil, B., Bakken, S., Bickford, C., & Warren, J. J. (2001). Toward comparable nursing data: American Nursing Association criteria for data sets, classification systems, and nomenclatures. *Computers in Nursing, 19*(6), 240–246.

Hardiker, N. (2001). Mediating between nursing intervention terminology systems. In S. Bakken (Ed.), *A medical informatics odyssey: Visions of the future and lessons from the past* (pp. 239–243). Philadelphia, PA: Hanley & Belfus, Inc.

Marin, H. F., Rodriques, R. J., Delaney, C., Nielsen, G. H., & Yan, J. (2001). *Building standard-based nursing information systems.* Washington, DC: Pan American Health Organization.

Peters, D. A., &. Saba, V. K. (2001). Community health applications. In V. K. Saba & K. A. McCormick (Eds.), *Essentials of computers for nurses: Informatics for the new millennium* (3rd ed., pp. 265–295). New York: McGraw–Hill, Inc.

Saba, V. K. (2001). Appendix A: Home Health Care Classification (HHCC) System: Two terminologies: HHCC of Nursing Diagnoses and HHCC of Nursing Interventions Classified by 20 care components. In V. K. Saba & K. A. McCormick (Eds.), *Essentials of computers for nurses: Informatics for the new millennium* (3rd ed., pp. 529–533). New York: McGraw–Hill.

Saba, V. K. (2001). Evidence-based practice, language, and documentation. International Council of Nurses (ICN) 22nd Quadrennial Congress, June 10–15, 2001. *Nursing: A new era for action: Abstract for concurrent sessions and symposia. List of Posters.* Geneva, Switzerland: ICN.

Saba, V. K. (2001). Nursing's languages: International terminologies, classifications and standards. In V. L. Patel, R. Rogers, & R. Haux (Eds.), *Medinfo 2001: Proceedings of the 10th World Congress on Medical Informatics* (p. 1544). Amsterdam, Netherlands: IOS Press.

Saba, V. K., & Irwin, R. G. (2001). An electronic system for home care protocols. In S. Bakken (Ed.), *Proceedings of the AMIA 2005 Annual Symposium* (p. 1013). Philadelphia, PA: Hanley & Belfus, Inc.

2000

Bakken, S., Campbell, K. E., Comino, J. J., Huff, S. M., & Hammond, W. E. (2000). Toward vocabulary domain specifications for Health Level 7-coded data elements. *Journal of the American Medical Informatics Association, 7*(4), 333–342.

Bakken, S., Cashen, M. S., Mendonca, E. A., O'Brien, A., & Zieniewicz, J. (2000). Representing nursing activities within a concept-oriented terminological system: Evaluation of a type definition. *Journal of the American Medical Informatics Association, 7*(1), 81–89.

Bakken, S., Cimino, J. J., Haskell, R., Kukafka, R., Matsumoto, C., Chan, G., & Huff, S. M. (2000). Evaluation of clinical LOINC (Logical Observation Identifiers, Names, and Codes). *Journal of the American Medical Informatics Association, 7*(6), 529–538.

Bakken, S., Parker, J., Konicek, D., & Campbell, K. (2000). An evaluation of ICNP intervention axes as terminology model components. In J. M. Overhage (Ed.), *Proceedings of the AMIA 2000 Annual Symposium* (pp. 42–46). Nashville, TN: Hanley & Belfus.

Bakken, S., Wage, G., Bain, C., Cashen, M. S., Sklar, B., & Kelber, C. (2000). Standardized terminology requirements for nurse practitioner documentation of clinical findings. In S. Bakken, P., Button, D., Konicek, S. Matney, K. A. McCormick, J. G. Ozbolt, V. K. Saba, et al. (Eds.), *Standardized terminologies for nursing concepts: Collaborative activities in the United States. In the 7th International Congress of Nursing Informatics: Post-congress workshop, Rotorua, New Zealand, May 3–6, 2000* (pp. 21–32). Auckland, New Zealand: Premier Print.

Park, H., & Cho, I. S. (2000). Standardisation of nursing classification systems in Korea. In V. K. Saba, R. Carr, W. Sermeus, & P. Rocha (Eds.), *Nursing informatics 2000. One step beyond: The evolution of technology and nursing. Proceedings of the 7th Nursing Informatics Congress* (pp. 277–282). Auckland, New Zealand, Adis International Limited.

Saba, V. K., Carr, R., Sermeus, W., Rocha, P., (Eds.). (2000). *7th International Congress: Nursing informatics one step beyond: The evolution of technology and nursing* (pp. 177–182). Auckland, New Zealand: Adis International Ltd.

Saba, V. K., & Irwin, R. G. (2000). An electronic tracking system for home care protocols. In V. K. Saba, R. Carr, W. Sermeus, & P. Rocha, (Eds.), *Nursing informatics 2000: One step beyond: The evolution of technology and nursing: Proceedings of the 7th Nursing Informatics Congress* (p. 779). Auckland, New Zealand: Adis International Ltd.

Strachan, H., Hoy, D., Moen, A., Park, H. A., Saba, V., & Skiba, D. (2000). Critical pathways and outcomes: Using evidence-based practice in community and home health care. In *The 7th International Congress on Nursing Informatics: Post-congress workshop.* Rotorua, New Zealand, May 3–6, 2000. Auckland, New Zealand: Premier Print.

1999

ANSI/HISB. (1998/1999). Home Health Care Classification (HHCC) of Nursing Diagnosis and Nursing Interventions. In *Inventory of Clinical Information Standards.* Washington, DC: ANSI.

Bakken, S., Button, P., Hardiker, N. R., Mead, C. N., Ozbolt, J. G., & Warren, J. J. (1999). On the path to a reference terminology for nursing concepts. In C. G. Chute (Ed.),

IMIA Working Group: 6th Conference on Natural Language and Medical Concept Representation. Phoenix, AZ: IOS Press.

Beyea, S. C. (1999). Standardized language: Making nursing practice count. *AORN Journal, 70*(5), 831–832, 834, 837, 838.

Sparks, S. M., Saba, V. K., & Rantz, M. J. (1999). Educational strategies for integrating diagnoses and care components. In *Classification of nursing diagnoses: Proceedings of the Thirteenth Conference, North American Nursing Diagnosis Association. Celebrating the 25th anniversary of NANDA* (pp. 366–371). St. Louis, MO: North American Nursing Diagnosis Association.

1998

Anderson, M. A., Pena, R. A., & Helms, L. B. (1998). Home care utilization by congestive heart failure patients: A pilot study. *Public Health Nursing, 15*(2), 126–162.

Button, P., Androwich, I., Hibben, L., Kern, V., Madden, G., Marek, K., Westra, B., et al. (1998). Challenges and issues related to implementation of nursing vocabularies in computer-based systems. *Journal of the American Medical Informatics Association, 5*(6), 332–334.

Coward, P. M. (1998). *Use of standardized nursing language in home care referral.* Cleveland, OH: Case Western Reserve University (Health Sciences).

Hardiker, N. R., & Rector, A. L. (1998). Modeling nursing terminology using the GRAIL representation language. *Journal of the American Medical Informatics Association, 5*(1), 120–128.

Henry, S. H., Warren, J. J., Lange, L., & Button, P. (1998). A review of major nursing vocabularies and the extent to which they have the characteristics required for implementation in computer-based systems. *Journal of the American Medical Informatics Association, 5*(4), 321–328.

McCormick, K. A., & Jones, C. B. (1998, Sept. 30). Is one taxonomy needed for health care vocabularies and classifications? *Online Journal of Issues in Nursing.* Retrieved from http://www.nursingworld.org/ojin/tpc7/tpc7_2htm

Parlocha, P. K., & Henry, S. B. (1998). The usefulness of the Georgetown Home Health Care Classification System for coding patient problems and nursing interventions in psychiatric home care. *Computers in Nursing, 16*(1), 45–52.

Saba, V. K. (1998). A new paradigm for computer-based nursing information systems: Twenty care components. In V. K. Saba, D. P. Pocklington, & K. P. Miller (Eds.), *Nursing and computers: An anthology, 1987–1996* (pp. 29–32). New York: Springer.

Saba, V. K., & Sparks, S. M. (1998). Twenty care components: An educational strategy to teach nursing science. In B. Cesnik, A. T. Cray, & J. R. Scherrer (Eds.), *Medinfo '98: Ninth World Congress on Medical Informatics* (pp. 756–759). Amsterdam, Netherlands: IOS Press.

Warren, J. J., & Coenen, A. (1998) International Classification for Nursing Practice (ICNP): Most-frequently asked questions. *Journal of the American Medical Informatics Association, 5*(4), 335–336.

Zielstorff, R. D. (1998). Characteristics of a good nursing nomenclature from an informatics perspective. *Online Journal of Issues in Nursing.* Retrieved from http://www.nursingworld.org/ojin/tpc7/tpc7_4htm

Zielstorff, R. D., Tronni, C., Basque, J., Griffin, L. R., & Welebob, E. M. (1998). Mapping nursing diagnosis nomenclatures for coordinated care. *Journal of Nursing Scholarship, 30*(4), 369–373.

1997

Burkhart, L. (1997). Nursing standardized language to promote professionalism. *Perspectives in Parish Nursing Practice, 1*, 3, 11.

Henry, S. H., & Mead, C. N. (1997). Nursing classifications systems; necessary but not sufficient for representing "what nurses do" for inclusion in computer-based patient record systems. *Journal of the American Medical Informatics Association, 4*(3), 222–232.

Henry, S. B., Morris, J. A., & Holzemer, W. L. (1997). Using structured text and templates to capture health status outcomes in the electronic health record. *Journal of Quality Improvement, 23*(12), 667–677.

Holzemer, W. L., Henry, S. B., Dawson, C., Sousa, K., Bain, C., & Hsieh, S. F. (1997). An evaluation of the utility of the Home Health Care Classification for categorizing patient problems and nursing interventions from the hospital setting. In U. Gerdin, M. Tallberg, & P. Wainwright (Eds.), *NI'97: Nursing informatics: The impact of nursing knowledge on health care informatics* (pp. 21–26). Stockholm, Sweden: IOS Press.

Hoskins, L. M., & Tantz, L. M. (1997). Linking nursing diagnoses across the NANDA, Home Health Care, and Omaha Classification Systems. In *Classification of nursing diagnoses: Proceedings of the Twelfth Conference, North American Nursing Diagnosis Association* (pp. 8–12). Glendale, CA: Cinahl Information Systems.

Saba, V. K. (1997). Georgetown University Home Care Project: Home Health Care Classification (HHCC) System. *Inventory of health care information standards pertaining to: The Health Insurance Portability and Accountability Act (HIPAA) of 1996* (Pub. L. No. 104-191). Washington, DC: American National Standards Institute: Healthcare Informatics Standards Board.

Saba, V. K. (1997). An innovative Home Health Care Classification System for continuity of care. In U. Gerdin, M. Tallberg, & P. Wainwright (Eds.), *Nursing informatics: The impact of nursing knowledge on healthcare informatics* (p. 607). Amsterdam, Netherlands: IOS Press.

Saba, V. K. (1997). An innovative Home Health Care Classification (HHCC) System. In *Classification of nursing diagnoses: Proceedings of the 12th Conference, April 11–14, 1996. NANDA* (pp. 13–15). Pasadena, CA: Western Adventist Health Services (CINAHL).

Saba, V. K. (1997). Home Health Care Classification (HHCC) System. In G. K. McFarland & E. A. McFarlane (Eds.), *Nursing diagnosis and intervention: Planning for patient care* (3rd ed., pp. 867–872). St. Louis: Mosby.

Saba, V. K. (1997). The Home Health Care Classification of Nursing Diagnoses and Interventions. In M. D. Harris (Ed.), *Handbook of home health care administration* (2nd ed., pp. 215–219). Gaithersburg, MD: Aspen Publications.

Saba, V. K. (1997). Why the Home Health Care Classification is a recognized nomenclature. *Computers in Nursing, 15*(2), S69–S76.

Sparks, S. M. (1997). Noun phrases for nursing diagnoses. *Nursing Diagnosis, 8*(2), 49–54.

1996

Saba, V. K. (1996). Community health applications. In V. K. Saba & K. A. McCormick (Eds.), *Essentials of computers for nurses* (2nd ed., pp. 429–484). New York: McGraw–Hill.

Saba, V. K. (1996). Appendix: Home Health Care Classification: Nursing diagnoses and nursing interventions. In V. K. Saba & K. A. McCormick, *Essentials of computers for nurses* (2nd ed., pp. 619–635). New York: McGraw–Hill.

Saba, V. K., & Hollers, K. (1996). An innovative Home Health Care Classification System for managing managed care. In J. J. Cimino (Ed.), *Proceedings: 1996 AMIA Annual Fall Symposium* (p. 936). Philadelphia, PA: Hanley & Belfus, Inc.

1995

Anderson, B., Hannah, K., Besner, J., et al. (1995). Classification systems for health information: Nursing components, Part 1. *AARN Newsletter, 51*(2), 10–11.

Lang, N. M., Hudgins, C., Jacox, A., Lancour, J., McClure, M. L., McCormick, K. A., Saba, V. K., et al. (1995). Toward a national database for nursing practice. In *American Nurses Association. Nursing data systems: The emerging framework* (pp. 7–18). Washington, DC: ANA.

Lang, N. M., & Marek, K. D. (1995). Quality assurance: The foundation of professional care. *Journal of the New York State Nurses Association, 26*(1), 48–50.

Lazerowich, V. (1995). Development of a patient classification system for a home-based hospice program. *Journal of Community Health Nursing, 12*(2), 121–126.

Mackenzie, W., Hannah, K., Anderson, B., et al. (1995). Classification systems for health information: Nursing components, Part 11. *AARN Newsletter, 51*(3), 32–33.

Saba, V. K. (1995). A new paradigm for computer-based nursing information systems twenty care components. In R. A. Greenes, H. E. Peterson, & D. J. Protti (Eds.), *Medinfo '95: Proceedings of the 8th World Congress on Medical Informatics* (pp. 1401–1406). Amsterdam, Netherlands: North–Holland.

[Reprinted in: Saba, V. K., Pocklington, D. B., & Miller, K. P. (1998). *Nursing and computers: An anthology* (pp. 29–32). New York: Springer Publishing.]

Saba, V. K. (1995). Home Health Care Classification (HHCC). In R. A. Mortensen (Ed.), Creating a European platform: *Proceedings of the 1st European Conference on Nursing*

Diagnoses (pp. 302–308). Copenhagen, Denmark: Danish Institute for Health and Nursing Research.

Saba, V. K. (1995). Home Health Care Classifications (HHCCs): Nursing diagnoses and nursing interventions. In N. M. Lang (Ed.), *Nursing data systems: The emerging framework* (pp. 61–103). Washington, DC: American Nurses Association.

Zielstorff, R. D., Lang, N. M., Saba, V. K., McCormick, K. A., & Milholland, D. K. (1995). Toward a uniform language for nursing in the US: Work of the American Nurses Association Steering Committee on Databases to Support Clinical Practice. In R. A. Greenes, H. E. Peterson, & D. J. Protti (Eds.), *Medinfo '95: Proceedings of the 8th World Congress on Medical Informatics* (pp. 1362–1366). Amsterdam, Netherlands: North–Holland. [Reprinted in: Saba, V. K., Pocklington, D. B., & Miller, K. P. (1998). *Nursing and computers: An anthology* (pp. 22–28). New York: Springer Publishing.]

1994

Henry, S. B., Holzemer, W. L., Reilly, C. A., & Campbell, K. E. (1994). Terms used by nurses to describe patient problems: Can SNOMED III represent nursing concepts in the patient record. *Journal of the American Medical Informatics Association, 1*(1), 61–74.

McCormick, K. A., Lang, N., Zielstorff, R., Milholland, D. K., Saba, V. K., & Jacox, A. (1994). Toward standard classification schemes for nursing languages: Recommendations of the American Nurses Association Steering Committee on Databases to Support Clinical Nursing Practice. *Journal of the American Medical Informatics Association, 1*(6), 421–427.

Miller, J. M., & Bakken, S. (1994). Toward a common healthcare language. *Computertalk, 2*, 40–42.

Ozbolt, J. Fruchtnicht, J. N., & Hayden, J. R. (1994). Toward data standards for clinical nursing information. *Journal of the American Medical Informatics Association, 1*(2), 175–185.

Saba, V. K. (1994). A home health classification system. In S. J. Grobe & E. S. P. Pluyter–Wenting (Eds.), *Nursing informatics: An international overview for nursing in a technological era* (pp. 697–701). Amsterdam, Netherlands: Elsevier.

Saba, V. K. (1994). Coding systems for nursing. In P. Waegeman (Ed.), *Toward an electronic patient record '94: 10th International Symposium on the Creation of Electronic Health Record System & 6th Global Congress on Patient Cards* (pp. 223–225). Newton, MA: Medical Records Institute.

Saba, V. K. (1994). *Home Health Care Classification (HHCC) of Nursing Diagnoses and Interventions, Revised.* Washington, DC: Georgetown University.

Saba, V. K. (1994). Twenty nursing diagnosis home health care components. In R. M. Carroll-Johnson & M. Paquette (Eds.), *Classification of nursing diagnoses: Proceedings of the 10th Conference* (p. 301). Philadelphia, PA: J. B. Lippincott Co.

Saba, V. K., & Zuckerman, A. E. (1994). Home Health Care Classification (HHCC) System. In J. G. Ozbolt (Ed.), *Transforming information, changing healthcare: Proceedings of the 18th Annual Symposium on Computer Applications in Medical Care* (p. 1046). Philadelphia, PA: Hanley & Belfus, Inc.

Zink, M. R. (1994). Nursing intervention classification: A comparison with the Omaha System and the Home Health Care Classification. *Home Healthcare Nurse, 12*(3), 63–4.

1993

Saba, V. K. (1993). Nursing diagnostic schemes. In Canadian Nurses Association (Ed.), *Proceedings: Nursing Minimum Data Set Conference. Alberta, Canada, December 1992* (pp. 54–63). Alberta, Canada: Canadian Nurses Association.

1992

Fuiper, M. (1992). Diagnose en interventie (Diagnosis and Interventions). In L. Regeer (Ed.), *Verpleegkundige diagnostiek in Nederland* (Nursing Diagnoses in Netherlands) (pp. 73–82). Amsterdam, Netherlands: LEO Verpleegkundig Management.

Gabrieli, E. R. (1992). *6-3-1-10 nursing terminology.* Buffalo, NY: Gabrieli Associates.

Milholland, D. K. (1992). Naming what we do: Nursing vocabularies. *Journal of AHIMA, 63*(10), 68–61.

Saba, V. K. (1992). A classification of home health care nursing diagnoses and interventions. *Caring, 11*(3), 50–57.

Saba, V. K. (1992). Home Health Care Classification. *Caring, 11*(5), 58–60.

Saba, V. K. (1992). *Home Health Care Classification (HHCC) of Nursing Diagnoses and Interventions.* Washington, DC: Georgetown University.

Saba, V. K. (1992). The classification of home health care nursing diagnoses and interventions. In L. Regeer (Ed.), *Verpleegkundige diagnostiek in Nederland* (Nursing Diagnoses in Netherlands) (pp. 62–82). Amsterdam, Netherlands: LEO Verpleegkundig (Nursing) Management.
[First translation of *HHCC Version 1.0* in Dutch by Marlou de Fuiper, RN, MsN, for conference proceedings.]

Saba, V. K., & Zuckerman, A. E. (1992). A Home Health Care Classification System. In K. C. Lun, P. DeGoulet, T. E. Piemme, & O. Reinhoff (Eds.), *MEDINFO 92: Proceedings of the 7th World Congress on Medical Informatics* (pp. 344–348). Amsterdam, Netherlands: North–Holland.

Saba, V. K., & Zuckerman, A. E. (1992). A new home health classification method. *Caring, 11*(10), 27–34.

1991

Saba, V. K. (1991). *Final report: Home Care Classification Project.* Washington, DC: Author.

Saba, V. K. (1991). Home Health Care Classification System. In *Computers in health care: 2nd Annual Conference & Exhibits* (pp. 19–20). Washington, DC: Georgetown University.

Saba, V. K. (1991). The international classification of diseases (ICD): Classification of nursing diagnosis. In R. M. Carroll-Johnson (Ed.), *Classification of nursing diagnoses: Proceedings of the Ninth Conference* (pp. 14–18). New York: J.B. Lippincott Co.

Saba, V. K., O'Hare, A., Zuckerman, A. E., Boondas, J., Levine, E., & Oatway, D. M. (1991). A nursing intervention taxonomy for home health care. *Nursing and Health Care, 12*(6), 296–299.

Index

In this index, the letters "f", "t" and "e" denote figures, tables and exhibits, respectively.

Made in the USA
Middletown, DE
28 April 2022

64939764R00155